The Treatment of Drinking Problems

In its third edition, *The Treatment of Drinking Problems* represents the further development of a highly successful clinical text that has been acclaimed internationally. Two new authors have been added to bring strong additional perspectives to this new edition. Major features of this book remain as before and it continues to address the real world directness which marked it out from other books in the literature. Revised throughout, the comprehensive subject matter of this edition comprises two parts; the first covering background issues essential to an understanding of alcohol problems, and the second, offering a very practical account of screening, assessment, and treatment strategies. Of particular note among the revisions are completely new chapters covering alcohol as a drug, causes of excessive drinking, drinking problems and the life course, and a new look at the physical complications associated with drinking and the organisation of treatment services. The everyday needs of the clinical front-line are addressed through presentations that are enlivened by the personal clinical experiences of the authors. Case vignettes are used to illustrate a range of common clinical dilemmas plus their effective solutions. *The Treatment of Drinking Problems* is intended for use by all whose responsibilities include helping people with alcohol problems. This comprehensive and timely new edition will ensure that it continues to be an essential and widely used classic, enhancing the clinical skills of students and professionals alike for many years to come.

The Treatment of Drinking Problems

A guide for the helping professions

Griffith Edwards CBE DSc DM FRCP FRCPsych
National Addiction Centre, London

E. Jane Marshall MRCP(I) MRCPsych
National Addiction Centre, London

Christopher C. Cook MD MRCPsych
Kent Institute of Medicine and Health Sciences, Canterbury

THIRD EDITION

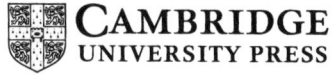

CAMBRIDGE
UNIVERSITY PRESS

PUBLISHED BY THE PRESS SYNDICATE OF THE UNIVERSITY OF CAMBRIDGE
The Pitt Building, Trumpington Street, Cambridge CB2 1RP, United Kingdom

CAMBRIDGE UNIVERSITY PRESS
The Edinburgh Building, Cambridge CB2 2RU, United Kingdom
40 West 20th Street, New York, NY 10011-4211, USA
10 Stamford Road, Oakleigh, Melbourne 3166, Australia

First published 1997

Printed in the United Kingdom at the University Press, Cambridge

Typeset in Palatino and Frutiger [SE]

A catalogue record for this book is available from the British Library

Library of Congress Cataloguing in Publication data

Edwards, Griffith.
The treatment of drinking problems : a guide for the helping
professions / Griffith Edwards, E. Jane Marshall, Christopher C.H.
Cook. – 3rd ed.
    p.   cm.
Includes bibliographical references and index.
ISBN 0-521-49696-9 (hc). – ISBN 0-521-49793-0 (pbk.)
1. Alcoholism – Treatment.   I. Marshall, E. Jane.   II. Cook,
Christopher C. H.   III. Title.
RC565.E38   1997
616.86'106–dc21   96–53577   CIP

ISBN 0 521 49696 9 hardback
ISBN 0 521 49793 0 paperback

100110141 9

This book is dedicated to

Sue, Daniel and Rose
François, David, Grace and Matthew
Joy, Andrew, Beth, Rachel and Jonathan

Contents

A note on the third edition

This book builds on a text which first appeared in 1982 and had its second edition in 1987. German, Japanese, Portuguese, Spanish and Swedish translations have been published. We have held onto the guiding principle that it is written for clinicians and in direct support of the practical business of treatment. With this commitment firmly maintained, something between revision and rewriting has been undertaken throughout, and four entirely new chapters (chapters 1, 2, 11 and 20) have been added. It has also been seen as useful to give fuller referencing than previously.

The first two editions had a single authorship and the senior author now takes great pleasure in welcoming as equal partners in the writing team Jane Marshall and Christopher Cook. Their scientific and clinical expertise gives valuable and complementary new strength.

We wish to thank Dr Jocelyn Foster, Medical Sciences Editor at Cambridge University Press, for her valued support. We are grateful to Esther Grant and Julie Barker for secretarial help, and our warm thanks are due to Patricia Davis for her invaluable secretarial and administrative support throughout the production of this book.

Introduction

When first opening any text the reasonable expectation of the reader is that the authors should declare what purpose the book in question aims to serve while also providing a signposting of the chapters to come. These are the matters which this introduction will now address.

A book intended to enhance clinical skills

This book is intended for anyone, generalist or specialist, whose responsibilities imply that they will sometimes or often be encountering people with drinking problems. It is written in the hope that it will be instrumentally useful in enhancing diagnostic and treatment skills in the alcohol arena for this wide variety of professionals. We have also tried to convey a sense of why this kind of work is so perpetually intriguing and worthwhile. We have employed the generic word 'therapist' to describe the person who does the helping and hope that the text will be equally relevant to the needs of psychiatrists and other medical practitioners, nurses, clinical psychologists, social workers, occupational therapists and counsellors. Different professions have their specific skills and roles, but in dealing with drinking problems there is much to be learnt which is relevant across all professions. We intend this book to be of multidisciplinary appeal, but Chapters 2 and 8 deal with matters which inevitably require a technical exposition in biological and medical language.

As for the question of how to refer to the person who is given the help, we have used the words 'patient', and 'client' as having much the same meaning. We have so far as possible eschewed the term 'alcoholic', feeling that this designation no longer has scientific meaning and too easily invites stereotyping and alienation, but we are aware that others (particularly members of Alcoholics Anonymous) still find this word useful. We prefer the phrases 'problem drinker' or 'person with a drinking problem', and more specifically and restrictively 'person suffering from alcohol dependence'. The term 'alcohol misuse' will for ease of communication now and then be employed, but within a stricter scientific framework we would argue that 'use' and 'misuse' of alcohol are not categorically separate behaviours.

Bridging the research and clinical worlds

The clinical position taken in this book is rooted in what science today has to say about the causes of drinking, the nature of alcohol-related problems and of alcohol-dependence, and the demonstrable efficacy of different treatment approaches. In staying close to the format of a clinical text we have felt that the right balance is struck by referencing key statements while not diverting into academic review for its own sake.

Internationalism

The way in which alcohol problems are defined and responded to is to an extent shaped by culturally and historically determined beliefs and by national health care provisions. The pattern of problems encountered and the appropriateness of different types of response must often be different between poorer and richer countries. There is much need for strengthened international support in training, technological development, and sharing of information. While hoping that this book will be useful in many different national settings we are aware that 'translation' of this kind of text into other cultural environments will require critical scrutiny and close local judgement.

Plan and Content

The chapters are grouped into two sections. Section 1, 'Background to Understanding', comprises Chapters 1 to 11, while Section 2 puts together Chapters 12 to 19 under the heading 'Screening, Assessment, and Treatment'. The content of these chapters will now be signposted.

Section 1. Background to understanding

Causes of drinking problems (Chapter 1)

Heavy drinking, and alcohol-related problems, arise as a result of multiple and interacting influences upon the individual. This chapter provides an overview of environmental factors, genetic predisposition, and psychological mechanisms which may lead to the development of drinking problems. Some indication of the clinical relevance of this material is also provided.

Alcohol as a drug (Chapter 2)

A knowledge of the biological effects of alcohol is basic to understanding many of the problems that arise from its use. This chapter brings together information on the absorption and metabolism of alcohol, its effect on several body systems, and in particular its action on the brain. The language is, of necessity, technical but we hope that the non-medical reader will find the chapter of value.

The alcohol dependence syndrome (Chapter 3)

Carrying on from discussion of alcohol as a drug with dependence potential (Chapter 2), this chapter describes the psycho-biological basis, profile, and clinical significance of the alcohol dependence syndrome. The question is discussed of whether dependence is one syndrome or a group of syndromes.

Alcohol-related problems (Chapters 4–8)

If alcohol dependence is one important dimension defining the concerns of this book, alcohol-related problems constitute a second and equally important dimension. Contributions deal in turn with drinking problems and the family (Chapter 4); social complications of excessive drinking (Chapter 5); drinking and psychiatric illness within a two-way connection (Chapter 6); drug problems and alcohol problems (Chapter 7); and physical complications of excessive drinking (Chapter 8).

Women with drinking problems (Chapter 9)

Alcohol problems are still a source of shame to women and they are under-represented in treatment settings. The reasons for this situation are discussed as are the risk factors for women across the life course.

Special presentations (Chapter 10)

This chapter again seeks to emphasise the clinical orientation of the book and will identify some of the special presentations which may be encountered in the clinic on any working day – the young drinker, the patient with violent propensities, the 'very important patient', and so on.

Drinking problems and the life course (Chapter 11)

Rounding off Section 1, the perspective developed in this chapter is fundamental to the stance taken throughout the treatment section which follows. It is argued that alcohol problems can only be understood as happenings within an ongoing life course, with treatment needing to be fashioned so as to support natural processes of recovery.

Section 2. Screening, assessment, and treatment

Screening and history taking (Chapters 12 and 13)

These chapters open the second section of the book. Case identification and screening are dealt with in Chapter 12 in terms of both laboratory and questionnaire approaches and this is followed by a discussion in Chapter 13 of how history taking is to be accomplished and used as an initiation of therapy. Separate sections of Chapter 13 describe the assessment interview with patient and spouse, and an approach to case formulation is outlined.

Withdrawal states and treatment of withdrawal (Chapter 14)

Detoxification is an important and necessary prelude to the further treatment of the dependent drinker. This chapter covers the medical and clinical basics of treatment, but it will also guide the non-medical reader as to the principles underlying the management of alcohol withdrawal. The diversity of withdrawal states, the choice between community and in-patient settings, and the proper use of medication, are all addressed.

The basic work of treatment (Chapter 15)

Here it is argued that what happens in the interactions between patient and therapist is often as important as the formalities of treatment, and attention is paid to such issues as the therapeutic relationship and the likely structure and content of a therapeutic interview.

Alcoholics Anonymous (Chapter 16)

This is an international self-help organisation which has helped millions of people with drinking problems. This chapter offers an introduction to its basic tenets and the essential processes by which it operates. The importance of effective co-operation between treatment professionals and Alcoholics Anonymous (AA) is emphasised. The 'Minnesota Model' and its relationship with AA are also described.

Special techniques (Chapter 17)

Chapter 17 provides a discussion on a range of special techniques, with a particular focus on cognitive-behavioural and pharmaceutical treatments that have proven efficacy. It emphasises our belief that treatment should increasingly be research based.

Working toward normal drinking (Chapter 18)

For patients who are not significantly alcohol dependent, normal drinking can with caution be a feasible and preferred goal. Criteria for supporting this choice are identified and relevant treatment approaches discussed.

When things go wrong and putting them right (Chapter 19)

Underlining once more this book's commitment to a practical, clinical orientation, Chapter 19 deals with a series of work-a-day situations where treatment can run up against difficulties and considers how the therapeutic processes can then be unjammed and got on course again.

Treatment settings, professional roles, and the organisation of treatment services (Chapter 20)

This chapter describes the diversity of treatment settings encountered, and the varied contributions that professionals can make, in the treatment of drinking problems. The aim is to show the ways in which such varied settings and differently trained professionals all have a valuable role to play in helping the drinker. The need for co-operation between agencies, and effective organisation and planning of services is stressed.

We would, of course, be happy if this book is seen as having a useful place on library shelves. Our happiness would be even greater if we found it lying around dog-eared and well-used in out-patient clinic rooms, ward side-rooms, nursing stations, doctors' offices and surgeries, and other places where treatment actually happens. The best use of this text will be if the reader is willing to move backwards and forwards between its chapters and that rich reality of clinical experience where the greatest learning is always to be done.

I

Background to understanding

1

Causes of drinking problems

Why do some people drink so much more than others? Why also are some people able to drink large amounts of alcohol with apparent impunity, while others remain moderate and yet suffer various problems as a result of their drinking? This chapter will attempt to provide answers to these two questions. However, the complexity of the individual case and the extensiveness of the research literature, both indicate that too simple answers should not be expected. Nor should it be imagined that any single factor can provide an adequate explanation. Drinking behaviour, and the problems with which it is associated, are determined by multiple, interacting, factors which concern both the individual and his or her environment.

'Normal' drinking, 'heavy' drinking, and drinking problems

The causes of 'heavy' drinking and drinking problems can only be properly understood within the context of an overall view of 'normal' drinking in the population as a whole. This is because there is no clear boundary between normal and heavy drinking, and because drinking problems occur in normal as well as heavy drinkers. A graph demonstrating the typical distribution of alcohol consumption within a population is shown in Figure 1.1. It may be seen that while the majority of people drink 'moderately', a small percentage drink very heavily indeed (but a small percentage can mean a lot of people). However, it is quite arbitrary (on the basis of quantity alone) to choose a point at which to draw the line separating 'normal' and 'heavy' drinkers.

Extensive research has shown that the higher the average consumption of alcohol in a population, the higher the population's incidence of alcohol related problems. This holds true for almost all types of alcohol

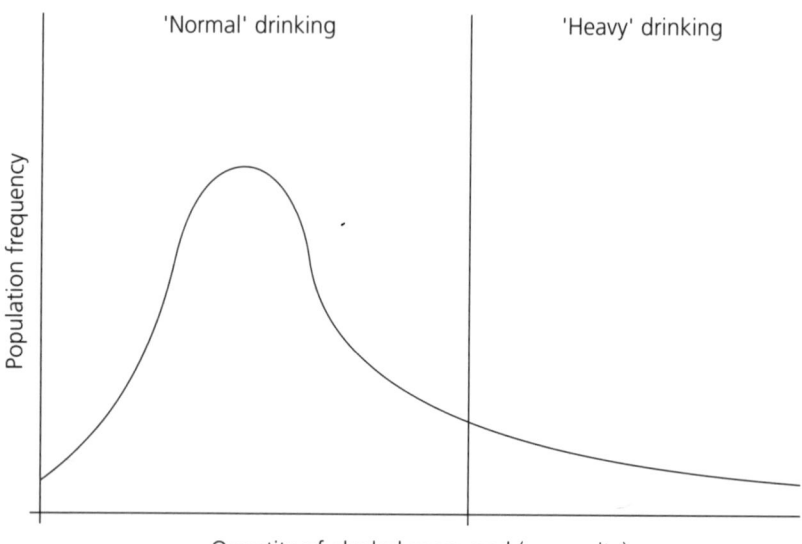

'Normal' drinking   'Heavy' drinking

Population frequency

Quantity of alcohol consumed (per capita)

Figure 1.1 Distribution of alcohol consumption in a general population

related problems – for example, drink driving offences, mortality due to cirrhosis of the liver, and crimes of violence all show such a relationship. This relationship also holds good at the individual level. Thus, for example, the risk of sustaining alcoholic liver disease, the risk of developing physical dependence upon alcohol, and the risk of breast cancer in females all vary in proportion to an individual's habitual level of alcohol consumption (Edwards *et al.*, 1994). With maximum benefit achieved at a low level of consumption (one drink a day or less) alcohol can reduce the risk of coronary heart disease among men aged over 40 years and post-menopausal women (see also p. 134).

Whilst heavy drinkers are at greater risk of various complications or problems arising from their drinking, Figure 1.1 reveals that (depending upon the arbitrary point at which we draw the line) there are many fewer heavy drinkers in the population than there are normal drinkers. Thus, although alcohol related problems are relatively rare amongst normal drinkers, the bulk of such problems in the population as a whole may still occur in normal drinkers, not in heavy drinkers. This has been referred to as the 'prevention paradox' because, paradoxically, preventive measures aimed at reducing such problems have to be directed at the whole population of drinkers – not just the heavy drinkers. In fact, the prevention paradox applies to some types of alcohol related problems, and not to others. The extent to which it applies depends upon the proportion of drinkers affected by a particular problem at each level of alcohol consumption (Edwards *et al.*, 1994). In general terms, the prevention paradox applies to the more immediate social problems such as drinking and driving. In contrast, very heavy drinkers contribute to the majority of chronic medical problems in a population (for instance cirrhosis).

Political and economic causes of drinking problems

Within individual countries over time, and in comparisons of different countries at any given time, it has been shown that reducing the real price of alcohol tends to increase the overall consumption of alcohol by a population. Similarly, measures which make alcohol more readily available by reducing restrictions on its supply also tend to increase consumption. Thus major influences upon per capita consumption in a population include factors amenable to political manipulation – such as taxation, licensing laws, and trade agreements. Manipulation of such influences can have enormous impact upon the level of alcohol consumption of a population. Conversely, failure to utilise such controls can allow alcohol consumption to escalate and related problems to reach epidemic proportions (Edwards *et al.*, 1994).

Many of the influences upon the economics of alcohol consumption are not deliberately manipulated, but follow in the wake of social change. Thus, for example, rapid socio-economic changes in Eastern Europe have led to increased availability of alcohol, increased consumption and increased drinking problems during the early 1990s. This would suggest that where possible, policy initiatives should be put in place as an intentional preventive measure, in advance of such changes. Equally, where controls on price and access already exist, they should not be removed for political, ideological, or trade reasons, with their public health significance ignored.

Socio-cultural causes of drinking problems

Availability of alcohol, and factors which influence availability (such as economic influences), are not the only factors of importance at a population level. Acceptability of alcohol consumption also plays an important part, and this is determined to a large degree by social and cultural values. However, these influences operate at various levels. For example, national and racial, religious, occupational, and family influences may all play a part.

Some cultures and societies promote total abstinence, for example Islamic culture, or the United States during the prohibition. In these cases the influence on drinking is explicitly negative, although there may be an associated counter-reaction towards illicit drinking, such that some members of the population still drink and the population as a whole may suffer from the associated criminal activity. At the other extreme are permissive cultures, including many Mediterranean countries, where drinking is actively endorsed. Such countries usually have high rates of morbidity attributable to, for example, alcoholic liver disease. In between these extremes there may be a mixture of cultural influences encouraging or discouraging drinking. In some cases, strongly opposing influences may be found in the same culture. Thus, for example, in Ireland there is a strong temperance movement within a culture that otherwise accepts and encourages drinking as a part of the general social order. In Jewish societies drinking is generally socially accepted, but strong negative connotations are attached to deviant drinking behaviour such as public drunkenness. Some would argue that this combination is responsible for the low incidence of alcohol related problems in Jewish societies (Bales, 1946).

Culture can influence the pattern and context, as well as the amount, of alcohol consumption. Pattern of alcohol consumption may in turn be an important determinant of drinking problems. Thus, in France habitual consumption of wine with meals is associated with a relatively high, but constant, per capita consumption which predisposes towards chronic medical complications such as cirrhosis and certain cancers. In urban centres in the UK and North America, particularly amongst working class men, alcohol is more likely to be consumed away from the home and often in relatively large quantity at a sitting. This pattern of drinking to intoxication seems to be more likely to be accompanied by adverse social consequences such as marital dysharmony, accidents, interpersonal violence, or drunkenness offences.

Culture may also influence the ways in which people behave when intoxicated. Thus drunken behaviour may be determined not only by the biological effects of alcohol as a drug, but also by social and cultural expectations as to how people will behave when drinking (MacAndrew & Edgerton, 1970). This may influence, for example, the likelihood of drunken antisocial behaviour.

There is a wide variation in drinking behaviour, and alcohol related problems, between different occupations. To some degree this may be a selection process which affects choice of occupation. However, there is also evidence that occupational environment itself influences drinking. Thus, for example, new employees in the drinks industry are likely to be relatively heavy drinkers, but there is evidence that they further increase their alcohol consumption after working in that industry (Plant, 1979). To some extent, as in this example, this may reflect ready availability of alcohol in a particular occupational environment. However, in different industries and occupations, a variety of other factors are also thought to be important, including for example, frequent absence from home, lack of supervision, long and irregular hours, social and peer pressures to drink (e.g. business lunches), and high stresses or hazards in the workplace.

Family 'culture' may also be an important influence upon drinking. In addition to any genetic influences, it seems likely that children will 'inherit' heavy drinking patterns by virtue of learning this behaviour, and any associated values or beliefs, from their parents. However, not all heavy drinking parents beget heavy drinking children. Where family rituals (including family traditions, ways of celebrating special occasions, and daily routines) are not disrupted by parental drinking, and where adult children deliberately establish new rituals when they marry, it seems that 'alcoholism' is less likely to be passed on to the next generation (Wolin et al., 1979; Bennett & Wolin, 1986). The importance of family factors will be further discussed in Chapter 4.

Stress and life events

Major life events and everyday hassles both appear to increase the amounts that people drink. This may be explained on the basis that alcohol relieves anxiety and is thus used as a means of coping with stress (the so called 'tension reduction' hypothesis). There is also evidence that an increased frequency of life events precedes the onset of alcohol misuse (Tatossian et al., 1983). These factors would therefore appear to be an important contributor to the development of drinking problems. However, the research evidence is not consistent and heavy drinking tends to cause further stress in the form of the problems that it generates (divorce, unemployment, ill health, and so on). There is also evidence that alcohol can exacerbate anxiety rather than relieve it. The association between heavy drinking and stress is therefore a complex one and should not be seen as simple cause and effect.

Contextual drinking problems

Drink-driving is an important example of a contextual drinking problem. Relatively modest alcohol consumption, which would cause no social, psychological, or medical problems in most other contexts,

13

may be the cause of serious injury or death when the drinker is also the driver of a car. Similar considerations also apply to other forms of transportation, as well as to a variety of other safety sensitive situations, particularly in the workplace.

Nature and nurture

Thus far, our analysis of the causes of heavy drinking and drinking problems may appear to indicate that the drinker is a victim of the environment, with individual factors having little part to play. (These environmental influences are summarised in Box 1.1.) Of course, this is at variance with our experience of the free will that we deploy in making decisions about our drinking, as well as the observation that some individuals in a heavy drinking environment drink moderately, or not at all. What part do individual factors play in the causes of heavy drinking and drinking problems?

Box 1.1. Some environmental determinants of drinking problems

- Individual and population levels of drinking

- Culture and religion

- Occupation

- Family experience of heavy drinking

- Stress and life events

- Safety sensitive environments, e.g. driving

It has long been observed that drinking problems tend to run in families (Cotton, 1979). The explanation for this was often assumed to be the effect of the family environment upon its members, tending in some way to produce uniformity of behaviour. There is almost certainly some truth to this hypothesis. However, more recent research has attempted to disentangle the effects of family environment from those of heredity. By studying identical and non-identical twins, and children raised in adoptive families and apart from their biological parents, it is possible to separate the effects of 'nature' and 'nurture'. With only a few exceptions, such studies have tended to confirm that there is a genetic component to drinking behaviour and drinking problems, in addition to the undeniably important influence of the environment (Cook, 1994).

What is it that is inherited, which in some way causes heavy drinking, alcohol related problems or alcohol dependence? In most cases we do not know the answer to this question. However, some clues are available and we may indulge in some informed speculation. For example, we know that in Oriental populations a genetic variant of one of the enzymes involved in alcohol metabolism (aldehyde dehydrogenase) is responsible for a 'flushing' syndrome which is manifested by an unpleasant physiological response to the ingestion of alcohol. Carriers of the mutant gene tend to drink little or no alcohol, since they feel unwell when they do. This genetic effect, due to a single gene mutation, dramatically reduces the incidence of heavy drinking and alcohol related problems amongst those affected by it. We might speculate that similar but more subtle effects may influence the amount that Caucasian individuals drink.

It would seem likely that particular organ systems (e.g. liver or brain) might be subject to genetic variation in vulnerability to alcohol induced damage. This hypothesis is supported, for example, by one of the twin studies of drinking problems, which showed evidence for a genetic influence upon both alcohol-induced liver disease and alcoholic psychosis (Hrubec & Omenn, 1981). There may also be biochemical traits, the inheritance of which predisposes to the development of alcohol dependence. For example, we know that alcohol dependence is associated with an increase in the number of voltage operated calcium channels in the cell membrane and that this is effected by gene activation (Harper et al., 1989). With a little more speculation, we may imagine that there are genetically determined differences in the extent to which the number of these channels is increased in response to heavy drinking.

How then can we understand the combined evidence supporting the importance of both genetic and environmental causes for heavy drinking and drinking problems? The truth is, of course, that a behaviour such as alcohol consumption cannot be totally understood either on the basis of genes or environment alone, but only as a product of the interaction between a variety of genetic and environmental influences. Thus we might see an individual as being more or less disposed to heavy drinking, or to particular alcohol related problems, or to dependence upon alcohol. This level of predisposition determines the risk, or probability of being a heavy drinker, or of suffering from a particular drink related problem. If a combination of environmental and genetic risk factors exceeds a certain hypothetical threshold, then that individual will drink heavily, or suffer a particular problem associated with their drinking.

We may now understand the enigma of the individual who drinks heavily, and escapes harm, or of the person who drinks moderately and suffers various complications. In the former case, the individual may be predisposed to heavy drinking by a combination of heredity and environmental factors. However, at the same time, they may have a (genetic) constitutional resilience which protects them from liver damage and they may learn (from their environment) social controls and patterns of behaviour which avoid public drunkenness, drink-driving or other alcohol related problems. In the latter case, the reverse may be true. Thus, the individual may drink moderately as a result of minimal genetic and environmental predisposition towards heavy drinking and yet be subject to, say, liver disease owing to genetic susceptibility of the liver to damage by alcohol.

Psychological explanations of drinking behaviour

The psychological characteristics of an individual may be seen as a product of their genetic constitution and the environment in which they live and grow. Psychological theories of drinking behaviour have been many and varied, but we can identify at least three main themes here. Firstly, there are psychodynamic theories which explain drinking as a result of early experiences and relationships, usually of a highly emotional nature. Secondly, cognitive and behavioural theories explain drinking as a learned behaviour. Thirdly, it has been suggested that certain personalities are particularly vulnerable, perhaps because of a tendency to use alcohol to deal with stress, anxiety, depression, or other problems.

It is often possible to apply all of these explanations to a given case. Take, for example, a woman with a drinking problem talking about her childhood:

> I can't think how I ever took to drinking myself when I remember what I went through in childhood. I hated the smell of the stuff. My father was more often drunk than sober, and my mother was stark terrified of him, would hide us away when she heard him coming home. What do I go and do? I follow exactly in his footsteps. I'm as nasty when drunk as ever my Dad used to be.

This woman may be drinking as a way of coping with the anger that she feels towards her father. She may also be drinking to relieve her feelings of guilt about the way that she treats her own family. As this causes more harm to the family, more guilt is generated and so a vicious cycle is set up, where guilt leads to drinking which leads to more guilt, and so on. The dynamic therapist might see this as a problem concerning unresolved anger towards her father. However, this scenario can also be understood on the basis of learnt patterns of behaviour copied from her father, or on the basis of a conditioning process whereby drinking is reinforced because (in the short-term) it relieves unpleasant experiences of anxiety, anger, and guilt.

The theory that there is a specific 'addictive personality' is now largely disproved. In so much as we can separate the consequences of drinking from its causes, it does not appear to be possible to predict 'addictive' personality traits which inevitably lead to alcohol misuse, drug addiction, or other problems of an addictive nature. However, some personality traits do seem to predispose to heavy drinking or alcohol misuse. Thus a tendency to experience anxiety or depression, or antisocial traits, may all increase the risk of heavy drinking. None of these traits inevitably lead to drinking problems, and not all heavy drinkers or problem drinkers manifest them.

In addition to these psychological explanations of the origins of heavy drinking, is the observation that heavy drinking may be associated with various psychiatric disorders. These disorders may be complications arising from the excessive consumption of alcohol, or they may be the underlying cause of heavy drinking, and often they are both. In such cases, it can be difficult to make judgements as to which problem came first. The relationship between psychiatric problems (including personality disorder) and drinking will be further explored in Chapter 6.

The lifetime perspective

'Alcoholism' is viewed by some as a chronic, progressive, and if left unchecked, inevitably fatal disease (Johnson, 1980). Certainly, a review of the life-history of a typical member of Alcoholics Anonymous (AA) would appear to support this contention:

> John started drinking in his early teens. He soon found that his friends were impressed by his ability to 'hold his drink', and as he grew older his social life increasingly revolved around pubs, bars, and clubs. Being naturally rather shy, he found that drinking not only relieved his anxieties about meeting people, but it also 'made him belong' within a social scene that revolved around alcohol. At the age of 18 he was charged with drinking and driving. His girlfriend left him a year later saying that she could

no longer tolerate the way that he behaved when he was drinking. Within five years he had also lost two jobs because of persistent lateness and poor performance. At the age of 24 years, when attending hospital for a head injury following a fall, he was noted to be severely alcohol dependent.

Such stories illustrate the combination of individual factors (e.g. personality) and environmental factors (e.g. social pressures and the 'youth culture') that lead to alcohol dependence, and appear to support the contention that 'alcoholism' is indeed qualitatively different from 'normal' drinking. Yet, as we have already seen, an epidemiological perspective does not appear to support this contention. In fact, many young people drink heavily, and experience some of the predictable alcohol related problems associated with such consumption, yet they do not inevitably progress to more serious or more frequent problems, or to alcohol dependence (Fillmore & Midanik, 1984; Temple & Fillmore, 1985). Indeed, increasing age generally seems to moderate the less restrained alcohol consumption of youth.

A person's age is, of course, simply another example of an individual characteristic which influences their liability to develop drinking problems. The importance of the lifetime perspective of heavy drinking is further emphasised by the interaction that occurs between age and environmental factors. Drink driving is a particularly poignant example of this. The young person is relatively inexperienced both in terms of driving and also in terms of drinking behaviour. At a given blood alcohol concentration, this combination results in a much higher risk of accidents for the younger driver.

We will return to a fuller consideration of the life course perspective in Chapter 11.

Application to the clinical context

Some of the research described in this chapter remains academic in day-to-day practice. For example, our efforts to help the problem drinker will be relatively uninfluenced by the knowledge that he or she has a strong family history of drinking problems. Nor will it be very important in practice to know whether that familiality is determined by genetic or cultural causes. However, neither should we imagine that such matters are irrelevant and there are two reasons for believing that they have an important bearing on work with our patients or clients.

Firstly, in relation to responsibilities which many professionals will accept for face-to-face health education (and community education), the question often arises as to what constitutes 'safe' or 'sensible' drinking. In truth, and as this chapter shows, the answer to this question will vary depending upon a range of individual and environmental vulnerability factors, many of which may be unknown. Because of this uncertainty, general guidelines for sensible drinking have been offered, which are estimated to be appropriate for most members of the population (Royal College of Psychiatrists, 1986; British Medical Association, 1995; Royal College of Physicians *et al.*, 1995). No drinking is, however, absolutely safe for all drinkers, on all occasions, and in all environments, and advice cannot properly be mechanistic. The child of the parent with a drinking problem, the person who is anxious or depressed, or the drinks industry employee are examples of people at particular risk, who may find it difficult to adhere to simple advice in practice, because of either constitutional susceptibility or environmental pressures, or both. A knowledge of the environmental and constitutional factors that make an individual vulnerable to drinking problems is therefore important both to the professional asked to advise on such matters and also to the individual wishing to make rational decisions about their own drinking.

The second area, where the matters discussed in this chapter are relevant to practice, is the logical basis that is very broadly provided for the approach to case assessment, as outlined in Chapter 13. There it will be suggested that whenever assessing a patient, or planning treatment, the requirement must be to look in detail both at the individual and the environment and to examine the multiple factors, both remote and current, which may bear on the genesis of that person's drinking problem. The research discussed in the present chapter gives that assessment approach its scientific underpinning.

It is also likely that, in future, different interventions will be offered to different groups of problem drinkers. Relapse prevention methods may be particularly appropriate for those people who drink to relieve anxiety. Particular drug treatments may be more beneficial for those with certain types of genetic predisposition (Lawford *et al.*, 1995). However, we currently know relatively little about how to achieve the optimum match of different treatments with different problem drinkers (Lindström, 1992).

References

Bales, R. F. (1946). Cultural differences in rates of alcoholism. *Quarterly Journal of Studies on Alcohol* **6**, 489–99.

Bennett, L. A. & Wolin, S. J. (1986). Daughters and sons of alcoholics: developmental paths in transmission. *Alcoholism* **22**, 3–15.

British Medical Association (1995). *Alcohol: Guidelines on Sensible Drinking*. London: British Medical Association.

Cook, C. C. H. (1994). Aetiology of alcohol misuse. Chap. 6. In *Seminars in Psychiatry: Alcohol and Drug Misuse*, ed. J. Chick & R. Cantwell, pp. 94–125 London: Royal College of Psychiatrists.

Cotton, N. S. (1979). The familial incidence of alcoholism. *Journal of Studies on Alcohol* **40**, 89–116.

Edwards, G., Anderson, P., Babor, T. F., Casswell, S., Ferrence, R., Giesbrecht, N., Godfrey, C., Holder, H. D., Lemmens, P., Mäkelä, K., Midanik, L. T., Norström, T., Österberg, E., Romelsjö, A., Room, R., Simpura, J. & Skog, O.-J. (1994). *Alcohol Policy and the Public Good*. Oxford: Oxford University Press.

Fillmore, K. M. & Midanik, L. (1984). Chronicity of drinking problems among men: a longitudinal study. *Journal of Studies on Alcohol* **45**, 228–36.

Harper, J. C., Brennan, C. H. & Littleton, J. M. (1989). Genetic up-regulation of calcium channels in a cellular model of ethanol dependence. *Neuropharmacology* **28**, 1299–302.

Hrubec, Z. & Omenn, G.S. (1981). Evidence of genetic predisposition to alcoholic psychosis and cirrhosis: twin concordances for alcoholism and its biological end points by zygosity among male veterans. *Alcoholism, Clinical and Experimental Research* **5**, 207–15.

Johnson, V. E. (1980). *I'll Quit Tomorrow*. New York: Harper and Row.

Lawford, B. R., Young, R. McD., Rowell, J. A., Qualichefski, J., Fletcher ,B. H., Syndulko, K. L., Ritchie, T. & Noble, E. P. (1995). Bromocriptine in the treatment of alcoholics with the D2 dopamine receptor A1 allele. *Nature Medicine* **1**, 337–41.

Lindström, L. (1992): *Managing Alcoholism: Matching Clients to Treatments*. Oxford: Oxford University Press.

MacAndrew, C. & Edgerton, R. B. (1970). *Drunken Comportment*. London: Nelson.

Plant, M. A. (1979). *Drinking Careers*. London: Tavistock.

Royal College of Physicians, Royal College of Psychiatrists & Royal College of General Practitioners (1995). *Alcohol and the Heart in Perspective: Sensible Limits Reaffirmed*. London: Royal Colleges of Physicians, Psychiatrists, and General Practitioners.

Royal College of Psychiatrists (1986). *Alcohol: Our Favourite Drug*. London: Tavistock.

Tatossian, A., Charpy, J. P., Remy, M., Prinquey, D. & Poinso, Y. (1983). Events in the lives of 120 chronic alcoholics: preliminary study. *Annales Medico-Psychologiques* **141**, 824–41.

Temple, M. T. & Fillmore, K. M. (1985). The variability of drinking patterns and problems among young men age 16–31: a longitudinal study. *International Journal of the Addictions* **20**, 1595–1620.

Wolin, S. J., Bennett, L. A. & Noonan, D. L. (1979). Family rituals and the recurrence of alcoholism over generations. *American Journal of Psychiatry* **136**, 589–93.

2

Alcohol as a drug

The purpose of this chapter

Alcohol is a beverage which is consumed as a food and sometimes as a medicine, and is rich with symbolic significance when used within social, cultural, and religious customs and rituals. Its properties have been familiar to countless peoples around the world for thousands of years. However, it is also a drug which has both important pharmacological and toxic effects upon the mind and upon almost every organ and system in the human body. A knowledge of these pharmacological effects is basic to understanding many of the problems that arise from its use, as well as to a consideration of how we may offer treatment for these problems. There is today considerable excitement among researchers about advances in understanding of the biological actions of alcohol and we hope that this chapter conveys that sense – much more is now known in this field than 10–20 years ago.

What is discussed here will inevitably make difficult reading for people whose expertise is in a discipline other than medicine. Some of those readers may prefer to move on to Chapter 3, but others may find it valuable to obtain at least a nodding acquaintance with what is happening at this pharmacological frontline. We are in no way seeking to imply that biological sciences provide the only or key insight into the determinants of drinking behaviour – in this book psychological and social influences on drinking and the genesis of drinking problems are fully discussed.

Absorption and distribution

Alcohol is rapidly absorbed into the circulation from the stomach, small intestine, and colon, and the time to maximum concentration in the

21

blood ranges from 30 to 90 minutes (Hobbs *et al.*, 1996). The rate of absorption is influenced by a number of factors. Higher alcohol concentrations (up to a maximum of 40% by volume) and the presence of carbon dioxide and bicarbonate in fizzy drinks increase absorption. The presence of food in the stomach slows absorption by delaying gastric emptying. Decreasing body temperature and physical exercise also reduce absorption, as does the presence of sugar in the alcohol. Peak blood levels are higher if the same quantity of alcohol is ingested in a single dose rather than in several small doses (Agarwal & Goedde, 1990). In women the stage of the menstrual cycle can influence absorption.

Following absorption, alcohol is distributed throughout the body. It is hydrophilic (water loving), accumulates in tissues with the highest water content, and can cross the placenta into the foetal circulation. Highly perfused organs such as the brain, lungs, and kidney, show the highest alcohol levels while in tissues with poor blood flow, such as muscle, alcohol concentrations are lower (Agarwal & Goedde, 1990).

Blood alcohol concentration (BAC) is very similar to tissue levels in most of the body except fat. The relatively higher body fat in women leads to a higher BAC than would occur in men after an equivalent dose of alcohol. This may explain, at least in part, the increased vulnerability of women to certain types of tissue damage.

Excretion and metabolism

Between 90 and 98% of ingested alcohol is eliminated from the body by oxidation to carbon dioxide and water. Most of the alcohol that escapes oxidation is excreted unchanged in expired air, urine, and sweat; elimination by these routes may increase after a heavy drinking bout or at elevated temperatures.

The amount of alcohol oxidised per unit time depends on body weight. In the healthy adult the average rate of metabolism is 120 mg per kg per hour, equivalent to 30 mls in three hours (Hobbs *et al.*, 1996). Breakdown can be faster in the heavier drinker (see below). Alcohol may undergo first pass metabolism in the stomach but 90–98% of ingested alcohol is metabolised in the liver. The major pathway is oxidation by alcohol dehydrogenase (ADH) to acetaldehyde. Acetaldehyde is, in turn, oxidised by aldehyde dehydrogenase (ALDH) to acetate. Both ADH and ALDH are NAD (nicotinamide adenine dinucleotide) dependent and the oxidations of alcohol and acetaldehyde reduce NAD to NADH. Excess NADH can cause hyperlacticacidaemia which can contribute to acidosis, reduce urinary excretion of uric acid and lead to secondary hyperuricaemia. NADH also contributes to hypoglycaemia and hyperlipidaemia (Lieber, 1995; see Chapter 8).

The enzymes ADH and ALDH are under genetic control. Three classes of ADH have been described and the class I variety is largely responsible for the first step in alcohol metabolism. At least four isozymes of ALDH have been detected in humans. ALDH2, the isozyme largely responsible for the oxidation of acetaldehyde exists in two forms, one of which is virtually inactive. Low activity ALDH2, which is common in Orientals, leads to a flush reaction when alcohol is taken. This reaction is unpleasant, therefore individuals with low activity ALDH2 are less inclined to drink and are thus less vulnerable to developing alcohol dependence. Low activity ALDH2 is also associated with a reduced rate of alcoholic liver disease (see Chapter 1). The acetate formed from acetaldehyde is released into the circulation and is largely taken up by muscle and heart for oxidation via the tricarboxylic acid cycle (Crabb, 1993). Although ADH is the major pathway for the oxidation of alcohol, it can be oxidised by two other enzyme systems, the microsomal ethanol-oxidising system (MEOS) located in the endoplasmic reticulum, and catalase, located in peroxisomes. The contribution of catalase is thought to be minimal. The MEOS is dependent on the cytochrome P450 system. It usually plays a small role in the metabolism of alcohol, but its role increases with increased consumption. Chronic alcohol intake enhances MEOS activity, increasing the rate of alcohol metabolism and increasing tolerance to alcohol. This process of 'induction' leads, in turn, to an increased production of acetaldehyde which is a toxic substance.

Induction of the MEOS also affects the metabolism of other drugs. Cytochrome P450 can convert many drugs, including anaesethetic agents, illicit drugs such as cocaine, other drugs such as isoniazid and phenylbutazone, and paracetamol, into toxic metabolites. Therapeutic amounts of paracetamol can cause hepatic damage in heavy drinkers (Lieber, 1995).

Pharmacological effects

Cardiovascular system

The effects of alcohol on the circulation are minor. Moderate doses cause a small transient increase in heart rate and vasodilatation, especially in the skin, with facial flushing. There is no increase in coronary blood flow. Blood pressure, cardiac output, and force of cardiac contractility are not significantly affected by moderate amounts of alcohol. Large doses produce an increase in cerebral blood flow, decreased cerebro-vascular resistance and reduced cerebral oxygen uptake.

Body Temperature

Moderate amounts of alcohol can lead to peripheral vasodilatation and sweating. Increased sweating can, in turn, lead to heat loss and a fall in body temperature. Large amounts of alcohol can depress the central temperature regulating mechanism causing a more pronounced fall in body temperature.

Gastro-intestinal tract

Alcohol can stimulate gastric secretion by reflex excitation of sensory endings in the buccal and gastric mucosa and by a direct action on the stomach, possibly involving release of gastrin. Strong alcoholic drinks cause inflammation of the stomach lining and produce an erosive gastritis. Alcohol intoxication causes cessation of gastro-intestinal secretory and motor functions.

Kidney

Alcohol itself produces a diuretic effect independent from the increased flow associated with the ingestion of large volumes of fluid. This diuretic effect is proportional to the blood alcohol concentration and occurs when levels are rising, but not when they are stable or falling.

Respiration

Moderate amounts of alcohol may stimulate or depress respiration, whereas large amounts (greater than 400 mg per 100 ml) produce depression of respiration.

Central nervous system (CNS)

The effects of alcohol on the brain are dependent on dose and the rate of rise in BAC. Driving skill is affected at 30 mg%. Mood and behavioural changes occur at levels of approximately 50–100 mg%. At levels of 150–300 mg% there is loss of self control, slurred speech, and clumsiness. Individuals unused to heavy drinking are moderately intoxicated at BAC levels of 150–250 mg% and obvious intoxication is usually evident at 300 mg%. At BACs of 300–500mg% individuals are usually severely intoxicated, and stupor and hypothermia may sometimes supervene. Hypoglycaemia and seizures are occasionally a feature of BACs in this range. Regular drinkers become tolerant to the CNS effects of alcohol and may have BAC levels of 500 mg% without obvious signs of intoxication. However, for non-tolerant drinkers, such levels are associated with depressed reflexes, respiratory depression, hypotension, hypothermia, and sometimes death.

The development of alcohol dependence

Individuals with drinking problems are a very diverse group yet share many commonalities, as is evident to anyone who takes a good drinking history (see Chapter 13).

There is increasing evidence that the evolution of alcohol dependence can be explained in terms of both psychological and pharmacological processes, and it appears likely that neuroadaptation changes in the brain underly the compulsion to drink, increased tolerance, alcohol withdrawal, and the other features of the syndrome. Not everyone who drinks heavily becomes dependent. Some may be more vulnerable than others by virtue of constitutional make-up or environmental influences. Hypothetical pathways into alcohol dependence might include the use of alcohol to relieve anxiety and stress, its use as a stimulant/euphoriant, or for sedation (Littleton & Little, 1994).

Pathways into alcohol dependence

Alcohol is a relatively non-specific psychoactive drug which alters neurotransmitter and receptor function. Until relatively recently, it was thought to act by entering neuronal membranes, altering the property of the lipids and increasing their 'fluidity' and permeability. Although this property may contribute to some of its effects, the action of alcohol on specific neurotransmitters and on the receptor-ion channel complex may be more important (Littleton & Little, 1994). Alcohol acts on several neuronal systems, which in turn interact with each other. It is, therefore, difficult to attribute the acute effects of alcohol to any specific system (Nutt & Peters, 1994; Nutt, 1996).

Anxiety reduction

Alcohol is a potent anxiolytic agent and this effect appears to be mediated largely by its action on the GABA-A receptor. Acutely, alcohol enhances the action of GABA (gamma aminobutyric acid), the major

25

inhibitory transmitter in the CNS, at the GABA-A receptor. Other mechanisms may contribute to alcohol's anxiolytic action including its ability to reduce the reuptake of adenosine in the brain and its effect on the 5-HT (5-hydroxytryptamine) system (Littleton & Little, 1994). The anxiolytic action of alcohol is theoretically a 'rewarding' effect and has the potential to reinforce further alcohol consumption and to contribute to the development of psychological dependence.

Stimulant/euphoriant effects

Alcohol has traditionally been described as a depressant drug. The view that it causes stimulation and euphoria has been controversial, but is now more widely accepted, though there is still debate as to whether this effect is separate from its anxiolytic or anaesthetic properties (Littleton & Little, 1994). The putative stimulant effect of alcohol can be explained by its action in the mesolimbic system of the brain, where it causes release of dopamine. This effect of alcohol may be mediated by an initial release of opioid peptides, via an action of alcohol on 5-HT receptors, or by interactions with GABA or other neurotransmitters in the ventral tegmental area where the dopamine neurones originate. Naltrexone, an opioid receptor antagonist, shown to reverse alcohol-induced dopamine release in the nucleus accumbens of rats, may have a place in the treatment of human alcohol dependence. This is discussed further in Chapter 17.

The stimulant/euphoriant effect of alcohol, mediated by increased release of dopamine, is less than that observed for the CNS stimulants amphetamine and cocaine. Nevertheless the positive reinforcement associated with the feeling of euphoria or 'reward' can also explain the development of a psychological dependence on alcohol.

Anaesthetic effects of alcohol

Alcohol also has an anaesthetic action and can induce amnesia for events that occur at sub-anaesthetic concentrations of the drug (Littleton & Little, 1994). These amnestic effects may be due to the inhibitory action of alcohol on the NMDA (N-methyl-D-aspartate) receptor. NMDA receptors are one subclass of receptors for glutamate, the major excitatory neurotransmitter in the human brain. When activated by large amounts of glutamate, NMDA receptors allow entry of calcium ions (Ca^{2+}) into the neuron, where they act as a second messenger, leading to changes in intracellular proteins that result in adaptations which underly learning and memory (Littleton & Little, 1994; Nutt & Peters, 1994). It could be postulated that alcohol-induced anaesthesia and amnesia are rewarding in the case of severe depression or in situations where alcohol is used to 'numb' traumatic memories, e.g. of childhood sexual abuse. The putative anaesthetic effects of alcohol are thought to be rare as a mechanism leading to psychological dependence. The quantities of alcohol consumed in order to obtain amnesia are more likely to lead to physical dependence.

Neuroadaptation

Chronic alcohol consumption leads to adaptive changes in the brain. Alcohol tolerance, physical dependence as manifest by the alcohol withdrawal syndrome, and psychological dependence manifest by the compulsion to drink, can be explained by neuroadaptation (Anton, 1996; Hoffman & Tabakoff, 1996). Although tolerance is one of the key elements of the alcohol dependence syndrome, the neuroadaptations underlying its development appear to be different from the neuroadaptations underlying the development of physical dependence and withdrawal. This would explain why some individuals manifest alcohol tolerance but not the components of the physical dependence syndrome.

Tolerance

Tolerance is defined as the decrease in sensitivity to the effects of alcohol that occurs as a result of previous exposure to it (Kalant, 1996). Three types of tolerance have been described – acute, rapid, and chronic. Acute tolerance occurs within the duration of a single exposure to alcohol. Tolerance to the effects of the second dose of alcohol, given between eight hours and three days after the effects of the first dose have disappeared, is termed rapid tolerance. Chronic tolerance occurs after repeated administrations of alcohol. It is not known whether acute, rapid, and chronic tolerance are mediated by the same process. However, there is probably a learned psychological component to acute tolerance (Vogel-Sprott, 1992).

Tolerance shares many of the features of learning and memory and it is thought that both operant learning and classical or Pavlovian conditioning play a major role in its development. Interactions between the serotoninergic, glutamatergic and vasopressinergic systems, forming a circuit in the limbic forebrain, are thought to play a central role in the development and maintenance of tolerance. More specifically, NMDA receptors, modulated by serotonin receptors in the septum or hippocampus, may play a direct role in the development of tolerance, whereas vasopressin V1 receptors, with help from 5-HT2 receptors in the same region maintain tolerance (Kalant, 1996).

Physical dependence and the alcohol withdrawal syndrome

Some types of neuroadaptation are associated with physical dependence. Neuroadaptation that opposes the action of alcohol and is reversed slowly on cessation of drinking can produce a withdrawal syndrome. These adaptations are effective while alcohol is present in the brain but when alcohol is removed, adaptations are made in the opposite direction, thus producing an alcohol withdrawal state.

Neuroadaptation within the CNS is a complex phenomenon and what follows is an attempt to simplify it for the non-medical reader. A fuller account can be found in reviews by Littleton & Little (1994) and Hoffman & Tabakoff (1996). Neuroadaptation can be divided into 'specific' and 'non-specific' components. 'Specific' neuroadaptation occurs in the transmitter/neuroreceptor system. 'Non-specific' neuroadaptation occurs 'downstream' of receptors and may involve second messenger systems to which receptors are coupled. This form of adaptation is likely to be widespread and can explain cross-tolerance and dependence on other classes of drugs, e.g. benzodiazepines.

Examples of 'specific' adaptation are seen in the NMDA and GABA-A systems. 'Acute' use of alcohol blocks the activation of the NMDA receptor by glutamate, the major excitatory amino acid, and reduces its function. Animal studies show that chronic alcohol use leads to 'upregulation' (increase) of the NMDA receptors in order to compensate for prolonged inhibition. Alcohol withdrawal is accompanied by glutamatergic hyperactivity which is thought to underly the various symptoms and signs, including withdrawal seizures (Grant et al., 1990), and to contribute to cell death and alcohol-related brain damage (Tsai et al., 1995).

Acutely, alcohol potentiates the effect of GABA at the GABA-A receptor. Here one would expect that the adaptive response would be a reduction ('down regulation') in the number of GABA-A receptors. The situation appears to be more complex, and is influenced by the fact that the GABA-A receptor is present in many isoforms with differential sensitivities to alcohol (Nutt & Peters, 1994). Animal studies suggest that the brain can modify its response to alcohol on GABA-A receptors without changing the total numbers of these receptors. Thus it currently appears unlikely that the GABA-A receptor plays a major role in the generation of withdrawal symptoms.

An example of 'non-specific' neuroadaptation implicated in alcohol withdrawal involves voltage-operated calcium channels. Alcohol inhibits the function of the 'L-type' (dihydropyridine-sensitive) calcium channel in the membrane of the neuronal cell body (Littleton & Little, 1994) thus reducing calcium entry and probably neurotransmitter release. Chronic alcohol administration increases the number of these channels in the neuronal membrane ('upregulation'). When alcohol is withdrawn the increased number of channels and increased calcium entry lead to excessive neurotransmitter release, and this contributes to the alcohol withdrawal state (Littleton & Little, 1994).

Reinstatement

How can we explain the process by which someone with alcohol dependence who has been abstinent for several years develops severe alcohol withdrawal symptoms days or weeks following relapse. This phenomenon is known as 'reinstatement' and is extraordinary because of the way the whole alcohol dependence syndrome re-emerges, as if there is an irreversible 'addiction memory' laid down in the brain.

Future directions

In recent years neuropharmacological research has helped to uncover the mechanisms underlying the actions of alcohol, 'appetite' for alcohol, and the biological basis of dependence. This has led to a renewed interest in pharmacotherapies for alcohol dependence already with some promising results. The challenge now is to integrate insights from neuropharmacology, molecular genetics, and clinical science with understanding from other and wider disciplines, particularly psychology. Drinking is a behaviour with multiple determinants and the truly crucial questions will in the long run yield only to multidisciplinary (and interdisciplinary) research.

References

Agarwal, D. P. & Goedde, H. W. (1990). *Alcohol Metabolism, Alcohol Intolerance and Alcoholism. Biochemical and Pharmacogenetic Aspects*. Berlin: Springer-Verlag.

Anton, R. F. (1996). Neurobehavioural basis for the pharmacotherapy of alcoholism: current and future directions. *Alcohol and Alcoholism* 31, 43–53.

Crabb, D. W. (1993). The liver. In *Recent Developments in Alcoholism*, ed. Galanter, M., vol. 11, pp. 207–30. New York: Plenum Press.

Grant, K. A., Valverius, P., Hudspith, M. & Tabakoff, B. (1990). Ethanol withdrawal seizures and the NMDA receptor complex. *European Journal of Pharmacology* 176, 289–96.

Hobbs, W. R., Rall, T. W. & Verdoon, T. A. (1996). Hypnotics and sedatives, ethanol. In *Goodman and Gilman's The Pharmacological Basis of Therapeutics*, ed. Hardman, J. G., Limberd, L. E., 9th edn, pp. 361–46. New York: McGraw Hill.

Hoffman, P. L. & Tabakoff, B. (1996). Alcohol dependence: a commentary on the mechanisms. *Alcohol and Alcoholism* **31**, 333–40.

Kalant, H. (1996). Current state of knowledge about the mechanisms of alcohol tolerance. *Addiction Biology* **1**, 133–41.

Lieber, C. S. (1995). Medical disorders of alcoholism. *The New England Journal of Medicine* **333**, 1058–65.

Littleton, J. & Little, H. (1994). Current concepts of ethanol dependence. Addiction **89**, 1397–412.

Nutt, D. J. (1996). Addiction: brain mechanisms and their treatment implications. *Lancet* **347**, 31–6.

Nutt, D. J. & Peters, T. J. (1994). Alcohol: the drug. In *Alcohol and Alcohol Problems*, ed. Edwards, G. & Peters, T. J., pp. 5–17. British Medical Bulletin No. 50. Edinburgh: Churchill Livingstone.

Tsai, G., Gastfriend, D. R. & Coyle, J. T. (1995). The glutamatergic basis of human alcoholism. *American Journal of Psychiatry* **152**, 332–40.

Vogel-Sprott, M. (1992). *Alcohol Tolerance and Social Drinking*. New York: Guilford Press.

3

The alcohol dependence syndrome

Dependence is an important clinical reality, and understanding of its implications is one essential part of the therapist's competence if they are to deal with drinking problems. Nothing which is being said should be misinterpreted as implying that dependence is everything, and many patients with drinking problems are not suffering from the dependence syndrome. That latter fact in itself is good reason for seeking to develop the skill to recognise the presence of dependence in any of its degrees; one needs to be able confidently to recognise when dependence is not present.

A mechanistic approach to the diagnosis of dependence is insufficient. Dependence cannot be conceived as 'not present' or 'present', with the diagnostic task then completed. The skill lies in being able to recognise the subtleties of symptomatology which will reveal not only whether this condition is there at all but, if it exists, the degree of its development. What has also to be learnt is how the syndrome's manifestations are moulded by personality, by environmental influence, or by cultural forces. It is the ability to recognise and understand the variations on these themes that constitutes the real art.

If the therapist cannot recognise *degrees* of dependence, they will not be able to fit their approach to the particular patient, and they may retreat into seeing 'addiction to alcohol' as a fixed entity from which all patients with drinking problems are presumed to suffer, for whom the universal goal must be total abstinence, and the treatment which is offered universally intensive. The needed skill is the development of a discriminating judgement which is able in each case to sense out the degree of dependence, identify the rational treatment goal for that person, and propose the treatment fitted to that particular individual's problem.

Dependence implies an altered relationship between a person and

31

their drinking. An individual may start to drink for many reasons, and when they are dependent many of these reasons will still pertain and are not necessarily wiped out because of the super-added fact of the dependence. However, the dependence now provides reasons for drinking which are truly super-added, and which may dominate the many preceding reasons for drinking and heavy drinking. Dependence becomes a self-perpetuating behaviour.

This chapter is organised as follows. Firstly, the clinical origin of the dependence syndrome concept will be discussed and its scientific underpinning outlined. Secondly, a detailed description of the individual elements within the syndrome is given. Thirdly, a case history is presented to illustrate the picture in the round and its coherence. Fourthly, the question of whether dependence is best viewed as a unitary condition with many and continuous variations, or alternatively as a family of disorders within a typology, will be considered.

The clinical concept and its scientific underpinning

Clinical genesis of the syndrome concept

The concept of a *syndrome* is used in medicine to designate a clustering of signs and symptoms. Not all the elements may be present in every instance, but the picture must be sufficiently regular and coherent to permit its clinical recognition and to allow distinction between syndrome and non-syndrome.

A syndrome is a descriptive clinical formulation which is initially likely to be agnostic as to causation or pathology. The existence of alcohol dependence has been evident to acute observers for many years (e.g. Trotter, 1804; Kerr, 1888), but in the 1970s a detailed clinical description was enunciated within a syndrome model (Edwards & Gross, 1976; Edwards *et al.*, 1977). It was suggested by Edwards and Gross that clinical observation revealed a repeated clustering of signs and symptoms in certain heavy drinkers. It was further suggested that the syndrome existed in degrees of severity rather than as a categorical absolute, that its presentation could be shaped by pathoplastic influences rather than its being concrete and invariable, and that alcohol dependence should be conceptually distinguished from alcohol-related problems. This clinically derived syndrome postulate was at that stage designated as only provisional, and within the general research tradition of psychiatric taxonomy the *validity* of the syndrome needed to be determined.

Establishing syndrome validity

Following the original description, research has tested multiple aspects of validity (Edwards, 1986). Studies have for instance been directed at determining the internal homogeneity of the syndrome and the degree to which its postulated elements co-occur (Stockwell *et al.*, 1979; Chick, 1980; Stockwell *et al.*, 1983; Meehan, 1985; Feingold & Rounsaville, 1995), and the related issues of construct validity (Heather *et al.*, 1983); concurrent validity (Stockwell *et al.*, 1983; Kivlahan *et al.*, 1989; Caetano, 1993); and finally predictive validity (Hodgson *et al.*, 1979; Rankin *et al.*, 1982). Added stimulus was given to this research by field trials which were conducted as background to the preparation of ICD-10, DSM-IIIR and DSM-IV (Grant *et al.*, 1992; Cottler, 1993; Rapaport *et al.*, 1993; Rounsaville *et al.*, 1993; American Psychiatric Association, 1994; Cottler *et al.*, 1995).

The overall conclusion to be drawn from this by now extensive body of research is that the syndrome is a reality rather than a chimera of the clinical eye. That is not to say that all elements are in psychometric terms equally well tied into the syndrome. Within the scientific perspective some elements may be redundant, and difficulties have been encountered in operationalising elements such as narrowing of repertoire, subjective change and reinstatement (Cottler *et al.*, 1995). With those provisos entered, the original syndrome description seems to be a formulation reasonably close to clinical actuality (Babor *et al.*,1990), and satisfactorily validated.

The neurobiological basis

If the clinical description of alcohol dependence was the first step and the establishment of its validity the second, the third stage in this sequential process must be to determine the nature of the underlying biological and psychological processes which are involved in the genesis, perpetuation, and reinstatement of the condition.

What *is* dependence? There has over recent years been progress on many fronts (White, 1996), but a comprehensive answer to that question is still not possible. We have bits of the answer, but the puzzle does not as yet entirely fit together. Although biological and psychological aspects of dependence can usefully be studied in their own right, the larger and outstanding challenge is to delineate the totality of the interactive psychobiological system which underlies dependence (Edwards & Lader, 1990).

At the biological level the systems which make alcohol behaviourally reinforcing are partly but not completely understood: it is likely that more than one transmitter system is involved, with both dopamine and serotonin release playing a part (Nutt & Peters, 1994). There have been many advances on the genetic front (Ball & Murray, 1994), and relevant biological and genetic aspects of dependence receive attention in Chapters 1 and 2. There is debate as to whether the primary drug effect on the brain is the dominant mechanism which reinforces the alcohol-seeking habit or whether relief of withdrawal is also a significant reinforcer (Edwards, 1990). The mechanisms which underly acquisition of tolerance and the underlying biology of withdrawal symptoms are increasingly understood (see Chapter 2). What is still missing is understanding of the mechanisms to explain why once a drinker has developed dependence, the condition is so readily reinstated if drinking is started again after a period of abstinence (Edwards, 1990).

At the psychological level, analysis has focused on identification of cues which trigger craving or alcohol-seeking behaviour, and the alteration in cue-responsivity which are a feature of dependence (Glautier & Drummond, 1992). The learning mechanisms involved in dependence include both classical and operant conditioning (Greeley *et al.*, 1993; Glautier & Drummond, 1994), and it is also likely that altered expectancies and other cognitive processes significantly contribute to the psychological basis of dependence (Stacy *et al.*, 1990; Leigh & Stacy, 1991; Jones & McMahon, 1996; Williams & Ricciardelli, 1996).

Further insights into the nature of dependence are likely to involve advances in understanding of relevant biological, behavioural, and cognitive processes and most importantly their interactions (Edwards *et al.*, 1981). It is not a condition that can be comprehended within any single-level reductionist model (Edwards, 1994), and it certainly comprises much more than the evident elements of tolerance and withdrawal (Carroll *et al.*, 1994).

Individual elements of the dependence syndrome

The elements of the syndrome, as originally formulated by Edwards and Gross (1976), are summarised in Box 3.1. It is these elements which will now be discussed sequentially below rather than only the more restrictive syndromal formulations described in ICD-10 or DSM-IV (see pp. 214–16).

Narrowing of repertoire

The ordinary drinker's consumption and choice of drink will vary from day to day and from week to week; they may have a beer at lunch on

---

Box 3.1. The alcohol dependence syndrome – key elements

- Narrowing of repertoire
- Salience of drinking
- Increased tolerance to alcohol
- Withdrawal symptoms
- Relief or avoidance of withdrawal symptoms by further drinking
- Subjective awareness of compulsion to drink
- Reinstatement after abstinence

---

one day, nothing to drink on another, share a bottle of wine at dinner one night, and then go to a party on a Saturday and have several drinks. Their drinking is patterned by varying internal cues and external circumstances.

At first, a person becoming caught up in heavy drinking may widen their repertoire and the range of cues that signal drinking. As dependence advances, the cues are increasingly related to relief or avoidance of alcohol withdrawal, and their personal drinking repertoire becomes increasingly narrowed. The dependent person begins to drink the same whether it is a workday, weekend, or holiday; the nature of the company or their own mood makes less and less difference. Questioning may distinguish earlier and later stages of dependence by the degree to which the repertoire is narrowed. With advanced dependence, the drinking may become scheduled to a strict daily timetable to maintain a high blood alcohol. More careful questioning will, however, show that even when dependence is well established, some capacity for variation remains. The syndrome must be pictured as subtle and plastic rather than as something set hard, but as dependence advances the patterns tend to become increasingly fixed.

Salience of drinking

The stereotyping of the drinking pattern as dependence advances leads to the individual giving priority to maintaining their alcohol intake. The wife's distressed scolding – once effective – is later neutralised by the drinker as evidence of a lack of understanding. Income which had previously to serve many needs now supports the drinking habit as the first demand. Gratification of the need for drink may become more important for the patient with liver damage than considerations of survival. Diagnostically, the progressive change in the salience given to alcohol is important, rather than behaviour at any one time. Typically, the patient relates that they used to be proud of their house, but now the paint is peeling; used always to take the children to football matches, but now spends no time with the family; used to have rather conventional moral standards, but will now beg, borrow, or steal to obtain money for alcohol.

Increased tolerance to alcohol

Alcohol is a drug to which the CNS develops tolerance (see Chapter 2). Patients themselves report on tolerance in terms of 'having a good head for liquor' or 'being able to drink the other person under the table'. Clinically, tolerance is shown by the dependent person being able to sustain an alcohol intake and go about their business at blood alcohol levels that would incapacitate the non-tolerant drinker. This does not mean that their functioning is not impaired – they will be a dangerous driver, but because of their tolerance they will (unfortunately) still be able to drive.

Cross-tolerance will extend to certain other drugs, notably general depressants such as barbiturates and benzodiazepines, which means that the person who has become tolerant to alcohol will also have a tolerance to these drugs and vice versa. The rate of development of tolerance is variable, but the heavy drinker who is not dependent can manifest tolerance. In later stages of dependence, for reasons which are unclear, the individual begins to lose their previously acquired tolerance and becomes incapacitated by quantities of alcohol which they could previously handle and they may then begin to fall down drunk in the street.

Withdrawal symptoms

At first these symptoms are intermittent and mild; they cause little incapacity, and one symptom may be experienced without others. As dependence increases so does the frequency and the severity of the withdrawal symptoms. When the picture is fully developed, typically the patient has severe multiple symptoms every morning on waking and perhaps even in the middle of the night. Questioning often reveals that the severely dependent patient experiences mild withdrawal symptoms (which they recognise as such) at any time during the day when their alcohol level falls. Complete withdrawal is therefore not necessary to precipitate disturbance.

The patient often remembers rather exactly the dating of the period when they first began to experience withdrawal, and there is no necessary association with a sudden increase in alcohol intake.

The spectrum of symptoms is wide and includes tremor, nausea, sweating, sensitivity to sound (hyperacusis), ringing in the ears (tinnitus), itching, muscle cramps, mood disturbance, sleep disturbance, hallucinations, *grand mal* seizures, and the fully developed picture of delirium tremens. There are four key symptoms:

(1) *Tremor*. This nicely illustrates that it is the *degree* of experience that is essential to clinical observation, rather than a recording in the case-notes simply that the patient does or does not experience withdrawal shakes. Shakiness may have been experienced only once or twice, or intermittently and mildly, or it may be experienced every morning and to a degree which is incapacitating, or with many intervening intensities and frequencies. As well as the hands shaking, there may be facial tremor or the whole body shaking. The therapist has to cultivate an awareness of something equivalent to the Beaufort scale for wind strength and look out for the patient saying that they rattle their morning teacup against the saucer. In the extreme case, a drinker may rely on the kindness of the barmaid to lift the day's first pint to his or her lips.

(2) *Nausea*. The patient or client who is asked only whether they vomit may well deny it. Their experience, however, may be that if they attempt to clean their teeth in the morning, they will retch; or they may never eat breakfast because they know it would be too risky. A common story is that most of the first drink of the day is vomited back.

(3) *Sweating*. This may be dramatic; the patient wakes regularly in the early hours of the morning with soaking sweats. At the earlier stages of dependence, the patient may report no more than feeling clammy.

(4) *Mood disturbance*. In the earlier stages patients may phrase the experience in terms of 'being a bit edgy' or 'nerves not too good', but when dependence is fully developed they may use vivid descriptions to indicate a state of appalling agitation and depression. Often the anxiety seems to be characterised by a frightened reaction to loud noises or traffic (sometimes with a phobia of crossing the road), a fear of a friend coming up suddenly from behind, fright at 'the twigs on the trees rubbing together'. The over-sensitivity can be like that of a gouty patient who fears a fly alighting on their toe.

37

An underlying anxiety disorder may at times exacerbate withdrawal symptoms (Johnston *et al.*, 1991).

Relief or avoidance of withdrawal symptoms by further drinking

In the earliest stages the patient may be aware that at lunchtime the first drink of the day 'helps to straighten me up a bit'. At the other extreme a patient may require a drink every morning before they get out of bed, as a matter of desperate need. As with withdrawal symptoms, relief drinking must not be conceived as only a morning event; the patient may wake in the middle of the night for the drink which will abort incipient withdrawal, and they may be aware that if they go three or four hours without a drink during the day, the next drink is valued especially for its relief effect. Relief drinking is cued not only by frank withdrawal but also by minimal symptoms of subacute withdrawal, which signal worse distress if drink is not taken. The dependent individual may try to maintain a steady alcohol level which they have learnt to recognise as comfortably above the danger level for withdrawal, and to this extent their drinking is cued by withdrawal avoidance as well as withdrawal relief.

Clues to the degree of a patient's dependence are often given by the small details they provide of the circumstances and timing of the first drink of the day, and their attitude towards it. If they get up, have a bath, dress, and read the paper before that drink, then dependence is not very advanced. A housewife who finishes her morning chores before having her first drink is at a different stage of dependence from the woman who is pouring whisky into her first cup of tea. Someone engaged in relief drinking may have ritualised the procedure. A man may go to the early-morning pub at 7 a.m., go straight up to the bar where the barman will know immediately to give him his pint of lager which he will grab at clumsily with both hands and drink down fast. He may go to the lavatory and vomit some of this pint back, but he can then drink the next pint at greater leisure, and he will know that within 20 or 30 minutes of walking into that pub 'the drink will have cured me'. A patient or client may relate that they know the exact quantity of alcohol required for this 'cure' and the exact time interval for the alcohol to take effect, and they report also that the 'cure' is repeatedly so complete as to be almost miraculous. Sometimes they describe what is presumably a conditioned effect: the mere fact of having a glass in their hand gives relief.

That the dependence syndrome is a plastic condition rather than something immutable is brought out again by the way this particular element is shaped by social and personal factors. For example, the building labourer for whom the idea of keeping drink in the house may be so against subcultural expectations that he will always wait for the pubs to open rather than 'keep a drink indoors'. The person of rigid personality may endure considerable withdrawal for some hours rather than take a drink before lunch. To understand fully what the patient reports always requires that these shaping factors are taken into account.

Subjective awareness of compulsion to drink

The conventional phrases used to describe the dependent person's subjective experience are not altogether satisfactory. For instance, awareness of 'loss of control' is said to be crucial to understanding abnormal drinking and patients sometimes say, 'If I have one or two, I'll go on', or 'If I go into the pub, promises don't mean anything', or 'Once I've really got the taste of it, I'm away'. It is unclear, however, whether the experience is truly one of losing control rather than one of deciding not to exercise control. Control is probably best seen as variably or intermittently impaired rather than 'lost'. Although 'loss of control' has in some of the classic texts been pictured as the touchstone for diagnosis of addiction to alcohol, it is obvious that many so-called 'social drinkers' at times drink too much and are sorry and embarrassed afterwards.

Another complex experience which can too easily be wrapped up in conventional phrasing is the experience of 'craving'. The patient may describe it in unambiguous terms – he or she may be 'gasping for a drink'. The subjective interpretation of the withdrawal may, however, be much influenced by environment, and the patient who is withdrawing on a ward may not experience any craving. Cues for craving may include the feeling of intoxication, as well as incipient or developed withdrawal, mood (anger, depression, elation) or situational cues (being in a pub or with a drinking friend).

The patient who is in a withdrawal state (or partial withdrawal) may report that they are compulsively ruminating on alcohol and that they have hit on the strategy of blocking these ruminations by bringing in other lines of thought. It is this feeling of being in the grip of something foreign, irrational, and unwanted, which for the severely dependent patient seems to be the private experience that is so difficult to convey.

Reinstatement after abstinence

If patients begin again to drink, relapse into the previous stage of the dependence syndrome follows an extremely variable time course. Typically, the person who had only a moderate degree of dependence will take weeks or months to reinstate dependence, perhaps pulling back once or twice on the way. A severely dependent patient typically reports that they are again 'hooked' within a few days of starting to drink, although even here there are exceptions: on the first day they may become abnormally drunk and be surprised to find that they have lost their tolerance. Within a few days they are, however, experiencing severe withdrawal symptoms and drinking for relief, the subjective experience of compulsion is reinstated, and their drinking is back in the old stereotyped pattern. A syndrome which had taken years to develop can be fully reinstated within perhaps 72 hours of drinking, and this is one of the most puzzling features of the condition.

A case history

A 45-year-old window cleaner gave the following story. He had grown up in a working class area of his city and identified himself with its culture. He saw the pub as being an essential part of that world, perhaps its centre. Before he had left school, he and his mates were going into pubs, and to brazen out the age question in the face of the barman's suspicions was proof of manhood. He had never worked other than as a window cleaner, and he said that a lot of his trade was picked up at the bar. When it rained, the pub was the place to which to retreat. He was married with three children and left the management of the home to his wife. Everything therefore was so set up as to enable a man who 'always liked his beer' to sustain a daily intake of 5 to 10 pints as compatible with his pattern of life.

About six years before he presented for treatment he had begun to notice that his hands were a little shaky in the morning – 'not too good for the job'. He started to call into the pub at 11 a.m. and would have a couple of pints which would relieve the shakiness and generally make him feel better. His daily intake of beer which had gradually increased over recent years, was now about 15–20 pints each day, but he never took any alcoholic drink other than beer. He was able to identify a transitional phase as occurring five to six years prior to presenting for help, and separating his previous lifetime of 'liking the beer' from the last five years of 'being bad like I am now'. The experience of withdrawal symptoms had during that phase itensified rapidly.

He had for three years experienced severe withdrawal symptoms every morning, and it was the retching and vomiting that worried him particularly – 'Alright when I'm lying flat, but as soon as I sit up in bed it starts, have to rush to the toilet, heave my heart out'. He had heavy night sweats. He did not at first directly mention the mood component in the withdrawal experience, and words like 'anxiety' or 'depression' were not part of his ordinary vocabulary. But he 'felt bad, sort of butterflies', and on closer questioning it was clear that each morning he was experiencing unpleasant mood disturbance, although he did not spontaneously differentiate between physical and mental symptoms; it was a matter of 'feeling bad, more than terrible'. Tremor was such that 'I'll knock over a milk bottle'. Withdrawal seemed only to be a morning experience, presumably because he otherwise kept his blood level constantly topped up.

Evidence for drinking to relieve withdrawal was present, but here a colouring due to class-related attitudes was to be seen. He never kept drink in his own home, and this was a taboo which despite the intensity of his dependence he was unwilling to break. So far as he was concerned, 'bringing drink indoors' would have been a depravity. He therefore tried to stay in bed almost until the pubs opened and would then be in the pub exactly at opening time. His needs were so well known that the barman would have two separate pints of beer drawn and waiting for him. He drank these pints straight down, and during the first hour he would have a third pint. But by the end of 30 minutes he was feeling much better, and within the hour he was 'guaranteed right as rain'.

The increased tolerance to alcohol had existed for many years before this man developed the dependence syndrome; no naïve drinker would be able to drink five or six pints of beer at lunchtime and then do an afternoon's work (and climb a ladder).

The narrowing of his drinking repertoire by the time he sought treatment had become extreme. From 11 a.m. to 2.30 p.m. he was in the pub and drank eight pints of beer during that time. He came home and slept, returned to the pub at 6 p.m. and drank another eight pints up to 10 p.m., after which he would always go home and take the dog out for a walk. He would get back to the pub before closing time, and have a final drink. Sometimes when he was short of money his daily intake would fall a little lower and if he was flush with money it might be a bit more. There had been occasions when he was ill with influenza and had spent a week or 10 days at home, and he had then been completely off drink (with some mild hallucinatory experience during the first few days).

The salience of drink-seeking over other considerations was witnessed by a number of features. Work would now have got in the way of his drinking so he had largely stopped working, and drinking had really become his occupation. Provided he had money for his beer nothing else mattered. He had previously always prided himself on 'giving the wife a good wage'; she now went out to work, and he took from her whatever money he could by wheedling or demanding. He would 'take the rent money' and had cashed an insurance policy. His drinking was also financed by welfare benefits.

The subjective awareness of compulsion was sensed. He contrasted 'the old days' with the present. In the old days if there was a job to do he went out and did it, and 'I drank but I didn't have to drink – now I have to drink'. He had recently promised himself to cut down on his drinking and get back to regular work, but 'it's no good, the beer's really got a grip of me, and if I go into that pub I can't get out again. When I've got a pint, I'm thinking of the next pint'. He did not spontaneously use the word 'craving', but he was aware of his need for the first drink of the day, 'If anyone stood between me and that beer I'd go mad'.

The fact that this man had on occasions been abstinent for 10 days or so because of minor illnesses made it possible to gain information on reinstatement. As soon as he was able to get out of the house, his first walk would be back to the pub. He would tell himself that he 'wasn't going to drink in that bad way again' but full reinstatement of the whole picture nowadays only seemed to take about a week, and within two or three days of restarting his drinking he was again experiencing severe withdrawal symptoms. He summed things up by saying 'Don't know what's happened really, but the drink's got on top of me'.

Dependence – interpreting the picture

Given an awareness of the basic elements of the syndrome, when confronted with a history such as that given by the window cleaner there is the task of bringing this theoretical knowledge to bear on the understanding of the individual story. Using this patient's history where appropriate as illustration, the matter can be discussed under a number of headings.

Sensitivity to language

Clinical work is dependent on being alert towards meanings of words and nuances of phrase which are partly idiosyncratic to that one patient, but often culturally endowed. There should be a willingness to play phrasings backwards and forwards until there is a flash of mutual comprehension. The possibility of understanding will often be destroyed if such conventional terms as 'craving' or 'loss of control' are prematurely introduced. The phrasing which is remembered from one patient's account may, however, on occasion seem immediately to reach another patient's experience; for instance, 'drinking one drink and thinking about the next one'.

Assessing the coherence of the picture

The picture which emerges of any patient's experience of the dependence syndrome ought to be coherent. If one element of the syndrome is well-established, another element should not be absent. For instance, if a patient or client reports that they are suffering from severe withdrawal symptoms, but their regular daily intake of alcohol is only the equivalent of six pints of beer (say 100–120 g ethanol), the story perhaps does not fit properly together. Either part of the information on which the picture is being built is inaccurate (the patient is perhaps underreporting their drinking), or morning symptoms of some other origin are being interpreted as alcohol withdrawal symptoms. Inconsistencies

42

are therefore valuable observations in their own right. They should alert the diagnostician to making a closer investigation of the case. Coexistent drug-taking may distort the picture. A seeming inconsistency may be accounted for by the influence of personality or culture, which are matters dealt with more fully below.

Influence of culture and environment

The picture given by the window cleaner is typical of alcohol dependence as manifested by an Englishman from his socio-economic background and of his age. As ever, there were personal as well as social causes for the drinking, but the social factors were in this instance important determinants of the years of heavy drinking which were the prelude to dependence, and these same factors then followed through to shape aspects of the dependence syndrome. For instance, an insistence on not drinking in the house meant that a degree of dependence which would normally have resulted in drink being kept by the bed for morning relief was characterised instead by the patient's waiting for the pubs to open. True to class drinking habits he drank only beer, despite the uncomfortable fluid intake. His stereotyped dependent drinking (like all his previous drinking) was centred round the pub. His whole present drinking pattern can be seen as an extension of 'pub drinking' rather than as something standing completely outside an accepted social pattern. This man's peculiar and makeshift but real economic stability (his wife's earnings and the welfare benefits), enabled his dependent drinking to be conducted in a steady fashion.

Influence of personality

Not much has so far been said about this man's personality, but there can be no doubt that there was play between his personality and features of his dependence. His responsiveness to cultural dictates is in itself evidence of a personality trait and he was basically a conventional person. The flat pattern of his dependent drinking, the rigidity of that narrowed drinking repertoire (the dog faithfully taken for a walk each evening), the exact daily repetition of the ritualised first two pints, might all be read as evidence of a rigid element in his temperament, and he had always been a methodical window cleaner. The salience that he gave to his drinking when he had become dependent on alcohol was understandable as an extension of what had always been his detachment from the family; he had never felt that responsibilities went beyond giving his wife a regular cash sum, and now he retreated from that one obligation.

Degrees of dependence

Although one element may be more, or less, developed than others (sometimes as a result of unexplained variation or sometimes because of the impact of modifying social or personal factors), the coherent picture which emerges should be of a certain *degree* of dependence, with each element more or less in step. Thus if, as with the window cleaner, withdrawal symptoms are severe and experienced every day, it is to be expected that there will be a well-established pattern of relief drinking. Tolerance will be well developed if severe withdrawal is experienced, although around this stage in the history some evidence of declining tolerance might begin to appear. The narrowing of drinking repertoire reported by this man was commensurate with his other symptoms, and it would, for instance, have been surprising if with this degree of dependence he had been drinking much less at weekends than on weekdays. The daily alcohol intake was commensurate and the salience he accorded his drinking fitted in with the total picture. The subjective awareness of compulsion was typical of this degree of development. And typically, the syndrome was rapidly reinstated after a few days abstinence.

It is not easy to set up absolute rules for grading the severity of dependence, but it would be a fair guide to say that if anyone has experienced withdrawal symptoms on a more or less daily basis for 6–12 months and engaged in regular relief drinking in response to those symptoms over the same period (with other elements congruently developed), they will be severely dependent on alcohol. If they have experienced withdrawal symptoms on no more than a few occasions, but been aware that alcohol usefully brings relief (even without intentionally bringing forward the first drink of the day), an early case of dependence can be diagnosed. Between those two pictures there are many gradations rather than fixed degrees. A history of an attack of delirium tremens is clinching evidence of severe dependence, but discussion of alcohol-related and dependence-related mental illness will be postponed to Chapter 6.

The time element

To discuss the severity of dependence inevitably introduces consideration of the significance of the time element. The longer someone has been putting themselves through repeated cycles of withdrawal and relief, the more severe the dependence they will have contracted. Note, however, has also to be taken of the rapidity or gradualness of the transition between heavy drinking and dependence, and of the age at which dependence developed. The window cleaner had sustained a pattern of heavy drinking for many years before the dependence syndrome started to be seen, and this is perhaps typical of a history where the determinants of drinking are largely cultural. Why dependence should at a certain phase in his life have become manifest is unexplained. Whatever the underlying causes, it is however rather typical for the man with a long-standing heavy alcohol intake to be able to identify a transition period of about 12 months during which the dependence symptoms had their onset and a quickly mounting severity. With other cultures, personalities, and patterns of drinking, dependence may arise earlier or later in life, after longer or shorter alcohol exposure, and may advance with greater or lesser rapidity.

In summary, to understand fully the individual's dependence, the present picture has to be related to its evolution over time, and the determinants of that evolution identified (see Chapter 11).

Dependence – the later stages

A patient may continue to drink dependently and at a heavy level for many years, and when one sees them again after a 10-year interval, the account in the old case-notes can seem, astonishingly, to be the description of the present – nothing has changed. If, however, the patient neither dies nor stops drinking, sooner or later the presentation is likely to evolve toward the breakdown of the old picture and a more fragmented type of drinking.

There are a number of themes within this evolution which can be identified:

(1) *Dependence becomes progressively worse.* We are referring here to the dependence disorder *per se* rather than to the surround of alcohol-related disabilities which are likely at this stage to occur with increasing severity. The withdrawal symptoms may have plateaued at the same level for many years or have gradually worsened, but at a certain phase there will probably be a rapidly mounting intensity of morning distress. The patient may, for example, report an appalling experience of shakes or almost suicidal disturbance in mood each morning. The immediate morning drink is a matter of terrifying urgency. Hearing voices, seeing things, frightening half-waking dreams, may all be experienced on a come-and-go basis, or the patient may experience attacks of frank delirium tremens.

(2) *Gross and incapacitating intoxication becomes more common.* Reference has already been made to the late-stage possibility of an actual

decline in tolerance. A patient reported his experience in the following terms: 'That last year, whenever I started to drink, I got so drunk that I literally didn't know night from day, just a haze. It would get so I couldn't go into any bar because I was just an embarrassment, and I was falling over in the street, brought home by strangers'.

The loss of tolerance can at the extreme be so severe that the patient is intoxicated after only a couple of drinks. Brain damage often underlies this picture. Gross and repeated amnesia becomes common. Although loss of tolerance and accompanying brain damage are usually the major factors lying behind this 'getting very drunk', other factors may also be involved, such as the fear of withdrawal leading to desperate and misjudged efforts to top up the blood alcohol, or a searching after the good feelings that alcohol used to give but no longer provides.

(3) *Drinking makes the patient feel very ill.* The patient or client finds that they can no longer drink in their previous continuous manner because after a few days of drinking they now feel so ill that, despite the threat of withdrawal symptoms, their suffering forces them to desist. The mounting intensity of the morning withdrawal contributes to this general feeling of distress, but it is likely to be compounded by the consequences of various alcohol-induced physical disorders, for instance, gastritis, liver disease, or chronic pancreatitis. Concomitant psychiatric disorder may also at this stage become more common.

The result of these various factors is that the patient moves towards a pattern of short, acute, and incapacitating bouts, each of them a chaotic and devastating experience. This end-result seems in large measure to be determined by the progression of the dependence itself – by the march of incompletely understood physiological and psycho-physiological processes. However, social and environmental factors must, as ever, also be taken into the analysis – marriage break-up and the loss of every constraint and support can make for further inevitability.

Many variations or a few species? The Jellinek typology

The window cleaner's story provides a history of one particular person's dependence, and it cannot adequately represent the whole range of pictures that can be encountered. There are an infinite number of ways in which the dependence syndrome and its degrees of development can be moulded in their manifestations by secondary factors, and it is not helpful to pick out sub-patterns and accord them the status of distinct 'species' of alcoholism. Setting up a segmented listing of 'types of dependence' would go against the central concept of one clearly identifiable syndrome that is moulded into different patterns by a variety of forces which have in each instance to be understood. Over time and with changing circumstances, an individual's presentation of the syndrome may vary greatly.

To reject the notion of 'species of alcoholism' is, however, to go against the Jellinek typology of alcoholism (Jellinek, 1960). E.M. Jellinek was an American scientist who made profoundly influential contributions to the study of drinking. As usually quoted and simplified, his system set out a five-fold species categorisation (see Box 3.2).

Box 3.2. Jellinek's typology of alcoholism

- *Alpha alcoholism*: excessive drinking for purely psychological reasons without evidence of 'tissue adaptation'.

- *Beta alcoholism*: excessive drinking which has led to tissue damage, but where there is no dependence on alcohol.

- *Gamma alcoholism*: excessive drinking where there is evidence of tolerance and withdrawal, a peaky and fluctuant alcohol intake, and marked 'loss of control'. Jellinek saw this as the pattern typical of Anglo-Saxon countries.

- *Delta alcoholism*: excessive drinking where there is evidence of tolerance and withdrawal, but with a much steadier level of alcohol intake. Rather than the patient manifesting 'loss of control', they would exhibit what was called 'inability to abstain'. The pattern was seen as typical of France and of other wine-drinking countries.

- *Epsilon alcoholism*: bout drinking, or what used to be termed dipsomania.

Jellinek's typology deserves scrutiny. Study of his original writing shows that his views on categorisation were more subtle than would be supposed from the oversimplified extracts from his thinking which later became the popular basis for a typology. For instance, the distinction he drew between gamma and delta alcoholism showed an awareness of the need to take into account the shaping influence of culture. When he discussed epsilon alcoholism he noted that the picture might be the result of the fragmentation of a previous pattern of continuous drinking by the influence of AA membership. He did not see his five-part typology as exhaustive, but said that all the other letters of the Greek alphabet might be needed in addition, and then some other alphabets besides. And yet, because of its attractive simplicity, it is the typology which is widely known, with Jellinek's insistence on the arbitrariness of a restricted focus on these few patterns usually ignored.

More orderly or more chaotic dependent drinking

Jellinek's contrasting identificates of gamma (loss of control) and delta (inability to abstain) species, point to an important aspect of drinking behaviour which shows variation between cases. He was, however, describing extreme types, and today the best use of his insights is to note the dimension of variation to which his ideas drew attention, rather than to accept the notion of contrasting ideal types with nothing inbetween. The relationship between the constructs of 'loss of control' and 'inability to abstain' has recently been investigated by Kachler et al. (1995).

Some alcohol-dependent patients drink predominantly in a chaotic fashion. When they start to drink they go on to a variable and uncertain upper limit of blood alcohol. Others, although suffering from alcohol dependence of similar severity, usually so order their drinking that they attain much the same high blood alcohol level every day and one with which their tolerance can cope; they do not overshoot the mark, albeit that the mark is an abnormally high one. Although it is possible to meet patients who seem to conform to one or other extreme stereotype (always losing control on the one hand, unable to abstain on the other), more careful enquiry usually reveals that even with the seemingly clear-cut and stereotyped case, patterns are more varied than first meets the eye. For example, a client who now appears to be drinking in a chaotic fashion is only doing so since losing their job and their marriage brake-up; before then their dependence manifested itself by heavy continuous drinking through the business day, followed by armchair drinking in the evening. Someone who appears to be drinking predominantly in a controlled fashion may reveal that there are patches when their drinking is more peaky and uncertain in its patterning. In addition to those cases that at the initial meeting appear extreme but then do not conform closely to a stereotype when more fully analysed, there are cases which even at first sight are obviously presenting with a mixed pattern. The true variety of patterns will be missed if all that is available to the diagnostician's thinking is a few pigeon-holes.

Continuous or intermittent drinking

Jellinek picked up another important dimension when he contrasted epsilon (bout) drinking with other types, but again the reality is degrees of variation rather than an absolute contrast between dependent patients who drink unfailingly every day and those who drink unfailingly in sharply demarcated bouts.

The degree of intermittency which often will be found to characterise supposedly 'continuous' drinking is surprising. Even the Skid Row drinker who is pictured as someone who drinks with relentless continuity, will usually be found to have several months of more or less voluntary abstinence during any year, even leaving aside the enforced abstinences during imprisonment; they may have abstained because they were 'too sick to drink', because they had temporarily settled in a job, or because they were living in a hostel where drinking was not allowed.

The person who at first presents with seemingly clear-cut bout drinking will often on closer questioning give a previous history of dependent drinking cast in a more continuous pattern. That a move towards a pattern of short bouts is common at the most advanced stages of dependence has already been noted, but bout drinking can also emerge as the predominant mode earlier in the drinking career. Remorse, mood swing, physical distress, mounting pressure from a spouse, the need to get back to work, running out of money, the general practitioner's calling at the house, AA friends coming to the rescue, may all mean that such a person may at any stage begin intermittently to pull out of their drinking. They relapse, pull out again, and hence 'bout drinking'.

The boutiness of the drinking is thus not witness to a patient suffering from a unique *species* of alcoholism, but to the many and complex influences which are moulding the presentation of the core dependence syndrome. Careful history-taking may reveal that bouts are beginning to be more or less frequent in occurrence, or more or less prolonged in duration, and enquiry may then also identify the shift in the play of influences which brings these changes about. The coherence of the dependence picture should be such that the patient who is highly dependent will be able to swing his drinking repertoire only between bouts of heavy dependent drinking and intervening periods of total or near-total abstinence. The less dependent person will have bouts with hazier edges, and intervening periods of non-dependent drinking which gradually edge again towards establishment of dependence.

What has been said here about patterns of drinking seeks squarely to meet the complexity of clinical reality as it will actually be found. The task is to describe each individual's drinking pattern as it exists in reality, and then to try as best as possible to identify the influences which shape this pattern.

Recent ideas on the typology question

Although this chapter argues that the most helpful clinical perspective is one which conceives alcohol dependence as a single core syndrome with infinitely varied patterning in individual presentation (see also Vaillant, 1994), other authors, particularly in the United States, favour the idea of typology (e.g. Babor *et al.*, 1994). Their opinions deserve respectful scrutiny, but the number of competing typologies which have resulted from that kind of approach might suggest that there is at present no conclusive empirical basis for this kind of syndrome splitting. For instance, Cloninger *et al.* (1981) and Cloninger (1987) have suggested a Type 1 versus Type 2 dichotomy on the basis of sex, family history, and age of onset. Babor *et al.* (1992a) have proposed a distinction between Types A and B on the basis of vulnerability and severity; Schuckit (1985) has differentiated between primary and secondary alcoholism. Others have distinguished between late and early onset alcoholism and between subjects with or without concurrent personality disorder or other psychopathology. All these approaches add to awareness of the multiple complexities with which the clinician is dealing (Babor *et al.*, 1992b) and there are many questions here that are still open to further investigation.

Why an understanding of dependence matters

Having outlined the diagnosis of dependence, the manner in which degrees of the syndrome's development are to be identified and the way in which personality and environment may shape the presentations, the question then arises – what is the practical purpose of such diagnostic work and what is the gain from developing this kind of diagnostic skill? The answers are both general and specific.

The dependence concept and the brokerage of understanding

The realisation that there exists such a condition as alcohol dependence, and an understanding of the personal implications of this diagnosis, may often assist in the relief of the patient's sense of muddle and bafflement. It can contribute to a helpful framework for personal understanding, and enable the patient to come to terms with a condition to which they had previously only reacted with confusion. The fact that alcohol is a drug which can produce dependence – 'a drug of addiction'

– often comes as a surprise to a patient's family as much as it does to the patients. The diagnosis if sensitively explained can, for the family too, mean a way of restructuring a reaction to a situation which previously engendered confusion, fear, or anger. The spouse begins to realise that there is more than 'weakness of the will' that has to be understood, that expecting their partner 'to drink like other people' is not possible.

For the therapist, what flows from understanding the nature of dependence lies partly in accurate empathy for that patient's or client's experience. To impart, baldly, no more than the diagnostic label – a sort of magisterial sentencing – is not what is meant by building up understanding.

Furthermore, it would be useful health education if the public in general were aware that alcohol has dependence potential. The public needs to know more of the dangers and the danger signals, what dependence can mean for themselves or someone in their family, for someone at work or someone they meet in the pub. Understanding of alcohol dependence should become part of ordinary social awareness, but it is equally important that society understands that alcohol problems also commonly occur without dependence.

The relevance of an understanding of dependence to the specifics of treatment

The ability to diagnose dependence and recognise the degrees is vital to setting the treatment goal (see Chapters 15 and 19). A severely dependent drinker is unlikely to be able to return to normal drinking (Edwards *et al.*, 1986) and the clinician's ability accurately to recognise the degree of dependence is vital to this important aspect of care. Assessment of the patient's degree of dependence is also relevant to choice of withdrawal regime and forewarning as to risk of delirium tremens or withdrawal fits (see Chapter 14). Understanding of the severity of relapse requires an ability to recognise whether dependence has been reinstated. Monitoring the progress of regression of dependence intensity over time is relevant to an understanding of the drinking career and drinking within the life course (Chapter 11).

There is also the question of whether intensity of dependence should be seen as indicating the intensity of the required treatment – a variant of the matching hypothesis (Glaser, 1980). There is commonsense appeal in the postulate that more heavily dependent drinkers should, for example, be given more therapeutic time, be more readily admitted to in-patient care, and be provided with more intensive follow-up. Some recent research does not, however, support that proposition (Edwards & Taylor, 1994).

References

American Psychiatric Association (1994). *Diagnostic and Statistical Manuall of Mental Disorders,* 4th edn. (DSM-IV). Washington DC: American Psychiatric Association.

Babor, T. F., Orrok, B., Liebowitz, N., Salomon, R. & Brown, J. (1990). From basic concepts to clinical reality: unresolved issues in the diagnosis of dependence. In *Recent Developments in Alcoholism,* vol. 8, *Combined Alcohol and Other Drug Dependence,* ed. Galanter, M., pp. 85–104. New York: Plenum Press.

Babor, T. F., Del Boca, F. K., Hesselbrock, V., Meyer, R. E., Dolinsky, Z. S. & Rounsaville, B. (1992a). Types of alcoholics 1: evidence for an empirically derived typology based on indicators of vulnerability and severity. *Archives of General Psychiatry* **49,** 599–608.

Babor, T. F., Dolinsky, Z. S., Meyer, R. E., Hesselbrook, M., Hoffman, M. & Tennen, H. (1992b). Types of alcoholics: concurrent and predictive validity of some common classification schemes. *British Journal of Addiction* **87,** 1415–31.

Babor, T. F., Hesselbrock, V., Meyer, R. E. & Shoemaker, W. (1994). *Types of Alcoholics: Evidence from Clinical, Experimental and Genetic Research.* Annals of the New York Academy of Sciences, vol. 708. New York: The New York Academy of Sciences.

Ball, D. M. & Murray, R. M. (1994). Genetics of alcohol misuse. In *Alcohol and Alcohol Problems,* ed. Edwards G. & Peters, T. J., pp. 18–35 British Medical Bulletin No.50. Edinburgh: Churchill Livingstone.

Caetano, R. (1993). The association between severity of DSM-III-R alcohol dependence and medical and social consequences. *Addiction* **88,** 631–42.

Carroll, K. M., Rounsaville, B. J. & Bryant, K. H. (1994). Should tolerance and withdrawal be required for substance dependence disorders? *Drug and Alcohol Dependence* **36,** 15–22.

Chick, J. (1980). Alcohol dependence: methodological issues in its measurement: reliability of the criteria. *British Journal of Addiction* **75,** 175–86.

Cloninger, C. R. (1987). Neurogenetic adaptive mechanisms in alcoholism. *Science* **236,** 410–16.

Cloninger, C. R., Bohman, M. & Sigvardsson, S. (1981). Inheritance of alcohol abuse. *Archives of General Psychiatry* **38,** 861–8.

Cottler, L .B. (1993). Comparing DSM-III-R and ICD10 substance use disorders. *Addiction* **88,** 689–96.

Cottler, L. B., Phelps, D. L. & Compton, W. M. (1995). Narrowing of the drinking repertoire criterion: should it have been dropped from ICD10? *Journal of Studies on Alcohol* **56,** 173–6.

Edwards, G. (1986) The alcohol dependence syndrome: a concept as stimulus to enquiry. *British Journal of Addiction* **81,** 171–83.

Edwards, G. (1990). Withdrawal symptoms and alcohol dependence: fruitful mysteries. *British Journal of Addiction* **85,** 447–61.

Edwards, G. (1994). Addiction, reductionism and Aaron's rod. *Addiction* **89,** 9–12.

Edwards, G. & Gross, M. M. (1976). Alcohol dependence: provisional description of a clinical syndrome. *British Medical Journal* **1**, 1058–61.

Edwards, G. & Lader, M. (eds.) (1990). *The Nature of Drug Dependence*. Society for the Study of Addiction Monograph No. 1. Oxford: Oxford University Press.

Edwards, G. & Taylor C. (1994). A test of the matching hypothesis: alcohol dependence, intensity of treatment and 12 month outcome. *Addiction* **89**, 553–61.

Edwards, G., Gross, M. M., Keller, M., Moser, J. & Room, R. (1977). *Alcohol-Related Disabilities*. WHO Offset Publication No.32. Geneva: WHO.

Edwards, G., Arif, A. & Hodgson, R. (1981). Nomenclature and classification of drug- and alcohol-related problems: a WHO memorandum. *Bulletin of the World Health Organization* **50**, 225–42.

Edwards, G., Brown, D., Duckitt, A., Oppenheimer, E., Sheehan, M. & Taylor, C. (1986). Normal drinking in a recovering alcohol addict. *British Journal of Addiction* **81**, 127–37.

Feingold, A. & Rounsaville, B. (1995). Construct validity of the dependence syndrome as measured by DSM-IV for different psycho-active substances. *Addiction* **90**, 1661–9.

Glaser, F. (1980). Anybody got a match? Treatment research and the matching hypothesis. In *Alcoholism Treatment in Transition*, ed. Edwards, G. & Grant, M., pp. 178–96. London: Croom Helm.

Glautier, S. & Drummond, D. C. (1992). Alcohol dependence and cue reactivity. *Journal of Studies on Alcohol* **55**, 224–9.

Glautier, S. & Drummond, D. C. (1994). Conditioning approaches: the analysis and treatment of drinking problems. In *Alcohol and Alcohol Problems*, ed. Edwards, G. & Peters, T. J., pp.186–99. British Medical Bulletin No.50. Edinburgh: Churchill Livingstone.

Grant, B. F., Harford, T. C., Chou, P. & Pickering, R. (1992). DSM-111–R and the proposed DSM-IV alcohol use disorders, United States 1988. A methodological comparison. *Alcoholism: Clinical and Experimental Research* **16**, 215–21.

Greeley, J. D., Swift, W., Prescott, J. & Heather, N. (1993). Reactivity to alcohol-related cues in heavy and light drinkers. *Journal of Studies on Alcohol* **54**, 359–68.

Heather, N., Rollnick, S. & Winston, M. (1983). A comparison of objective and subjective measures of alcohol dependence as predictors of relapse following treatment. *British Journal of Clinical Psychiatry* **22**, 11–17.

Hodgson, R., Rankin, H. J. & Stockwell, T. (1979). Alcohol dependence and the primary effect. *Behaviour Research and Therapy* **17**, 379–87.

Jellinek, E. M. (1960). *The Disease Concept of Alcoholism*. New Brunswick: Hillhouse Press.

Johnston, A. L., Thevos, A. K., Randall, C. L. & Anton, R. F. (1991). Increased severity of alcohol withdrawal in in-patient alcoholics with a co-existing anxiety diagnosis. *British Journal of Addiction* **86**, 719–25.

Jones, B. T. & McMahon, J. (1996). A comparison of positive and negative alcohol expectancy and value and their multiplicative composite as predictors of post-abstinence survivorship. *Addiction* **91**, 89–99.

Kachler, C. W., Epstein, E. E. & McCrady, B.S. (1995). Loss of control and inability to abstain: the measurement of and relationship between two constructs in male alcoholics. *Addiction* **90**, 1025–36.

Kerr, N. (1888). *Inebriety, Its Etiology, Pathology, Treatment and Jurisprudence.* Edinburgh: H. K. Lewis.

Kivlahan, D., Sher K. J. & Donovan, D. M. (1989). The Alcohol Dependence Scale: a validation study among inpatient alcoholics. *Journal of Studies on Alcohol* **50**, 170–5.

Leigh, B. C. & Stacy, A. W. (1991). On the scope of alcohol expectancy research: remaining issues of measurement and meaning. *Psychological Bulletin* **110**, 147–54.

Meehan, J. P., Webb, M. G. T. & Unwin, A. R. (1985). The severity of alcohol dependence questionnaire (SADQ) in a sample of Irish problem drinkers. *British Journal of Addiction* **80**, 57–63.

Nutt, D. J. & Peters, T. J. (1994). Alcohol: the drug. In *Alcohol and Alcohol Problems,* ed. Edwards, G. & Peters, T. J., pp.5–17. British Medical Bulletin No.50. Edinburgh: Churchill Livingstone.

Rankin, H., Stockwell, T. & Hodgson, R. (1982). Cues for drinking and degrees of alcohol dependence. *British Journal of Addiction* **77**, 287–96.

Rapaport, M. H., Tipp, J. E. & Schuckit, M. A. (1993). A comparison of ICD10 and DSM-III-R criteria for substance abuse and dependence. *American Journal of Drug and Alcohol Abuse* **19**, 143–51.

Rounsaville, B. J., Bryant, K., Babor, T., Kranzler, H. & Kadden, R. (1993). Cross system agreement for substance use disorders: DSM-III-R, DSM-IV and ICD10. *Addiction* **88**, 337–48.

Schuckit, M. A. (1985). The clinical implications of primary diagnostic groups among alcoholics. *Archives of General Psychiatry* **41**, 1043–9.

Stacy, A. W., Widaman, K. F. & Marlatt, G. A. (1990). Expectancy models of alcohol use. *Journal of Personality and Social Psychology* **58**, 918–28.

Stockwell, T., Hodgson, R., Edwards, G., Taylor, C. & Rankin, H. (1979). The development of a questionnaire to measure alcohol dependence. *British Journal of Addiction* **74**, 79–87.

Stockwell, T., Murphy, D. & Hodgson, R. (1983). The severity of alcohol dependence questionnaire: its use, reliability and validity. *British Journal of Addiction* **78**, 145–55.

Trotter, T. (1804). *An Essay on Drunkenness and its Effects on the Human Body.* London: Longman, Hurst, Rees and Orvine.

Vaillant, G. E. (1994). Evidence that the Type1/Type 2 dichotomy in alcoholism must be re-examined. *Addiction* **89**, 1049–57.

White, N. M. (1996). Addictive drugs as reinforcers: multiple partial action on memory systems. *Addiction* **91**, 921–49.

Williams, R. J. & Ricciardelli, A. (1996). Expectancies related to symptoms of alcohol dependence in young adults. *Addiction* **91**, 1031–9.

4

Drinking problems and the family

Drinking problems generally have a profound effect upon the family of the drinker. The spouse and the children are the people commonly drawn into the play, but parents, brothers, sisters, uncles or aunts, or grandparents may in some way be involved. The nature of the involvement can be in terms of: that person experiencing the adverse impact of the drinker's behaviour; the family's interaction in the genesis of the drinking problem; the family member's unhelpful connivance with or encouragement of the drinking problem; or most positively in terms of that person being able to aid the process of recovery.

A person with a drinking problem may appear to have lost all links with their family. Even so, they may harbour strong emotions in respect of those relationships which have been severed by death, dysharmony, or neglect and it is likely that similar feelings are experienced by the estranged relatives. Where these relatives are alive, and if they can be traced, the question of renewing contact may arise. This can present a major challenge both to the coping skills of the client and to the professional skills of the therapist.

This chapter will give a groundwork description of certain important aspects of family interaction, but fuller discussions of therapeutic implications are presented in chapters 15 and 17. Readers seeking a more detailed review of the impact of parental drinking problems upon children should refer to Sher, 1991.

The spouse

At the outset, it is necessary to emphasise that the spouse may be the husband of the woman with a drinking problem, as well as the wife of the man who is drinking. Although the initial discussion will largely be in terms of the wife of the problem drinker – for this is the commoner situation – many of the considerations would apply equally to the reverse circumstances. (A later section will focus on the husband of the woman with alcohol related problems, p. 60.)

A history from the spouse in her own right

The assumption is too often made that the purpose of taking a history from the spouse is solely that of obtaining 'independent information'. What is frequently forgotten is the need to take a history from the spouse as a person in her own right. The result is that after months have gone by it is suddenly realised that treatment is proceeding on the basis of much being known about the patient while the wife remains a cipher, and their interaction is hence inexplicable. No one has bothered to see this woman in terms of her own being, and her own needs and expectations. Treatment of the patient is handicapped, and the fact that the wife herself needs help is overlooked.

What has to be overcome is a subconscious social constraint – the feeling that it is embarrassing to ask a woman whose role is presumed to be that of someone coming to the clinic to talk about her husband, then within that definition to talk about herself. Indeed, the interview may soon reveal that the wife has a great pressure of need to talk about herself. How the initial history is to be taken from the spouse in terms that honour her in her own right is discussed fully in Chapter 13.

Theories of the 'alcoholic marriage'

A number of different theories have been put forward to explain what may happen in a marriage where one partner is an alcoholic. (The term 'alcoholic' will be retained here, as it has been employed by most of the proponents of these theories.) Each of these approaches can at times give useful understanding, but stereotyped descriptions of the alcoholic's wife have no general validity.

One of these theories is that the wife actually wishes her husband to be an alcoholic. The fact is noted that a proportion of wives had a father who was an alcoholic, and it is argued that the wife then marries an alcoholic with whom she can continue to enact her unresolved dynamic problems. She will subtly or overtly hamper treatment, persuade her husband to discharge himself prematurely from hospital, and tell him that a few drinks will not do him any harm. She will even buy the drink for him and bring it back to the house, and she will indicate to him that 'he's horrid now he's sober'. If the husband persists in his recovery, the wife herself may in terms of this theory then decompensate and develop a depressive illness.

There can be no doubt that marriages are occasionally encountered which astonishingly resemble such a bizarre picture as that just given, and where it is a reasonable supposition that the wife is subconsciously willing the husband's drinking. She married him knowing he was an alcoholic, she gains from seeing him as weak and despicable, has enjoyed taking over the management of home and finance, and wishes to have her expectations confirmed that men are dirt. She likes to show how badly she is used, enjoys mothering or dominating, and so on. But cruel mistakes result if the assumption is made that this is the common picture of *the* alcoholic marriage, and from forcing all such marriages into interpretations in these terms. For instance, the truth of the matter may be that when the husband began to drink excessively the wife inevitably then had to make the choice between letting the home go to rack and ruin or taking much of its running into her own hands; her seeming 'dominance' is merely adjustive.

Some research has suggested that the wife's and family's reactions go through a predictable sequence of stages (Jackson, 1954). The evidence does not in fact support the notion that all wives follow exactly the same pathway, but certain phases can sometimes be recognised. At the beginning there is the reluctant admission that drinking is indeed a problem, and then the first attempts to control or prevent the problem behaviour. The family begins to be socially isolated, partly as a protective strategy; invitations are refused, people are not encouraged to call, relatives are not visited. Later, the wife may go into a phase where she begins to realise her strategies are not working, that things are getting worse rather than better, that her reserves are being worn down. She may start to fear for her own sanity, and a feeling of hopelessness sets in. Sexual contact is diminished or ceases, and there is a general and continuing sense of estrangement, fear or anger. At this stage or earlier, the wife may begin to feel that 'something must be done'; she tries to persuade her husband to look for help. If no improvement follows, the marriage may either break up or continue for years in a phase characterised by strategies which might be called *circumvention*:

> It's terrible really, but I suppose we've all got used to it. We'll all go to bed before he comes in at night and I'll pretend to be asleep when he comes into the room. I tell the kids to keep out of his way. Sometimes he gets back early but if we're in the sitting room watching the television, more often than not he just goes out to the kitchen. I take the children on holiday, he doesn't come, and frankly we don't ask him.

Given that the ordering of phases may vary widely, it is still useful to try to make an assessment of the *coping style* which the wife is at any stage employing (Orford & Edwards, 1977), and this knowledge can be useful in therapy. One such style is exactly the circumvention (or with-drawal) employed by the woman who has just been quoted. Contact is so far as possible minimised, and there is emotional as well as physical avoidance. Another style is that of *attack* – the wife tries to control her husband's behaviour by scolding, shouting, threatening to leave him, or on occasions even by physical assault. She lets him know that she is con-tacting a solicitor. Drink is poured down the sink. *Manipulation* embraces a number of behaviours, such as seeking to shame the drinker, with the woman showing her own distress or emphasizing the chil-dren's suffering, while the wife herself may get purposely drunk 'to show him what it's like'. *Spoiling* may be another approach – the spouse nurses him through his hangovers, keeps the dinner warm for him whether he is drunk or sober, or promises him treats if he will amelio-rate his behaviour. A further style is that of *constructive management* – she retains her own sense of worth and protects and looks after the family by making sure that finances are in as good order as possible while she goes out to work. She makes sure that the children go short of nothing, and herself paints the house and cares for the front garden. *Constructive help seeking* is a pattern characterised by behaviour such as the wife going to see the family doctor and asking him to speak to the husband, she finds out about AA and leaves some pamphlets around for the husband to come upon, or goes along to the public library and reads books on alcoholism, so as to help her own understanding.

Box 4.1. Coping styles employed by partners of problem drinkers

- Circumvention

- Attack

- Manipulation

- Spoiling

- Constructive management

- Constructive help seeking

These various styles (summarised in Box 4.1) seldom exist in pure form, and there are other types of behaviour which do not go under any of these headings. The choice of style may be influenced by the way in which this woman generally copes with life, by class expectations, by the type of behaviour which the husband is manifesting, and by the duration of the problem. The coping style employed at a particular time may be a response in a sequence of experiments in which the wife is searching around, trying first one tack and then another.

What is the wife having to cope with?

The special stressfulness of a situation where there may often be social isolation rather than social support, and where there are no guidelines, has already been noted. A frequent additional feature is the stress imposed by the unpredictability of what is going to happen; the wife does not know whether when the husband gets back from the pub he will be in a sentimental or maudlin mood, or whether he will be in a raging temper and threaten her with his fists. The exhaustion which can be engendered by the experience of dealing with continuing distress and peaks of crisis over a period of years can be the wife's dominant complaint.

Fundamentally the wife is having to cope with the problems both at the emotional and at the reality level (Orford & Edwards, 1977). The emotional problems include anxiety, fearfulness, and misery. Often there is an element of self-doubt or self-blame; she wonders whether the problem has arisen because she is a bad wife and has sexually or in some other way failed her husband. She may also be perplexed by the acute conflict in the feelings which she develops towards her husband; she married this man because she loved him, and yet now she at times feels almost murderous towards him. There is often also a sense of emotional deprivation and of loss – the man she married has disappeared. She herself begins to feel in some way diminished in her worth, or disgraced.

At the reality level the problems can be tangibly threatening; there is the risk of eviction if the rent is not paid, or his violence may result in serious personal damage. More commonly it is the host of minor reality problems which have to be coped with – no housekeeping money this week, no money to pay the electricity, the neighbours complaining about the doors being slammed when he got home last night, constant rowing, his jealousy, his dirtiness, or his wetting the bed.

It would, however, be a mistake always to picture such marriages only in extreme terms. Extremes of suffering certainly occur with sad frequency, but there are all gradations. Sometimes the husband's deportment when drunk causes little distress; he is a bit silly and argumentative, tends to fall asleep in the chair after supper and can be difficult to get to bed, but in a drunken sort of way he remains polite and is never violent. He regularly hands over the housekeeping money, and if there are the finances to cushion the effects of his drinking and a job which is secure, some of the more distressing reality problems will not be so evident.

The types of hardship that the wife may encounter are discussed in more detail in relation to taking the 'independent history' from the spouse (Chapter 13).

Marriages where the wife is the problem drinker

As was stated at the beginning of this chapter, most of the principles which apply to understanding the situation where the husband has the drinking problem apply equally well when it is the wife who is the patient or client. There are, however, certain additional aspects to the marriage problem which may then develop, many of these relating to the generally punitive attitudes towards the female heavy drinker which many cultures display, and which are more fully discussed in Chapter 9. The husband's reaction may be coloured by a primitive disgust at his wife's behaviour, or by fear of social disapprobation, and of the family being disgraced by a drunken woman. His feelings can lead to violence. To work through these feelings so that the husband is less frightened of what is happening and less blindly condemnatory may be the necessary prelude to any constructive changes.

If the husband is employed and the woman is the housewife and mother, he may find himself drawn into a managing role within the family to compensate for the wife's impaired competence. If he is also trying to keep going in a demanding job, he may find the double demands difficult to cope with, and the welfare of the children may be a particular worry. Failure of the woman to fulfil her expected roles sets neither greater nor lesser problems, though in some ways different, than a man's role failures. Sometimes the husband will seek to solve the family's plight by rather purposely promoting an elder daughter to the central female role within the household.

Another difference relates to the fact that economically it is often easier for a man to leave his drinking wife than for a wife to leave her drinking husband. Despite continued suffering she may hold back from separation because she does not see an alternative way of providing a roof to shelter herself and the children. The husband can more readily see separation from his wife as an option, either taking the children with him or surrendering his responsibilities.

Marriages where both partners have a drinking problem

This extraordinarily difficult situation is sometimes encountered. The story is usually that of a person with a drinking problem marrying someone else with an established and evident drinking problem. For one or both partners it may be a second marriage. They met perhaps in a bar or even in a hospital ward, and it is a marriage of convenience between drinkers. Their only shared interest is drinking, they have no knowledge of each other's sober beings, and are, sadly, likely to drag each other down further. Alcohol related problems do sometimes develop in both partners in an already established marriage. Quite often the development is not simultaneous, but the wife seems to follow in the husband's footsteps, her drinking being in part perhaps a reaction to the stress of the husband's behaviour. Another type of marriage is where the partners have met at AA, are both committed to 'recovery', and are able to give each other much support.

In general, where both husband and wife have a serious problem, it can be difficult to reach them with any effective help. If they met in a pub and each purposefully married a drinking partner, the therapist may encounter a baffling pack of pathological motivations. In such instances all that may be possible is to make the offer of help, try to maintain some sort of monitoring contact, and wait for the happening which can provide the therapeutic opening – for example, one partner going into hospital with a physical illness. Where the heavy drinking has developed during the marriage, rather than being the foundation of the marriage, the possibilities for therapy are usually more hopeful. Both partners may then simultaneously be able to seek help, or it may be necessary to start with the partner who is more motivated. If therapy can capture the potential for mutual understanding which can exist between partners who have shared the same problem, an initially difficult situation can be turned to special advantage.

Gay and lesbian couples

Problems similar to those which occur in a heterosexual marriage are encountered when one partner in a homosexual liaison has a drinking problem. A rather common story seems to be of the partner who is more emotionally dependent and more insecure beginning to drink heavily at a period when they fear that the relationship is going to break up:

> I'd get home from work, and after I'd had a drink I'd start doing the cooking. All the time I was cooking the dinner I'd be wondering – is he coming home tonight? Who is he with? What lies is he going to tell? Not like the old days! So while I was cooking I'd have a few more drinks. By the time he came in I'd be all ready for a row.

The therapist may find that they are helping such people through the dissolution of their relationship or assisting in the exploration of basic and previously unresolved issues relating to sexuality and identity.

Children

For the children of the problem drinker to be entirely forgotten by the therapeutic team is sadly all too easy. Their names and ages are noted in the initial history-taking, out of the corner of an eye there is the awareness of their continued existence, but the parents are the focus of attention and are taking up all the therapeutic time. There is the vague feeling that 'more ought to be done about the children', but the intention is all too seldom honoured.

Damages that can be inflicted

The variety and extent of damages that can be inflicted are varied and must depend on the personality of the child, the degree of emotional support provided by either parent, the variety of other social and emotional supports which may be available, and the age of the child when the parent developed the drinking problem. Of great importance is the actual behaviour of the parent when intoxicated; if there is continued rowdiness, arguments or violence, the impact will be far more adverse than in those instances where drunkenness is not associated with verbal or physical aggression. A drinking problem of whatever degree or nature which as its end-result produces what can in summary be described as a bad home atmosphere is attacking the centre of what family life should be able to give to a child. This is the kind of family where the social worker will report that 'you know there is something wrong as soon as you go in at the door'. Whether it is more damaging for the mother rather than the father to be the person with the drinking problem is uncertain, and there may be a different impact on the boys and the girls in the family. If a parent when drunk continuously picks on a particular child, scolding them, finding fault, demeaning, or hitting, then that child is immensely at risk.

At the psychological level, one effect may be a general and non-specific raising of the anxiety level in that child. In girls especially, there is also a higher incidence of depression, and in both sexes self-esteem is likely to be low (Zeitlin, 1994). But as well as this general impact on psychological health, a variety of important dynamic processes related to psychological growth can be affected. The child may, for instance, be very basically deprived of a satisfactory role model when the same-sex parent is the drinker, and a disturbed or ambivalent relationship with the parent of the opposite sex may result in feelings which are later going to be acted out in other relationships.

The psychological damages, and the social disabilities which can result, will interact. In the school setting, anxiety may lead to social disability, poor academic performance, and other problems. Boys are especially likely to display antisocial behaviour. Children of both sexes may display temper tantrums, or get involved in problems which come to the attention of the police (Zeitlin, 1994).

There is, however, little which is absolutely specific to the damaging psychological experience of this kind of home, and much the same types of disturbance must often result in homes where, for instance, one parent is chronically or repeatedly psychiatrically ill. What may be more specific is that the experience of intense family conflict centred on alcohol leaves the child with conflicting attitudes towards drinking and drunkenness which are built into their psychological being as highly charged determinants of later feelings and behaviours (see p. 292). Part of the emotional damage is latently the risk of drinking problems in later life.

The absence of emotional regard within the home can mean that a child will as an adolescent develop particularly rejecting attitudes towards the parents, and enter precipitously into identification with an adolescent peer group. Such an extreme version of a normal process is not necessarily harmful, but the children from this disturbed home can be vulnerable to involvement with groups which are themselves disturbed and engaging in drug-taking or delinquency. These associations may in part represent a revenge on the parents, or substitute comfort or excitement to replace the good inner feelings which are so lacking. There can, however, be no fixed predictions as to how a child from a drinking home will meet adolescence. Another outcome may be that the child is clinging, desperately and anxiously involved in the home, tied to protecting the non-drinking parent, and unable to make any identification with other young people.

At any stage of childhood the possibility of actual physical damage must be considered. There is an association between drinking problems and baby battering, and in childhood and adolescence the risk of physical assault may continue; the damage is often no more than bruising, but the risk of more serious injury is not to be discounted. Sexual abuse of children is also more likely, as is accidental injury due inadequate supervision. Help for the child is discussed in Chapter 15.

There is less information on the long-term outlook for children who come from homes that have been severely or chronically afflicted by a parent's abnormal drinking. However, research has suggested that in adult life, children of parents with drinking problems are more likely to display low self-esteem, depression, anxiety, antisocial behaviour, marital dysharmony, and generally poor strategies for coping with life (Box 4.2).

Box 4.2. Problems experienced by children of problem drinkers

- Anxiety

- Depression

- Low self-esteem

- Relationship difficulties

- Poor school performance

- Anti-social behaviour

- Physical and sexual abuse

- Accidental injury

- Risk of alcohol-related problems in later life

- Other problems in later life (depression, marital dysharmony, etc.)

Drinking problems and the family

Whether discussing the marriage or the children, what has essentially been argued in this Chapter is that drinking problems will inevitably be embedded in a network of family interactions. Those interactions are in terms both of overt communications and direct impacts, and dynamic processes of great subtlety. Heavy and problematic drinking influences the spouse's behaviour, which in turn influences the drinker's behaviour, so that a sort of resonance is set up. Plus, the children are not just passive recipients of what is done to them, but may themselves actively participate. Not only are parents and children and other family members involved, but so also perhaps the wife's friend 'who is always dropping in'. Ever to become focused only on a single actor is to lose sight of the play.

However, a play comprises a stage set and script, as well as the actors. So in family life, the 'script' that the actors learn is a vital ingredient to the success of the play. A couple who come together in marriage, or in a partnership outside of marriage, bring with them all kinds of expectations based upon their different experiences of family life. In each area of family life, some of these scripts will come from one side of the family, and some from the other. If one family of origin was adversely affected by the drinking of one or more of its members, then this may significantly influence the script that conveys the identity of the new family.

An established family is likely to display a range of behaviours which regulate daily life. Family therapists recognise these behaviours as including problem solving strategies, routines, and rituals (Steinglass *et al.*, 1987). In 'alcoholic families', these processes may become unduly concerned with the need to accommodate the adverse consequences of chronic drinking. There is evidence that the extent to which family rituals become influenced by alcohol is important not only in determining the successful adjustment of that family in the face of chronic drinking, but also the risk of drinking problems occurring in the next generation. Where rituals are not sacrificed to the salient priority of heavy drinking, or where a new family makes a conscious decision not to perpetuate rituals that have been so sacrificed, the family identity is less likely to suffer, and drinking problems are less likely to be continued through into the next generation. Where a new family perpetuates rituals which are subordinate to drinking, drinking problems are also likely to be perpetuated (Steinglass *et al.*, 1987).

> Christmas celebrations were frequently spoiled during Kate's childhood, as a result of her father's invariable drunkenness. Similarly her memories of family holidays were dominated by alcohol, and most birthdays or anniversaries were associated with anxiety about her father's drunkenness. Even the normal routine of daily life had accommodated his unpredictable behaviour after 'a drink with colleagues' on the way home from work. When Kate married and started a family of her own, she and her husband determined that they would never let drinking spoil their family life.

References

Jackson, J. K. (1954). The adjustment of the family to the crisis of alcoholism. *Quarterly Journal of Studies on Alcohol* **4**, 562–86.

Orford, J. & Edwards, G. (1977). *Alcoholism: A Comparison of Treatment and Advice, with a Study of the Influence of Marriage*. Maudsley Monograph, 26. Oxford: Oxford University Press.

Sher, K. J. (1991). *Children of Alcoholics*. Chicago: University of Chicago Press.
Steinglass, P., Bennett, L. A., Wolin, S. J. & Reiss, D. (1987). *The Alcoholic Family*. London: Hutchinson.
Zeitlin, H. (1994). Children with alcohol misusing parents. In *Alcohol and Alcohol Problems*, ed. Edwards, G. & Peters, T. J., pp. 139–51. British Medical Bulletin 50. Edinburgh: Churchill Livingstone.

5

Social complications of excessive drinking

In this chapter what is meant by 'social complications' of drinking will be explored and specific types of complication then considered under headings. Complications that occur within the family – an important type of social problem – have been discussed in Chapter 4.

Convenient though it is to think in terms of three classical problem dimensions – physical, mental, and social – this must not be allowed to obscure the fact that in the real lives of patients the dimensions are not separate at all. Problems in any one area lead to, and are exacerbated by problems in the other areas. By and large the more severe the dependence, the greater the likelihood of alcohol-related problems of all three kinds (Caetano, 1993). The clinical skill lies not only in making the detailed, one-dimensional assessment, but in putting the dimensions together.

Even as the social worker may be tempted by training or habit of mind to neglect the importance of the physical considerations in the equation, so may the physician be guilty of too narrow a concern with the patient's physical well-being at the cost of a proper awareness of the other issues. This chapter will seek to provide a checklist of what should be borne in mind in the social sphere, which should be useful whatever one's professional affiliation.

The concept of social complication

The idea of 'social complication' often implies a *failure to fulfil adequately an expected social role*. The failure may be in meeting expectations as, for example, family member, employer or employee, good neighbour, or law-abiding citizen. The result may be detrimental both to the individual and to those around them. A social complication may also mean *tangible alcohol-related loss of damage in the social dimension* – the driving licence forfeited for instance, the doctor's loss of right to practise, the house gone, and so on.

As for the alcohol-mediated processes that lead to functional impairments, several factors usually interact. Excessive drinking can at an early stage result in a hangover which makes it difficult to get to work, while intoxication may impair ability to manage the complexities of the job, and physical and mental impairment later make work impossible. More subtly, the drink-centredness of the individual and the salience which dependent drinking begins to acquire over other demands can mean that work ceases to matter, and this person moves into *an 'alcoholic role' which competes with any pre-existing roles.*

A secondary process is likely to arise in terms of *loss of reputation* and the way that others now think about and react to the drinker and confirm them in the alcoholic role. These reactions will be influenced by the background of social attitudes toward drinking and drunkenness and public perspectives of possibilities for recovery. A series of self-fulfilling prophecies may be set up with a process of amplification getting underway:

> I wrote 30 job application letters to various firms and told them I had been treated for a drink problem, was now sober and wanted to find my way back with everything in the open. Didn't get a single interview. So next time I kept quiet about my drinking, spun a yarn about that year off work, handed in two out-of-date references, lied on the medical form, and got the job. And then? They checked things out, I was fired on Friday, and yes, it's stupid, but I've been drinking. Just what they expected.

Social complications will almost inevitably spread to involve the *family and other people*, rather than ever affecting only the one individual. Such impacts on other people are in the economist's language referred to as *externalities*. In the United States and for the year 1988 the total financial cost of alcohol-related problems was estimated at US $85.8 billion (Rice *et al.*, 1991).

So much for general principles. The list of headings that follows attempts to deal with major areas of social problem experience and a summary is given in Box 5.1. The ordering does not indicate precedence of importance, and the list is not exhaustive. Social complications range from the trivial and the ephemeral to the major and are widely distributed in the drinking population (Clark & Hilton, 1991; Edwards *et al.*, 1994).

Box 5.1. Social complications of excessive drinking

- Family

- Problems at work

- Housing

- Financial difficulties

- Homelessness and vagrancy

- Crime, including violent, and sexual crime

- Drink-driving

- Victimisation

- Impact on education and training

Problems at work

The difficulty that a person with a drinking problem may encounter when seeking employment has just been instanced, and this example shows how stigmatisation may compound the objective difficulties. The varieties of adverse influence that excessive drinking may have on work performance are many and costly (Jones *et al.*; 1995, Romelsjö, 1995). The impact is not limited to any one level of seniority in the employment hierarchy, and drinking problems are as likely to be found in the boardroom as on the shopfloor.

The drinking doctor (Brooke, 1996)) provides an instance of a profession where alcohol-induced impairment can set special kinds of problems, but occupations and alcohol can interact in many different ways and, whatever the job, result in impaired efficiency or cause inconvenience, loss, or danger to other people. In senior positions in industry or the armed services, in the diplomatic service, or in the legal profession (Goodliffe, 1994), drunken indiscretion, irascibility, or bad judgement at a crucial meeting may be the major problems. For the bus or train driver, the aeroplane pilot (Holdener, 1993), or the ship's officer drunk on the bridge, intoxication carries enormous dangers for the public. In professions such as the church or teaching, the hint of scandal may be specially damaging, although it is surprising how tolerant or blind-eyed those in the individual's environment often appear to be. The seriousness with

69

which excessive drinking is officially viewed by the medical profession is evidenced by the disciplinary procedures which in many countries may be called into action if a doctor's drinking comes to official notice, although the story is again often one of complicity and cover-up. The conclusion to be drawn from this paragraph must therefore be that, whoever the individual we are trying to assess and help, the analysis of their alcohol-related social problems requires a job-specific enquiry.

Housing

Urban housing problems and urban drinking problems often go together (each exacerbating the other), and where there are great concentrations of substandard housing and social deprivation, drinking is one of many endemic disorders contributing to, and deriving from, the totality of social disorganisation.

However, cases are frequently encountered where drinking is leading directly to a housing problem. In this latter type of instance the patient's claim that they are 'drinking because of their unsatisfactory surroundings' has a hollow ring – theirs is the only house in the street which is shabby and unpainted and with, perhaps, an old sofa lying in the front garden. Housing problems of this kind will be more acute the more marginal the family's income. Bad relationships with neighbours, gross evidence of poor house maintenance, failure to meet the rent, services cut off, eviction, the sojourn into 'temporary accommodation', and multiple changes of address are familiar elements in the housing history as the drinking problem becomes more extreme.

Financial problems

An awareness of the possible financial complications of drinking problems and of the family's financial position, is necessary for any complete case assessment. To maintain a major drinking habit is expensive and large additional sums are often spent without the drinker knowing how the money has gone – drinks for friends, or drinks grandly offered to strangers, meals out and taxis home, a massive cigarette consumption, gambling, and so on. As with housing problems and many other social complications, the well-moneyed will be better protected for a longer time.

The financial balance is determined not only by the cost of the drinking and associated spendings, but also by the inflow of cash. Demotion, sickness and unemployment add to the stringencies. Complicated and devious stratagems may be engaged in to maintain the cash flow. 'Moonlighting' or the second job is common (often in a bar so as further to aid the drinking), loans are negotiated on preposterous terms, goods are pawned, houses re-mortgaged. The employee 'works a bit of a racket' and a load of bricks disappear from the builder's yard. It becomes vital to evade income tax and to defraud Social Security. The rent is not paid and hire purchase payments fall behind.

The family may have reached the stage where financial chaos has become the central and pressing pain. From the social work angle, sorting out that chaos may be the necessary first-aid, but it will be very temporary aid if the drinking problem is not radically met.

Homelessness and vagrancy

The vagrant way of life offers many pressures towards drinking, and at the same time the man or woman with a serious drinking problem may move towards vagrancy (Braumohl, 1989; Fischer, 1991). Professionals with a special interest in alcohol do well also to remember that 'the homeless single person' may be homeless for many other reasons than their drinking. Economic hardship and unemployment vary in the contribution they make to vagrancy from decade to decade, while mental illness, physical incapacity, epilepsy, and personality disorders contribute continually to the genesis of a city problem which in many countries still seems intractable, come boom or slump.

With those provisos noted, it is still true that the vagrant who is sleeping under the railway arch may be manifesting the end-result of a drinking career – a 'social complication' of highly visible and dramatic nature, and the concern of the social reformer from the nineteenth century onwards (McDermott 1994). The elements of this 'complication' constitute a complex system of related problems: the homelessness itself, the difficulty in getting a wash, the lack of clothes, the lack of fixed employment, the breakdown in family contacts and lack of any kinship or friendship supports, the petty criminal involvement, the poor nutrition, and the risks of illness and accident. Drinking is what particularly contributes to the ultimate core characteristic of this situation – its seeming inescapableness, the sense of the treadmill. It is easier to find a way into that degradation than a way out. On leaving hospital or the detoxification centre the only friendship or support readily available may be that offered by a return to the company of the drinkers in the park.

What is the likely background of the man or woman who is begging at the street corner and hoping to raise funds for the next bottle of cheap wine? There are many routes into that situation but with the need to avoid constructing a picture in terms of any stereotype again noted, the average story is as follows. That individual is more frequently a man than a woman, although women do reach this plight. The parents were often themselves holding onto socio-economic survival tenuously – the father an unskilled worker living in poor urban conditions or rural poverty, and the childhood family often large and lacking in care. Gross disruption of the childhood home is a frequent finding; education is likely to have been meagre and job-training nil. The picture is therefore typically of someone who has started with few advantages and many handicaps. The vagrant drinker is with overwhelming frequency a casualty with origins in the underprivileged working class; the shop-keeper or skilled tradesman who becomes involved in drink and falls on hard times seldom goes in that direction. The geographical origins may be well-known and typical in a particular country – in London the casualties will usually not be London-based, but have come from Scotland or Ireland.

After leaving school the story tends to be of a few short-term jobs in the home town, a period perhaps in the armed forces or the merchant navy, a short-lived marriage and an unsuccessful attempt to settle down, and then probably the mobility and rootlessness of the casual labourer who moves from town to town, and who follows the construction work and the big wages. Contacts with family and friends are lost. As the drinking becomes more incapacitating, there is a drift towards low-grade work such as kitchen portering and with periods of unemployment, spells in prison and psychiatric hospitals, and the final arrival at that disorganised way of life which is often referred to as Skid Row. That term was originally used in the United States to indicate the downtown tract of rooming houses, cheap hotels, blood banks, rescue missions, winos, and bottle-gangs found in many North American cities. In the UK and other European countries clearly segmented patches of social disorganisation generally do not exist. Skid Row refers more to a way of life than to particular streets.

As for the involvement of drinking in this unfolding story, excessive drinking has often started at an early age and then followed an accelerated course. Soon after the age of 30, drink has become a dominantly destructive influence, and this man is now beginning to stand apart even from other heavy drinking members of the casual workforce, is beginning to be picked up for drunkenness with alarming frequency, is violently shaky every morning, and is finally drawn into companionship with the bottle-gang and to sharing their cider, wine, or industrial spirits. The Skid Row way of life may appear to be chaos and disorder, but it has its own social organisation and sub-culture; it becomes the

individual's only support system and gives them values and expectations as well as drink. The pathways through which women move
toward a life of alcohol and vagrancy may overlap with the typical male
routing, but can often involve more evidently individual negative life
experience, with a history of spousal violence a common feature.

Accurate and sympathetic understanding of this extreme social
complication of drinking is needed if we are to be able to cope with such
problems. Too often the person in this condition tends to be even further
alienated and his or her pessimism further reinforced by responses
which indicate that we do indeed regard them as alien, hopeless, and
beyond the pale. One of the lessons of close experience is in fact that this
condition is recoverable, and that there are pathways off Skid Row,
however difficult to find (Cook, 1975).

Crime

Multiple relationships

The relationship between crime and drinking is as complex as with any
other social complications of alcohol. Simple, direct, and one-way
causality is seldom a sufficient analysis and various models of understanding have been proposed (Collins, 1981). Personality, background,
and social circumstances which predispose to crime may as much and
independently predispose to drinking. Genetic influences may need to
be considered. Alcohol and criminality are both then symptoms of an
underlying nexus of disorders. A drinking problem may also in passing
affect a dedicated and professional criminal, perhaps at a later stage of
their career. Alternatively, one may see the person who is alcohol dependent and who at a much later age than the usual 'first offender' falls foul
of the law, or is caught up in a flurry of recidivism. Sometimes the
person is seen who suddenly shifts from a circulation around the
prisons to a hospital and voluntary agency circuit: their drinking
remains much the same, but they have learnt to present themselves and
their problems differently. The offence may by definition involve the
actual intoxication itself – for instance, 'the drunkenness offender'
(Greenfield & Weisner, 1995) and 'the drink driver' (National Institute
on Alcohol Abuse and Alcoholism, 1996). The drunkenness offender
overlaps with the vagrant drinking population.

The variations on the alcohol-crime connection are legion. There is no
type of offence that will not sometimes be related to drinking, and many
types of offence that will often be so related. The problems load at the
'petty' end of the spectrum – petty theft, minor assault, travelling on

public transport without a ticket, failing to pay for the meal in the cheap café, urinating in the subway, begging. The person with a drinking problem may know that when they are drunk (and only when they are drunk), they are apt to engage in their own particular offence, for example, taking cars and driving them away, 'going burgling' in a clumsy sort of fashion, or passing dud cheques. Drinking may be the story behind an embezzlement.

Alcohol, violence, and sexual crime

To the judge or the magistrate the relationship between drinking and violence may appear to be evident and to make a repeated contribution to the offences coming before the courts. We describe on page 88 an example of an alcohol-related assault. All too often drinking seems to be responsible for disinhibition and release of violent or sexually violent behaviour. A Skid Row drinker hits a fellow member of a bottle-gang on the head with an iron bar; a man comes out of a pub and follows a woman down an alleyway and rapes and murders her; three drunken youths brutally assault and rob the owner of an off licence.

Although to the courts and the ordinary citizen it may appear evident that alcohol causes or considerably contributes to the genesis of these kinds of serious crime, researchers have repeatedly pointed out the dangers in assuming an identity between correlation and causality in this arena (Collins, 1991; Shepherd, 1994). Many case series have shown a high frequency of intoxication among violent offenders at the time of the criminal act (Roslund & Larson, 1979), but that does not prove that the drinking *caused* the crime. People bent on violence may coincidentally choose to drink, drinking can be a mere adjunct to intrinsically dangerous situations and confrontations, and alcohol may be used for excuse.

Several different research approaches have been used to examine the validity of the assumption that alcohol can contribute to the genesis of these types of offence, and the inherent difficulties in the interpretation of simple cross-sectional studies has been referred to above. One approach has come from anthropological research which has suggested that the degree to which people behave violently or sexually when drunk is not so much determined by their drinking, but the way in which society and culture believes or proposes that people will behave when intoxicated (MacAndrew & Edgerton, 1969). Psychologists have explored the influence of alcohol on aggression within experimental paradigms (Gustafson, 1993). From the various lines of work mentioned above it is reasonable to infer that culture and set and setting will influence the individual's response to alcohol, but these studies still leave unanswered the question of whether alcohol is likely significantly and directly to contribute to violent crime in an industrial society.

Further light has, however, been thrown on an issue where everyday experience and rational analysis have previously sometimes seemed to be at odds, by research which explores the correlation over time in national per capita alcohol consumption and rates for assault or homicide (Lenke, 1990; Edwards et al., 1994). For some, but not all, countries the correlations are positive. Other recent research has looked specifically at the relationship between drinking and offending among juveniles and has shown that with correction for shared risk factors there is in this age group a significant association between drinking and violent offending (Fergusson et al., 1996). Despite the intrinsic complexity of the question being asked it is thus more possible to give answers than was earlier the case. The relationships are indeed multiple and varied, but alcohol consumption plays a direct part in the cause of violent crime. Whether this conclusion can be extended to sexual crime is still unclear.

A rather similar literature has been developing on the relationship between drinking, self-harm, and suicide (Murphy & Wetzel, 1990; Rossow, 1996). That a true causal link exists here of some significance is becoming increasingly evident.

Drink-driving offenders

The bulk of drink-driving offences are committed by the generality of the drinking population and it is to that broad target that counter-measures should predominantly be directed (Edwards et al., 1994). The factors which predict involvement in this kind of offence include not only drinking behaviour (quantity and frequency of drinking), but also other groups of variables such as socio-demographic factors, drinking behaviour, and psychological characteristics (National Institute on Alcohol Abuse and Alcoholism, 1996).

Estimates for the proportion of subjects among drink-driving offenders variously defined as 'alcoholics' or 'problem drinkers' have varied from 4% to 87% across samples and jurisdictions, with incidence rates influenced by operational definition and tending to be lower when definitions are more tightly drawn. Alcohol dependence is likely to have a stronger association with drink driving the higher the BAC at the time of offence and among repeat offenders, and a research literature attempts to identify the differential characteristics of drinkers in treatment who are likely to offend (Macdonald & Pederson, 1990). Multiple offenders are not only likely to be more alcohol involved but to show wider personality and background disturbance.

From the clinical angle the conclusion must be that enquiry into driving behaviour and drink-driving offences should be an integral part of any assessment. By no means everyone who has been convicted of driving while intoxicated will have an otherwise manifest drinking problem (Gruenewald *et al.*, 1990), but among clinical populations there will be a significant proportion of individuals whose driving poses a threat to themselves and other people, with that fact putting distinct responsibility on the clinician.

The individual's drinking and their risk of being a victim of crime

There is a positive relationship in the general population between the quantity an individual drinks and the likelihood of being assaulted (Room, 1983; Edwards *et al.*, 1994). A grossly intoxicated person will easily fall prey to having their pockets turned out, or be deprived of capacity to resist violence or rape. Thus victimisation is a common social complication of heavy drinking.

Impact on education and training

An aspect of social complication that deserves greater note is the long-term handicap which results when an educational or training opportunity is partly wasted or totally lost. Being sent down from university, failing to complete a postgraduate degree, or the abandonment of an apprenticeship because of a drinking problem, may all have serious long-term consequences.

The essential themes

Having started this chapter with a general discussion of the nature and genesis of social complications and having then worked through a listing of specific problem areas, it is useful finally to re-emphasise certain essential themes. Drinking can impair many aspects of social adjustment and lead to many types of social loss or damage, but is usually an element which *contributes* to causality. The social impact of excessive drinking can seldom be understood in uni-causal and single-directional terms. Impairment of social well-being is as real and important as the physical and mental impairments with which it may interact, and concern for this dimension is therefore fundamental both to the initial assessment and the work of recovery.

References

Braumohl, J. (ed.) (1989). Alcohol, homelessness and public policy. *Contemporary Drug Problems* **16**(3), Special Issue, 281–526.

Brooke, D. (1996). Why do some doctors become addicted? *Addiction* **91**, 317–19.

Caetano, R. (1993). The association between severity of DSM-III-R alcohol dependence and medical and social consequences. *Addiction* **88**, 631–42.

Clark, W. B. & Hilton M. F. (eds.) (1991). *Alcohol in America: Drinking Practises and Problems.* Albany: State University of New York Press.

Collins, J. J. (ed.) (1981). *Drinking and Crime.* London: Tavistock.

Cook, T. (1975). *Vagrant Alcoholics.* Boston: Routledge and Kegan Paul.

Edwards, G., Anderson, P., Babor, T. F., Casswell, S., Ferrence R., Giesbrecht, N. *et al.* (1994). *Alcohol Policy and the Public Good.* Oxford: Oxford University Press.

Fergusson, D. M., Lynskey, M. T. & Horwood, L. J. (1996). Alcohol misuse and juvenile offending in adolescence. *Addiction* **91**, 483–4.

Fischer, P. (1991). *Alcohol, Drug Abuse and Mental Health Problems among Homeless Persons: A Review of the Literature 1980–1990.* Rockville: National Institute on Alcohol Abuse and Alcoholism.

Goodliffe, J. (1994). Alcohol and depression in England and American lawyer disciplinary proceedings. *Addiction* **89**, 1237–44.

Greenfield, T. K. & Weisner, C. (1995). Drinking problems and self-reported criminal behavior, arrests, and convictions: 1990 US national and 1989 county surveys. *Addiction* **90**, 361–74.

Gruenewald, P. J., Stewart, K. & Klitzner M. (1990). Alcohol use and the appearance of alcohol problems among first offender drunk drivers. *British Journal of Addiction* **85**, 107–17.

Gustafson, R. (1993). What do experimental paradigms tell us about alcohol-related aggressive responses? *Journal of Studies on Alcohol (Suppl. 11)* 20–9.

Holdener, F. O. (1993). Alcohol and civil aviation. *Addiction* **88** (Suppl), 953–8.

Jones, S., Casswell S. & Zhang, J-F. (1995). The economic costs of alcohol-related absenteeism and reduced productivity in the working population of New Zealand. *Addiction* **90**, 1453–62.

Lenke, L. (1990). *Alcohol and Criminal Violence – Time Series Analyses in a Comparative Perspective.* Stockholm: Almqvist and Wiksell.

MacAndrew, C. & Edgerton, R .B. (1969). *Drunken Comportment.* Chicago: Aldine.

MacDonald, S. & Pederson, L. L. (1990). The characteristics of alcoholics in treatment arrested for driving while impaired. *British Journal of Addiction* **85**, 97–105.

McDermott, I. (1994) Journal Interview 34. Conversation with Monsignor Ignatius McDermott. *Addiction* **89**, 791–8.

Murphy, G. E. & Wetzel, R. D. (1990). The lifetime risk of suicide in alcoholism. *Archives of General Psychiatry* **47**, 383–92.

National Institute on Alcohol Abuse and Alcoholism (1996). Drinking and driving. *Alcohol Alert* **31**, 1–3.

Rice, D. P., Kelman, S. & Miller, L. S. (1991). The economic cost of alcohol abuse. *Alcohol Health and Research World* **15**, 307–16.

Romelsjö, A. (1995). Alcohol consumption and unintentional injury, suicide, violence, work performance and intergenerational effects. In *Alcohol and Public Policy: Evidence and Issues*, pp.114–42. Holder, H. D. & Edwards, G. Oxford: Oxford University Press.

Room, R. (1983). Alcohol and crime, behavioural aspects. In *Encyclopedia of Crime and Justice*, ed. Kadish, S., vol.1, pp.35–44. New York: The Free Press.

Roslund, B. & Larson, C. A. (1979). Crimes of violence and alcohol abuse in Sweden. *International Journal of the Addictions* **14**, 1103–15.

Rossow, I. (1996). Alcohol and suicide. *Addiction* **91**, 1413–16.

Shepherd, J. (1994). Violent crime: the role of alcohol and new approaches to the prevention of injury. *Alcohol and Alcoholism* **29**, 5–10.

6

Drinking problems and psychiatric illness

Anyone working in the field of drinking problems must cultivate an awareness of the range of mental illnesses that may result from, or lie behind, the drinking. Very serious issues will otherwise be overlooked. Alcohol problems and mental disorders are both common, and are therefore bound to overlap in any population. More importantly, alcohol is a readily available medication for many types of mental distress, and in these cases drinking is a complication of the underlying and primary pathology. Some aspects of the relationship between personality, mental illness, and alcohol problems have already been touched on briefly in Chapter 1 when discussing the causes of excessive drinking. Yet another facet of the relationship is that in some instances the drinking actually causes the mental illness. This chapter will not deal with the treatment issues in detail, but will mention them in passing.

In the US, the Epidemiologic Catchment Area (ECA) Study investigated the prevalence of alcohol, drug, and mental disorders in over 20,000 people, across a range of community and institutional settings (Regier *et al.*, 1990). The estimated US population life-time prevalence rates were 13.5% for DSM-III alcohol dependence and abuse and 22.5% for any non-substance-abuse mental disorder. Individuals with a life-time history of an alcohol disorder had high rates of co-morbid psychiatric disorder (37%); this included anxiety disorder (19.4%), antisocial personality disorder (14.3%), mood disorder (13.4%), and schizophrenia (3.8%). The odds of having an anxiety disorder if one had an alcohol disorder were only 1.5 times greater than those of a person without an alcohol disorder. The odds ratios for the other diagnostic groups were as follows: mood disorder (1.9), antisocial personality disorder (21), schizophrenia (3.3). Relevant data are summarised in Table 6.1

Prevalence rates for comorbid alcohol problems and mental disorders

Table 6.1. *Life-time prevalence and odds ratios (ORs) of various mental disorders among persons with any alcohol disorder diagnosis (five-site Epidemiologic Catchment Area Study combined community and institutional sample standardised to the US population).*

| | Any alcohol disorder | | |
	%	(SE)	OR
Comorbid Disorder			
Any mental	36.6*	(1.4)	2.3
Any anxiety	19.4*	(1.0)	1.5
Antisocial personality disorder	14.3*	(1.1)	21.0
Any affective (mood)	13.4*	(0.9)	1.9
Schizophrenia	3.8*	(0.6)	3.3

Note:
*p<.001 prevalence in exposed versus non-exposed group.
Source: From Regier *et al.*, 1990.

will depend on the setting within which the patients are seen. The probation service, social work office, primary care, general or psychiatric hospital, and prison, will all draw a different type of caseload. Individuals seeking treatment for an alcohol disorder have higher rates of comorbid mental disorder than those with an alcohol problem who are not seeking treatment (Regier *et al.*, 1990).

We will look firstly at alcohol-related hallucinatory states as exemplifying conditions where drinking or withdrawal of alcohol are of undoubted and central causality, and then go on to discuss the relationship between drinking problems and types of general psychiatric disorder. Alcohol-related brain damage and the Wernicke-Korsakoff Syndrome are discussed in Chapter 8.

Transient hallucinatory experience

Transient hallucinatory experience deserves note for two reasons. Firstly, it may herald the onset of delirium tremens or alcoholic hallucinosis, and can often give early warning of the likelihood of these much more serious illnesses. It may therefore be viewed as continuous with those states, rather than an altogether discrete clinical entity. Secondly, it is important to be aware that transient hallucinations may occur without the illness progressing to either of the major presentations. The diagnostician who is unfamiliar with these transient phenomena may be tempted to record incorrectly that the patient has 'suffered from delirium tremens' when this was not the case.

The essence of this condition is that the patient fleetingly and suddenly experiences any one of a variety of perceptual disturbances, often very much to their surprise and consternation, and with the episode then immediately over. These occurrences may be experienced during periods of continued, heavy, and chaotic dependent drinking or during withdrawal. There is no delirium or evidence of severe physiological disturbance as seen in delirium tremens. Here are some examples of how patients described such experiences:

> I would be driving along the road and suddenly something would run across in front of the car – a dog, a cat, I couldn't be sure – and I would slam on the brakes. A real fright. And then I'd realise there was nothing there.

> I would be walking down the road and, ZOOM, a car would come up behind me and I'd jump on the pavement. Frightened out of my life. But it was all imagination.

> What used to happen was that I would turn around thinking someone had called my name.

The degree of insight is often characteristic; the patient immediately disconfirms the reality of the hallucination. A relatively stereotyped and limited kind of hallucinatory experience is also typical; for one patient it is nearly always the car coming up from behind, for another a pigeon flying into the room. It is important to realise that some patients can experience such discomforting happenings for many months without progressing to a major disturbance. The meaning and significance of 'continuity' will immediately become clear as we go on below to discuss delirium tremens and alcoholic hallucinosis.

Delirium tremens

The clinical picture

Delirium tremens is a short-lived toxic confusional state, which usually occurs as a result of reduced alcohol intake in alcohol dependent individuals with a long history of use (World Health Organisation, 1992).

Delirium tremens can produce a variety of clinical pictures, but it is best viewed as a unitary syndrome with a continuum of severities and a variation in symptom clustering. The disturbance is often fluctuating, with the patient's condition worsening in the evening or when the room is unlit and shadowy. The classical triad of symptoms includes clouding of consciousness and confusion, vivid hallucinations affecting any sensory modality and marked tremor. Delusions, agitation, sleeplessness, and autonomic arousal are frequently also present.

Symptoms of delirium usually occur from about 24 to 150 hours after the last drink (within this band earlier rather than later onset is more typical), peaking between 72 to 96 hours later (Naranjo & Sellers, 1986). Prodromal symptoms are usually evident, but may be overlooked. The onset is often at night with restlessness, insomnia, and fear (Lishman, 1987).

Delirium

The patient is more or less out of contact with reality and potentially disorientated as to person, place, and time. For instance, they may believe that they are cruising on a liner, mistake the nurse for a steward and order a drink, but five minutes later know that they are in hospital and correctly identify the people around them.

Hallucinations and Illusions

Hallucinations and illusions are characteristically vivid, chaotic, and bizarre and occur in any sensory modality – the patient may see visions, hear things, smell gases, or feel animals crawling over them. The classical visual hallucinations are vivid and horrifying and typically include snakes and rats and other small animals which may appear to attack the patient as they lie in bed. They may also take a 'microscopic' form (small furry men dancing on the floor), but any type of visual hallucination can occur. These visions are often brightly coloured and have been described by Hemmingsen and Kramp (1988) as 'kaleidoscopic with a niavistic, animated, cartoon-like flavour'. One patient in their series had visual hallucinations of soldiers outside the window, Marilyn Monroe on the roof, policemen selling flowers, and insects. Patients often become completely preoccupied by, and interact with, the hallucinated objects. Thus, they feed the dogs or argue with the little men.

Hallucinatory voices or bursts of music may be heard, or the threatening screams of animals. Hallucinations are often based on a ready tendency to illusional misrepresentation – the wrinkles in the bedclothes become snakes, patterns in the wallpaper become faces.

Tremor

As the illness develops the patient becomes anxious and more fearful and develops tremor. At worst they may be shaking so severely that the bed is rattling, but as with other symptoms there can be a continuum of severity and the tremor may not be very noticeable unless the patient is asked to stretch out their hands.

Fear
The patient may be experiencing extremes of horror in reaction, for instance, to the snakes which writhe all over their bed, but on other occasions the hallucinations appear to be enjoyable or entertaining, and the patient is perhaps happily watching a private cinema show.

Paranoid delusions
The illness often has a degree of paranoid flavouring – enemies are blowing poisonous gas into the room, assassins lurk at the window, and there is a nameless conspiracy afoot. The mood can in fact be paranoid, with every happening and stimulus being misrepresented as it comes along, but the patient's mental state is too muddled for the delusional ideas to become systematised.

Occupational delusions or hallucinations
The barman, for instance, may believe that he is serving in his cocktail bar and pour out imaginary drinks, or the bricklayer may be building an imaginary wall.

Restlessness and agitation
Partly as a consequence of the fearfulness of the hallucinatory experiences, the patient is often highly restless, clutching and pulling at the bed clothes, starting at any sound, or attempting to jump out of bed and run down the ward. This over-activity, when combined with a degree of weakness and unsteadiness, can put the patient seriously at risk of falls and other accidents.

Heightened suggestibility
The patient who is suffering from delirium tremens can show a heightened susceptibility to suggestion, which occasionally becomes evident spontaneously but may only come out on testing. The older text books often mention such stories as the patient agreeing to deal from an imaginery pack of cards or 'drinking' from a proffered but empty glass.

Physical disturbances
Heavy sweating is typical, with risk therefore of dehydration. Appetite is usually lacking, the pulse is rapid and the blood pressure is likely to be raised, and the patient feverish. If the illness continues over many days, the picture gradually becomes that of dehydration, exhaustion, and collapse, with the possibility of a sudden and disastrously steep rise in temperature.

Aetiology and course

Delirium tremens is today generally viewed as essentially an alcohol withdrawal state, although it is conceded that other factors such as infection or trauma sometimes play an ancillary part. The withdrawal, which precipitates the attack, may have been occasioned by admission to hospital, arrest and incarceration, or a self-determined effort to give up drinking. Often, though, there is no history of abrupt withdrawal and the illness starts while the patient is still drinking, but there has probably been at least partial withdrawal. In some instances the patient seems to have hovered on the brink of delirium tremens for many preceding weeks, with much evidence of transient hallucinatory experience, whereas in other instances the illness has a more explosive onset. It is unusual for a patient to experience delirium tremens without a history of at least several years of severe alcohol dependence and many years of excessive drinking, but an attack may occur even after one or two weeks if a previously abstinent patient rapidly reinstates dependence. Recurrent attacks are common once a patient has had one such episode.

The condition usually lasts for three to five days, with gradual resolution. On rare occasions the illness drags on for some weeks, fluctuating between recovery and relapse. The possibility of severe physical complications has been mentioned and before the advent of antibiotics, intercurrent chest infection or pneumonia constituted serious risks. Reported mortality rates have varied from centre to centre and even with skilled care a degree of risk remains, with death occurring in about 5% of admissions (Cushman, 1987; Chick, 1989). Death is typically due to cardiovascular collapse, hypothermia, or intercurrent infection.

Possibilities of diagnostic confusion

It might be supposed that delirium tremens would give a picture so vivid and distinct as to make diagnostic mistakes unlikely. There is always the possibility that an underlying condition which is contributing to the picture is being overlooked. Liver failure, pneumonia, and head injury should always be borne in mind. Confusion may also occur when the possibility of delirium tremens is entirely overlooked, although in retrospect the diagnosis was plainly evident. This is often the case in the setting of a general hospital ward, where the patient is noted to be suffering from 'confusion', to be 'rambling a bit', or to be trying to get out of bed at night. In this situation the condition may be put down to the non-specific effects of infection, trauma, or operation. The diagnosis is at times overlooked in the psychiatric hospital setting when it may be misdiagnosed as an 'acute schizophrenic reaction', for instance when the acutely disturbed person with delirium tremens has florid paranoid ideas and is found running up the street with a knife in their hand and presents as an emergency admission from the police. (The treatment of delirium tremens is outlined on p. 242.)

Alcohol withdrawal seizures

Alcohol withdrawal seizures occur in about 5–15% of alcohol dependent individuals, approximately 7 to 48 hours after cessation of drinking (Brennan & Lyttle, 1987). The seizures are generalised, tonic-clonic (grand mal) and are thus associated with a loss of consciousness, followed by convulsive movements in all four limbs. During a particular withdrawal episode the patient may have only one seizure, but more commonly there will be three or four seizures over a couple of days. Very rarely, status epilepticus will supervene. This is a continuous run of seizures, one merging into another, which is associated with risk to life. Alcohol withdrawal seizures have sometimes been termed 'rum fits' but they are not associated with any one type of beverage.

Alcohol dependent individuals who have experienced seizures due to alcohol withdrawal may be more prone to developing further seizures in future withdrawal episodes. For them any projected detoxification should therefore be carried out in an in-patient setting.

Predisposing factors to alcohol withdrawal seizures include hypokalaemia, hypomagnesaemia, a previous history of withdrawal seizures, and concurrent epilepsy. The EEG is generally unhelpful but computerised tomography will help to rule out intracranial lesions (Earnest et al., 1988).

Tragedies have sometimes occurred when a severely dependent patient has stopped drinking on their own initiative and sustained a withdrawal seizure which has led to an accident. For example, the driver of a heavy goods vehicle had, after a long period of sobriety, relapsed into dependent drinking, but after two to three months he determined abruptly to put a stop to his drinking. He had a seizure, his truck went out of control and mounted a pavement and killed a woman who was standing by a bus stop. There are thus a number of reasons for taking withdrawal seizures and the risks of such seizures very seriously.

Other possible reasons for seizures are discussed on pp. 137–8.

Alcoholic hallucinosis

The term alcoholic hallucinosis is used to describe auditory or visual hallucinations that occur either during or after a period of heavy alcohol consumption (Glass, 1989a,b; Tsuang *et al.*, 1994). The hallucinations are vivid, of acute onset, and typically occur in the setting of clear consciousness (World Health Organisation, 1992). They may be accompanied by misidentifications, delusions, ideas of reference and an abnormal affect. Alcoholic hallucinosis typically resolves over a period of weeks, but can occasionally persist for months. Delirium tremens and psychotic disorders must be ruled out before diagnosis of alcoholic hallucinosis can be made.

In alcoholic hallucinosis, the auditory hallucinations may consist of unformed noises or snatches of music, but usually take the form of voices. These voices may be talking to the patient directly, but more often take the form of a running commentary about them. Sometimes there is only one voice but often several engage in discussion, and the same voice may come back again on different occasions. The commentary may be favourable and friendly, or accusatory and threatening. Sometimes the voices command the patient to do things against their will and this may result in acting-out behaviour or a suicide attempt. There is a lack of insight and the voices are considered as real, but the patient will seldom elaborate any complex explanation as to the supposed mechanism by which the voices are reaching them. The voices may come and go or haunt the patient more or less incessantly.

The majority of studies of alcoholic hallucinosis were carried out before the widespread use of operational criteria and standardised assessment and were therefore based on mixed samples of patients having hallucinations associated with alcohol withdrawal, schizophrenia, major depression, and psycho-stimulant use such as amphetamines or cocaine. Tsuang *et al.* (1994) have shown that the prevalence of 'alcoholic hallucinosis' varies according to the diagnostic criteria used.

There is little evidence to support the view that alcoholic hallucinosis is a form of latent schizophrenia. Nevertheless, it may superficially resemble acute paranoid schizophrenia and the differential diagnosis may be difficult. The delusions associated with alcoholic hallucinosis are usually attempts to explain the hallucinations. There is no evidence of a complicated delusional system, schizophrenic thought disorder, or incongruity of affect, and insight is regained as the voices diminish (Lishman, 1987). While these guidelines provide useful indications, it can still in practice be difficult to make the distinction, and in such circumstances the sensible course of action is to admit the patient to hospital, withdraw them from alcohol and observe what happens.

Recovery may take place abruptly, but more often there is a slow fading of the symptoms. The voices become less persistent, do not make such an urgent demand on attention and their reality begins to be doubted. The possibility that the illness will finally declare itself to be schizophrenia has, of course, to be borne in mind, and if symptoms have not ceased within a couple of months, the latter diagnosis becomes more likely, although it has been reported that alcoholic hallucinosis may sometimes require even six months for complete recovery. Some drug intoxications, including most noteably amphetamine psychosis, can also result in a picture mimicking alcoholic hallucinosis and with a presentation of this sort it is always wise to carry out urine testing for drugs.

When a patient has experienced one attack of alcoholic hallucinosis they are at risk of recurrence of this condition if they drink again, although such reinstatement is not inevitable.

The possible pathophysiological mechanisms underlying alcoholic hallucinosis are described by Soyka (1995). The acute onset of hallucinations during alcohol withdrawal may reflect increased dopamine activity and decreased serotonin (5-HT) in the brain (see Chapter 2). More recent work points to the role of beta-carbolines and essential fatty acids.

Alcohol-induced psychotic disorder with delusions

The category alcohol-induced psychotic disorders with delusions has been included in DSM-IV (American Psychiatric Association, 1994) and deserves mention here. Although few studies have systematically focused on this clinical condition, it has been reported in the literature for at least 150 years. Such patients typically develop paranoid or grandiose delusions in the context of heavy drinking, but remain alert, and do not display any confusion or clouding of consciousness. Although psychiatric hospitalisation may be required, the prognosis is generally good, and the delusional syndrome clears within days to weeks of abstinence. As with alcoholic hallucinosis, there appears to be no association with schizophrenia.

'Pathological intoxication'

Pathological intoxication, sometimes referred to as *mania à potu*, is a term used to describe a sudden onset of aggressive and often violent behaviour, not typical of the individual when sober, and occurring soon

after drinking small amounts of alcohol that would not produce intoxication in most people (Coid, 1979). There is classically an amnesia for
the event and it is alleged that the aggressor was in a trance state or displaying automatism. The episode is usually followed by a long sleep.
There may be an association with EEG abnormalities and other signs of
brain damage, particularly frontal lobe dysfunction.

Pathological intoxication is an ill-defined entity (Coid, 1979) and it is
doubtful whether such a distinct entity deserves recognition. Clearly a
relationship between drinking and crime does exist (see p. 73), and the
aggressor in such circumstances often manifests an alcohol-induced
amnesia if there has been a high blood-alcohol level at the time of the
offence. Careful questioning will usually reveal that the amount of
alcohol ingested was more than a 'small amount' and that there has
been previous evidence of propensity to violence. This is borne out by
Maletzky's (1976) work which demonstrated that large amounts of
alcohol were required before disturbed behaviour was evident. Other
instances of supposed pathological intoxication may be attributable to
alcohol-induced hypoglycaemia, organic brain damage, or personality
disorder.

Here is an account of the type of case which frequently comes before
the courts:

> A young man, aged 23 years, had a pattern of frequent but intermittent
> heavy drinking. At his brother's wedding he became very drunk and
> argumentative. The best man tried to quieten him down but a quarrel
> ensued, and without warning this young drinker picked up a knife and
> stabbed a bystander, narrowly missing the victim's heart. The assailant
> said that he had 'only taken a drink or two', but this was clearly untrue.
> He displayed a patchy amnesia for the surrounding events. Enquiry
> revealed that he had on several previous occasions been involved in
> dangerous fights, both when drunk and when sober.

It can hardly be doubted that this young man's intoxication contributed
to his loss of impulse control, and it was probably the crucial additional
factor which sparked off his violence, given also the background importance of predisposition and circumstance. The position taken here is not
that intoxication is irrelevant to understanding such events, but rather
that it is unproductive to segment cases into those due to 'intoxication',
as opposed to instances where 'pathological intoxication' is deemed to
be the cause. This distinction is encouraged by legal systems which give
simple drunkeness no standing, and which therefore lead defence
lawyers to search for a medical basis on which to argue that their client's
intoxication was a disease manifestation. From the strictly medical
point of view 'pathological drunkeness' is a very uncertain concept.

Alcoholic blackouts (alcohol-induced amnestic episodes)

The widely used but somewhat confusing lay-term 'alcoholic blackout' refers to transient memory loss which may be induced by intoxication. Although such occurrences are reported in some two-thirds or more of alcohol dependent individuals (Goodwin et al., 1969a; Schuckit et al., 1993) alcoholic memory blackouts are also relatively common in social drinkers after incidents of heavy indulgence. Approximately one-third of young men in the general population are likely to have experienced memory blackouts (Goodwin et al., 1969a). Thus, while they are an important warning sign of problem drinking, they are not pathognomonic of alcohol dependence.

Blackouts have been described as being of two types (Goodwin et al., 1969a,b). The en bloc variety is characterised by a dense and total amnesia with abrupt points of onset and recovery, and with no subsequent recall of events for the amnesic period, either spontaneously or with prompting. This period may extend from 30 to 60 minutes up to as long as two or three days. In contrast, 'fragmentary' blackouts or 'greyouts' are patchy episodes of amnesia, with indistinct boundaries and islands of memory within these boundaries. They are often characterised by partial or complete subsequent recall, and usually extend over a shorter period than the 'en bloc' variety. In reality, alcoholic memory blackouts can occur with every degree of gradation, and although it is useful to recognise the two types, the experience of each patient has to be described separately.

Blackouts may begin to occur at a late stage in a career of excessive drinking or never at all. Once they start to be experienced with any frequency, they tend to recur, and a patient may often be able to identify the phase at which they 'began to get bad blackouts'. The reason for such varied susceptibility to the disorder is unknown, but blackouts are associated with an early onset of drinking, high peak levels of alcohol, and a past history of head injury (Kopelman, 1991). Concurrent use of sedatives and hypnotics may increase the likelihood of amnesia. Blackouts are not predictive of long-term cognitive impairment.

During an alcoholic blackout the individual can engage in any type of activity. To the observer, the drinker will not obviously be in an abnormal state of mind (other than being intoxicated), although a spouse or someone else who knows them well, may claim to recognise subtle changes – for instance, 'they get that glazed look'.

The journey syndrome

Patients sometimes report that during an amnesic period they wandered away from home, later 'waking up' in a strange place, an event which is described as a 'fugue state' in psychiatric terms. For example:

> When I came round I was sitting in a barber's chair having a shave. Hadn't a clue where I'd got to this time, terribly embarrassed, didn't like to ask. I had to go outside and look at the shop signs until I found the answer, and then to my amazement I discovered I was in this town 150 miles from home. To this day I don't know how I got there. That was the worst experience of this kind, but time after time I woke up in strange places or found myself sitting on a train going to the coast.

Blackouts and their significance to the patient

One patient may mention their blackouts only on direct questioning and appear not to be at all worried about such experiences, while another patient may be very worried about these experiences and see them as a leading reason for seeking help. Blackouts for that type of patient are often a matter of dread with, for instance, recurrent anguished fear that they may have hurt or killed someone while driving home; they do not remember getting their car into the garage the previous night, and they go out in the morning fearfully to check the paint work.

This discussion of alcohol-related hallucinatory states, withdrawal seizures, and alcoholic blackouts, when taken together with the account given in Chapter 8 of alcohol-related brain damage (p. 140), covers the spectrum of conditions making up the classical list of mental disorders which can result from drinking. We now go on to look at the many practical ways in which problem drinking and syndromes of general psychiatry can interlock. The issue of comorbidity is widely recognised and has diagnostic and treatment implications.

Depression

This is common amongst individuals with drinking problems and may be the decisive factor in seeking treatment. However, the nature of the relationship between the two is still poorly understood. What seems, on the surface, to be a simple association, is in fact extremely complex. Part of the problem is a lack of clarity in terminology. The word 'depression' has a variety of meanings and a distinction has to be made between the experience of being depressed and depressive illness.

The experience of being depressed

The ordinary range of experience
Feelings of sadness and unhappiness can occur as a normal reaction to

adversity. Individuals vary greatly in temperament and response to psychological stress.

Persistent mood disorder

Some individuals experience persistent but fluctuating depression of mood which is not severe enough to merit a diagnosis of depressive illness. This usually begins in early and adult life and lasts for several years, sometimes for the greater part of the individual's adult life, causing considerable distress.

Depression associated with other psychiatric syndromes

Depressive symptoms are often evident in other psychiatric syndromes, for instance, schizophrenia, obsessional illness, or dementia.

Depressive illness

Depression as a psychiatric illness must be distinguished from feelings of depression which have been described above. The essential feature of a depressive episode is a period of at least two weeks during which there is depressed mood and loss of interest or pleasure in nearly all activities. The mood disturbance is often worse at a particular time of day, usually the morning. Loss of energy, fatigue, and diminished activity are common, as is marked tiredness after slight effort. Other symptoms include reduced concentration and attention, reduced self-esteem and self-confidence, ideas of guilt and unworthiness, bleak and pessimistic views of the future, disturbed sleep and early morning wakening, diminished appetite and weight loss, and ideas of self harm and suicide (World Health Organisation, 1992). Sexual interest is lost. Somatic complaints, rather than feelings of sadness may be emphasised and the patient thinks that they are physically ill. There is often increased irritability, an impaired ability to think or make decisions, and poor concentration. The patient may be agitated or slowed down. Psychotic symptoms such as delusions, hallucinations or depressive stupor can occur in a severe depressive episode.

Depressive illness exists in degrees, and there are many variations in which symptoms cluster and present. No one description can do justice to the true variety of presentations. The picture will be influenced by culture and the patient's age and personality. There have been many attempts to typologise this disorder – endogenous versus reactive, 'neurotic depression' versus true depressive illness, and so on. The most up-to-date classification can be found in ICD-10 (World Health Organisation, 1992) and DSM-IV (American Psychiatric Association, 1994). A distinction is made between unipolar affective disorder and bipolar affective disorder, the latter characterised by repeated episodes in which the patient's mood and activity levels are significantly disturbed, sometimes in terms of elevation of mood (elation), increased energy and activity (mania or hypomania), and at other times by episodes of depression.

So much for the basic concepts. Deciding whether a person is just miserable or on the contrary ill with depression can, however, be extraordinarily difficult when they are drinking, and there is the ever-looming possibility of suicide as the price of a mistake. Depressive illness is often over-diagnosed in problem drinkers, with consequent needless prescribing of drugs or pointless administration of ECT (electroconvulsive therapy), while on other occasions the diagnosis may be overlooked. This is an instance where correct diagnosis will speak very importantly to correct management. If the patient is suffering from non-specific unhappiness rather than a depressive illness, that aspect of their situation may require skilled help, but not the same type of help as would be indicated for the undoubted illness. A picture of drinking problems together with a complaint of depression is illustrated by the following case abstract:

> A married woman, aged 35 years, had been drinking excessively for three or four years. Visited at home by a social worker, the house was in a terrible state and the children much neglected. The patient herself was dishevelled, obviously rather drunk, and declaring in a maudlin fashion that she was no good and that the family might as well be rid of her.

How should the social worker respond to this situation? Quite certainly an entirely inadequate course of action would be simply to arrange for a prescription of anti-depressant drugs, and let the patient mix these drugs with the drinking. Treatment cannot be intelligently and usefully started until it is known what there is to treat. The obverse approach, and one as misguided as the ill thought out use of drugs, is to assume that all problem drinkers can be a bit maudlin at times, and to dismiss this woman's complaint as 'just the alcoholic miseries' – later perhaps to hear that she killed herself.

How is the question as to whether such a patient as this is suffering from a depressive illness in practice to be decided? Assessment of the history is very important – a previous history of depressive illness, an event such as childbirth or bereavement which might have precipitated the illness, a sense of some more or less demarcated point where 'things changed' and the patient knew that whatever the previous ups and downs of mood, something was now being experienced which was fixed and of a different degree. A family history of depression can also be an important indicator. Integrated with the history has to be any details that can be observed of present behaviour and mental state. But it is also true that many problem drinkers will, when drinking, show emotional lability, will cry easily, will talk of the hopelessness of their lives. Immediately in all such instances to leap to a diagnosis of depressive illness would result in a great deal of over-diagnosis. The dilemma can be very real, and even experienced clinical judgement may be unable to resolve this diagnostic question while that patient is intoxicated. The patient's account may be inconstant, it may seem to be over-dramatised, the immediate life situation may be distressingly fraught and chaotic, but it is still unclear whether or not behind this drinking lies a depressive illness.

In such circumstances the sensible rule is to admit that diagnosis cannot be made in the presence of drinking, and to see the patient's stopping drinking as the prerequisite to a resolution of the diagnostic difficulty. After a week of sobriety it may be obvious that the misery has almost miraculously faded away – such often happens. Alternatively, it may become very apparent that a classical depressive illness now stands out as certainly as a rock left by the tide. Sometimes, however, even after a few weeks of in-patient observation and continued sobriety, it may be difficult to know whether what is emerging is a depressive illness, or a personality chronically prone to unhappy feelings and explosive declarations of misery. The ultimate resolution of the diagnostic problem might, for instance, be that the woman described above had always been a rather unhappy and insecure person, that in this setting and to relieve these feelings she had gradually started to drink and had been drinking heavily for five or more years, but that against all this background she had undoubtedly a year previously and following childbirth developed a true and severe depressive illness which had been untreated. The unravelling of such a story may require a lot of time, but arriving at a proper understanding is no optional extra if the depressed drinker is effectively to be helped.

Drinking problems and depression – their relationship

In many cases, depression is secondary to the drinking problem. However, it is worth noting that the ECA study already mentioned reported that depression preceded DSM-III alcohol dependence or abuse in 66% of women (Helzer & Pryzbeck, 1988). Depression is more common in women drinkers, and in problem drinkers who have a family history of alcohol problems, an earlier onset of heavy drinking, are divorced, and of lower social status (O'Sullivan et al., 1983). Other predisposing factors include a history of anxiety, other drug misuse, and previous suicide attempts (Roy et al., 1991). Depressive symptoms are common during alcohol withdrawal, particularly following a period of heavy consumption. Clinically significant levels of depression are found among in-patients with drinking problems during the early stages of admission (Brown & Schuckit, 1988; Davidson, 1995), but typically improve after two to three weeks of abstinence. However, depressive symptoms may persist, or even emerge during abstinence and the astute clinician should always be on the look out for this. Long-term follow-up studies also suggest that depressive experience declines with continued abstinence.

The frequent co-occurrence of depression and alcohol dependence has raised the question whether these two disorders might be genetically linked. Current research suggests that, although both disorders are to an extent familial, they are transmitted independently in families (Merikangas *et al.*, 1985; Maier *et al.*, 1994). However, a recent general population-based twin study by Kendler *et al.* (1993) proposes a partial genetic link between the two disorders in women.

Box 6.1. Drinking problems and depression

- Drinking problems are a major cause of depression

- Abstinence from alcohol alleviates depression

- A small proportion of problem drinkers will benefit from anti-depressants but the alcohol problem must be tackled first

---

Depression and drinking problems – the practical importance of the diagnostic question

The reasons for it being of practical importance to determine whether a patient with drinking problems is suffering from a depressive illness are several (Box 6.1). If such an illness exists, it of course deserves treatment as well as whatever psychological or social help may be necessary – the illness may respond to an antidepressant drug, or ECT may still sometimes be indicated if the patient does not respond to drug treatment. The second important reason for believing that every effort must be made not to miss this diagnosis is that if depression is untreated, any attempts to treat the drinking problem will be grossly handicapped (Mueller *et al.*, 1994). A depressed patient may find it extremely difficult to stop drinking, and untreated depression can on occasion run on for two or three years, or even longer, perhaps then with partial remissions and further relapses making the time course even more blurred and extended. A further important reason for taking the diagnostic question extremely seriously is the influence, which the answer must have, on assessment of suicidal risk (see below). Problem drinkers who are not suffering from depressive illness may kill themselves, but the risk is certainly enhanced if this illness is present.

For the long-term management, knowledge that there has been a depressive illness has a bearing which must be openly discussed with the patient. Once someone has suffered from one such illness they are at some risk of later again developing depression after a shorter or longer interval, and if they can recognise early signs and seek appropriate help, a lot of trouble may be averted. A depression is not an uncommon cause of relapse into drinking after a longish period of sobriety. Paradoxically, the development of an underlying depression may be the reason after many years for the drinker's eventually seeking help. It may be an expression of their depressive illness when they say they 'can't carry on any more', start to blame themselves rather than others for their drinking, or makes the suicidal gesture which gets them into hospital.

Summing the matter up, it can fairly be said that an awareness of the significance of depressive illness is so essential to working with problem drinkers that anyone who is going to take a close interest in drinking problems will also need to develop a good understanding of depression. If in relation to this question there exists a golden rule, it is that when a drinker is suffering from depressive illness, the therapeutic priority is to aid and persuade that patient first to stop drinking (offering perhaps immediate admission to achieve this purpose). Treating the depression is then the second phase of help and the immediate follow-through. It is generally messy and ineffective to try to treat a depressive illness when the patient is still drinking.

Suicide

The life-time risk of suicide in 'alcoholism' has previously been reported to be 11–15% (a detailed discussion is provided by Murphy & Wetzel, 1990). However, these rates have been derived from methodologically flawed studies and have overestimated the life-time risk which is now thought to be in the order of 3–4% for the United States and other Western countries. This is between 60 and 120 times that of the general population. Comorbidity plays an important role in the suicide of problem drinkers, with depression being the most substantial risk factor. Interpersonal losses and social isolation are also important.

Hypomania

Pathological elevation of mood is not so common a condition as pathological depression, and when it occurs does not carry a particularly high risk of being associated with drinking. Occasionally the hypomanic patient may, however, find that alcohol relieves unpleasant elements in their feelings: accompanying the basic elevation of mood, the hypomanic state may be characterised by considerable admixture of anxiety, irritability, and suspicousness. Mixed affective illnesses exist where the patient is both excited and tearful, with a confusing presentation that moves within minutes from elation to depression. A patient with repeated hypomanic bouts may give the appearance of 'bout drinking'. In an attack they are likely to lose their social judgement, and to spend large sums of money and live things up, and this general disinhibition, as well as the more specific seeking of relief from unpleasant feelings, may contribute to the drinking. The treatment is primarily that of the underlying illness.

A more difficult diagnostic problem arises when there is a suspicion that the patient's mood may phasically become slightly elevated but with the condition not approaching a hypomanic illness in severity. This slight elevation and disinhibition may appear to be sufficient to spark off some weeks of drinking, and on occasion this is a plausible explanation of 'periodic drinking', although there are many other explanations for such a drinking pattern (see p. 49). What is being discussed here is a mood disturbance, which would usually be seen as a character trait (cyclothymic personality) rather than as an illness, but there is no absolute demarcation between this sort of state and hypomania. In turn, hypomania merges with mania, with the latter term indicating a state of appalling over-excitement, or the traditional picture of 'raving madness'. A patient with fully developed mania is far too disordered to be other than rapidly admitted to hospital, and drinking as a complication of this illness is not a question which arises other than in the very short-term.

Anxiety

Clinical studies consistently report an association between alcohol problems and anxiety disorders (Mullaney & Trippett 1979; Stockwell & Bolderston, 1987; Kushner et al., 1990; Allan, 1995). Estimates vary, but among a clinical population up to about one-third of problem drinkers may have significant anxiety experience. This kind of comorbidity has also been reported in community samples. Alcohol problems can sometimes develop as a result of agoraphobia and social phobia, and may reflect attempts at self-medication (Mullaney & Trippett, 1979; Stockwell *et al.*, 1984). The association with panic disorder is less clearcut (Ross *et al.*, 1988).

Paradoxically, alcohol appears to increase or exacerbate clinical anxiety in alcohol-dependent individuals who have prolonged histories of heavy drinking. This seems to be particularly prominent after a bout of heavy drinking and during alcohol withdrawal (Schuckit *et al.*, 1990; Brown *et al.*, 1991). Alcohol withdrawal symptoms can mimic anxiety and panic disorder, and it is possible that a common neurochemical process underlies both (George *et al.*, 1990). As noted earlier (p. 38), individuals with alcohol dependence and anxiety disorder have been found to experience more severe alcohol withdrawal symptoms than a non-anxious control group, even though the two groups had similar drinking histories (Johnston, 1991).

Here is a case example that illustrates one kind of possible clinical relationship between alcohol and anxiety:

> A woman, aged 50 years, was admitted to hospital with a long history of drinking. Her immediate presentation was that of a working woman who earned her living by getting up early and going out to do office cleaning. She would have a drink at 6.00 a.m. before leaving the house, and then put a couple of bottles of wine into her bag. What was found in her old notes was that many years previously her first presentation to the hospital was as someone with a phobic state who found great difficulty in leaving her house. Careful questioning revealed that phobic anxiety symptoms still very much persisted, although alcohol dependence had now been contracted as a problem in its own right.

The practical clinical approach when a problem drinker appears to be suffering from a phobic anxiety state is usually to arrange hospital admission, both for purposes of diagnosis and of treatment. It is difficult to assess the true severity or fixedness of the phobic symptoms until the patient has been completely off alcohol for some weeks, and sometimes a longer period of observation is required. What may then happen is that seemingly rather severe phobic symptoms fade away, and in the event there is no phobic anxiety to be treated. The symptoms were part of general 'bad nerves' related to alcohol dependence.

If, however, phobic symptoms persist in severe degree, an effort then has to be made to treat them, with treatment started while the patient is in hospital. Treatment of the underlying condition requires sobriety, and an attempt to treat these symptoms when the patient is still drinking is a hopeless undertaking. Treatment will today usually involve the planned application of behaviour therapy, and the response is often excellent provided that the patient can co-operate, that there is not a too high background level of anxiety, and that the phobic situations are not too universal. It would, however, be optimistic to suppose that behaviour therapy is a panacea and those favourable conditions are not always fulfilled. The use of minor tranquillisers or hypnotics with such patients has to be approached with extreme caution. To treat the phobic alcohol dependent patient while they are still drinking, by giving them a minor tranquilliser, is likely to be both dangerous and ineffective. Drugs and alcohol will be haphazardly mixed, with risk of super-added drug dependence. Indeed, by the time the severely phobic problem drinker presents for treatment, it is not uncommon to find that they have a medically-induced drug problem, as well as their alcohol dependence.

Damage to the brain tissue

The question often arises as to whether the patient with a drinking problem is suffering from brain damage. If the damage is gross there will be no diagnostic difficulty, but the diagnosis (and significance) of lesser degrees of damage commonly set problems.

The most familiar picture is that of an associated alcoholic 'dementia', and this condition is discussed more fully on p. 140 in relation to the physical damages that can result from drinking. Much the same sort of picture is to be seen when the patient is developing a dementia for any other reason (pre-senile dementia, for instance, or senile or multi-infarct dementia). The patient with alcoholic dementia will typically give a history of many years heavy drinking with ultimate development of brain damage. With non-alcoholic dementia the sequence of events is the other way round – the patient develops dementia and, as a result of the ensuing disinhibition and personality deterioration, becomes involved in drinking.

The fact that brain damage can be cause as well as consequence of drinking needs to be written into any diagnostic checklist. Besides brain damage due to degenerative processes such as those already mentioned, the significance of a history of brain injury should be specially borne in mind. Instances occur where personality change as a sequel to head injury is disproportionate to any fall-off in intellectual functioning, and this type of personality change may for example result in drinking problems as a late sequel of a road accident. The following brief case extracts show some of the many possible organic relationships that should be on such a checklist:

> A young man, aged 23 years, of previously stable personality, sustained a severe head injury in a car crash, and was unconscious for several days. He appeared to make a good recovery and there was no paralysis.

However, his concentration seemed rather impaired, and his wife complained about his irritability, and although he went back to clerical work his performance had fallen off. Five years later he was drinking very heavily.

A woman civil servant, aged 50 years, of previously unblemished record, suffered a subarachnoid haemorrhage (a bleed into the space around the brain). The leaking blood vessel was operated on and she 'recovered completely' but she had in fact sustained a degree of brain damage. Work habits which had for a life time been almost over-meticulous now deteriorated, and she was found to be drinking secretly in the office.

A boy, aged 16 years, developed a severe viral brain infection (encephalitis) and was for a time desperately ill. Within a few years he was involved in criminal behaviour and was drinking heavily. He came from a stable home, and his two brothers and his sister grew up to lead settled and happy lives.

A man, aged 40 years, suffered from crippling obsessional symptoms, and a leucotomy was performed. His obsessional symptoms were relieved, but although up to the time of his operation he had been a very moderate drinker, he now rapidly developed alcohol dependence.

A woman of 60 years of age presented with alcohol dependence, seemingly of recent onset. She was found to have a brain tumour.

Some of these case histories illustrate only rather rare associations and the precise part that brain damage played in the aetiology of the drinking is in some instances difficult to establish. The general picture which is being built up by listing these diverse cases, however, is valid and important. Some associations between brain damage and alcohol dependence are relatively common (for example, post-traumatic personality deterioration), while others, such as tumour, are rare, but the general message that no diagnostic assessment is complete without thinking about the possible significance of brain involvement has to be stressed. Alcohol dependence can also supervene as a complication of learning disability (mental subnormality) of any origin.

Whatever the underlying brain syndrome associated with alcohol dependence, the clinical features can be grouped under a number of headings. There are, of course, firstly the primary symptoms of the brain damage itself. Features of the drinking problem will also stand in their own right, but it is the interaction of the underlying brain damage and the drinking that gives these cases their colouring. Personal and social deterioration may seem to be disproportionate to the drinking or suddenly to have accelerated. Drunken behaviour where there is underlying brain damage often appears to be particularly heedless of consequences or is anti-social. There are, for example, increasing episodes of violence or the patient sets their lodgings on fire. There is also an increased sensitivity to alcohol; the patient gets drunk on less drink, and with relatively little alcohol becomes disinhibited or begins to fall about.

Given proper alertness to the possibility of such underlying problems, what are then the practical implications? If brain involvement is in any way suspected, this usually constitutes an indication for hospital admission so that appropriate neurological and psychological investigations can be carried out with a sober patient. The sad fact is that most of the possibly relevant brain conditions are going to prove more diagnosable than treatable, but even so an accurate diagnostic formulation is the necessary basis for working out what is best to be done. If, for instance, an individual with alcohol dependence is severely brain damaged, the only kind and safe policy may be to propose long-term hospital care, or care in a supportive residential community. If there is milder damage, the patient will be able to keep going outside an institution, but brain damage can adversely affect the course of alcohol problems, and relapse and further troubles are probably to be expected. The continuing treatment policy must be set up so as to be able to meet these sorts of eventuality, and be designed to support the family in what may well be a difficult situation. The emphasis may sometimes have to be on rather directive intervention such as ensuring that money is properly handled or that the local publicans will not serve drinks. But even here there is no cause for absolute pessimism for sometimes a patient with brain damage will be able to stop drinking, the progression of alcoholic dementia will be arrested and the patient's behaviour will improve. Treatment implications are discussed further on pp. 158, 258).

Pathological jealousy

Jealousy is a normal human emotion, and it is not easy to set a cutting point between the normal and the pathological. At one end of the spectrum there are, however, a group of people whose lives are plagued and corrupted by their jealous feelings, and who make life miserable for the objects of their jealousy. For reasons which will be discussed below, this condition is likely to be met quite frequently in the treatment of drinking problems, and one should know how to recognise its features.

A 34-year-old garage owner said that he had been painfully jealous ever since his adolescence. His jealousy was now threatening to break up his marriage. He would repeatedly charge his wife with infidelity, taunting her and threatening her, as well as accusing her. His mental state when he made these charges was one of extreme distress – an overwhelming sense of being betrayed, of not being loved, of having a secret kept from him. There would then be explosive rows, and sometimes violence resulted. Later he would be desperately sorry, and transiently realise the falseness and cruelty of his accusations. But very shortly worrying doubts would again return. He would come home secretly and keep watch on the house, and sometimes he would follow his wife down the road. He would cross-question his children as to whether any other man had been into the house. He went through the ashtrays to see whether an unfamiliar brand of stub-end was to be found in the litter. His wife's handbag was regularly searched, and he checked on her underclothes for seminal stains. Recently he had thought of hiring a detective. He remained sexually potent, and wanted to keep his wife pregnant so as to make her uninteresting to other men. His drinking appeared to be inextricably mixed with the jealousy story, but his jealousy only came to light when his wife was interviewed.

The essential characteristics of this syndrome suggest that it may some-times parallel an obsessional disorder, although this is not a view of the condition which finds approval in the standard psychiatric texts. The constant rumination, the fact that there is frequent (if only short-lived and partial) realisation of the falseness of the belief, the unpleasantness of the associated feelings, the compulsive need to check, and the tran-sient relief from the active checking, are features very reminiscent of obsession. But it seems certain that pathological jealousy cannot be related to any one all-embracing psychiatric diagnosis, and underlying the common presenting features may be any one of several psychiatric disorders, including paranoid schizophrenia.

The usual view is that alcohol dependence is a cause of jealousy rather than jealousy a cause of alcohol dependence. The psychodynamic explanations offered for this chain of events are complex, but can be sketched out in very abbreviated terms as the individual doubting his own masculinity and therefore drinking, drinking leading to impo-tence, and the reaction to impotence being jealousy. Impotence and pathological jealousy are thus alleged frequently to coexist. Pathological jealousy is also sometimes vaguely subsumed (if not explained) under the general heading of 'alcoholic paranoia'. There is much still to be found out about this condition, but it may be questioned whether the conventional view that alcohol dependence causes pathological jealousy is too simple. The story which the patient gives more often suggests that jealousy has been in some degree a life-long feature, perhaps even with manifestations in childhood, and very early family dynamics can be rather obviously related to the genesis of the problem. The distress which is associated with the experience of jeal-ousy may be appalling, and the patient in adulthood discovers that this distress is at least temporarily relieved by drinking. This may therefore sometimes provide just another illustration of the fact that anyone for whom drink is available, and who suffers from any kind of chronic psychological distress, may be led into excessive drinking as a result of self-medication. The general level of heightened anxiety so often associated with alcohol dependence may then make the jealousy more intractable, and the situation becomes circular.

However, by the time the patient comes for help both jealousy and drinking have probably been going on for many years, and it can be extremely difficult to untangle the true, historical relationship of the two elements. In the here-and-now they are usually best seen as mutually interacting, as exacerbating each other, rather than as either taking precedence. The practical approach is to try somehow to persuade the patient to stop drinking, and then assess the severity of the jealousy. What happened to the garage owner is fairly typical, and shows that pessimism is by no means always well founded if drinking can be got out of the way.

> He 'realised that something had to be done about it', and as an act of faith he stopped drinking. He immediately needed to talk about his jealousy, which was at first very painful for him. But the terrible scenes of destructive accusation forthwith ceased. He was able to realise that drinking had been making matters worse, and been leading to drunken acting-out of his anxieties. He and his wife were, for the first time, able safely to discuss his jealousy, both admitting its irrationality, but agreeing that his feelings were a serious and painful problem for both of them. Over the next few months he then reported that 'my nerves are much better, not all jumpy the way I used to be when I was drinking'. As his mood lifted, the intensity of his jealously considerably faded, and to his surprise he and his wife settled on a rather joking way of dealing with the problem, and one which helped them both. 'Come on, love, I say to him, none of that old nonsense, you're my one and only and you know it'. Seen a year later he still on occasion had a surge of jealous feelings (he would not take his wife to a party), but these feelings were less severe than they had been for many years and his wife could live with the situation.

The extracts from this case history illustrate an approach that focused initially on the drinking, in the hope that the jealousy would then become more manageable. This is almost inevitably the best approach, for unless one is dealing with an underlying psychotic illness (which is seldom the case), there is no specific treatment available for the jealousy. Drugs have no part to play, and behavioural treatments are largely untried. Talking the matter through in sympathetic and common sense fashion, bringing husband and wife together to work on the problem, encouraging a sense of optimism, may, if the patient stays off alcohol, often bring good results. Sometimes, however, the condition is intractable. The patient simply cannot stop drinking, and the result is break-up of the marriage (with the husband still haunting the doorstep), or even a tragic drunken murder.

The reasons for giving this space to what has often been termed a rare syndrome, are several. It may be doubted whether the condition is in fact all that rare; with an open eye and alert questioning, many more cases will come to light. Although the basic description of the syndrome is to be found in the textbooks, the clinical handling of this problem seldom receives due attention. It is a condition easily missed, but very real once recognised, and it needs to be given a definite place on the checklists of any one working with alcohol problems.

Personality disorder

The relationship between alcohol problems and personality factors is complex and still poorly understood. It is impossible to work with drinking problems without becoming aware of the relevance of person-ality to an understanding of the genesis of drinking and the treatment of excessive drinking and dependence. Personality has multiple dimen-sions and is influenced by genetic, environmental, and cultural factors. Cross-sectional studies of male 'alcoholics' in treatment have suggested that they are 'anti-social, rebellious and impulsive individuals who have difficulty delaying gratification' (Bates, 1993). However, these studies are flawed, because such characteristics may either predate or follow the development of excessive alcohol use, and are not unique to it.

More recent behavioural genetic research suggests that certain per-sonality subtypes and temperaments may increase the risk for develop-ing alcohol problems in adulthood. Tarter (1991) proposed that there are heritable dimensions of temperament which render individuals vulner-able to the development of alcohol problems in adulthood. Zuckerman (1991) postulated a sensation-seeking trait based on inherited, biolog-ical traits of reactivity to stimulation. Cloninger (1987) hypothesised a typological classification. His theory implies inheritance of a predis-posing personality type manifesting high levels of impulsivity and novelty seeking and low harm avoidance. This personality type in turn predisposes to type II 'alcoholism' which occurs exclusively in men, has an early age of onset (under 25 years) and is associated with childhood antisocial behaviour and criminality in the father. Although this typology has been validated empirically in some studies (Babor *et al.*, 1992), and the traits of impulsivity and novelty seeking are closely related to Zuckerman's sensation-seeking traits, this concept remains controversial. The question of typologies has been discussed earlier (p. 46).

While the association between antisocial personality disorder and alcohol problems has gained acceptance in the United States, it has not been taken up with as much enthusiasm in UK, largely perhaps because it is seen as potentially unhelpful in working with individuals troubled by their drinking. Studies suggest poor outcomes for individuals with antisocial personality and alcohol problems, but do not take into account the heterogeneity within this population. The consequence of a rigid categorical approach may be therapeutic nihilism.

So far as this chapter is concerned there is common ground between the two seemingly divergent schools of thought in that both parties would agree that patients with drinking problems are sometimes, and to various degrees, angry, unhappy, non-conformist, rule-breaking, aggressive, and handicapped in their ability to deal with social demands and expectations. It would also be common ground that when a patient is first met it can be difficult to determine how much such seeming disturbances are cause and how much are the consequence of excessive drinking. Furthermore it would be widely agreed that personality disturbance can make treatment difficult and has to be dealt with therapeutically as a significant issue.

Eating disorders

The most common disorders of body weight which result from excessive drinking are obesity, due to the high calorie content of the alcohol which is being consumed, and paradoxically the loss of weight and general malnutrition that are consequent on the dietary neglect which frequently accompanies heavy drinking.

It is those two common types of disorder to which the diagnostician is likely to be very properly alert. There is, however, increasing evidence that certain eating disorders, that were until recently considered to be only rare accompaniments of alcohol problems, are not, in fact, uncommon. These conditions are anorexia nervosa and bulimia nervosa.

Eckert et al. (1979) reported a 6.7% life-time prevalence of 'alcohol problems' among patients with anorexia nervosa. However, a controlled 10-year follow-up study of women with anorexia nervosa found no significant relationship with drinking problems (Halmi et al., 1991). Higher rates of 'alcoholism' were found in the first degree relatives of patients with anorexia nervosa, compared with relatives of the controls. Prevalence rates of alcohol misuse in bulimic subjects vary from 9 to 49% (Goldbloom, 1993).

Fewer studies have explored the prevalence of eating disorders in patients referred for treatment of drinking problems (Lacey & Moureli 1986; Peveler & Fairburn 1990). Depending on sampling and the criteria employed, it seems possible that up to about 30% of women with drinking problems may at some time experience a significant eating disorder. The problem of eating disorders in Japan is lower than that reported in Western countries, and yet 11% of an in-patient sample of women 'alcoholics' fulfilled DSM-III-R criteria for eating disorders, especially bulimia nervosa (Higuchi et al., 1993). Clinical research suggests that eating disorders complicated by drinking problems respond as well to treatment as those in which alcohol is not a problem (Goldbloom, 1993). However, individuals with eating and drinking problems may also have a predisposition towards other 'impulse' disorders such as self-mutilation, parasuicide, misuse of illicit or prescribed drugs, and shoplifting (Lacey, 1993).

Schizophrenia

The relationship between schizophrenia and alcohol problems is an important one. As mentioned earlier the ECA study reported a 3.8% prevalence of schizophrenia in individuals with any DSM-III alcohol disorder (Regier et al., 1990). High rates of alcohol problems have been reported in individuals with schizophrenia (22.1%, Duke et al., 1994) and psychosis (31.6%, Menezes et al., 1996). The term 'dual diagnosis' has been used to describe patients with co-existent severe mental illness and substance misuse disorders. The concept of 'dual diagnosis' is established in the USA but is less widely employed in the UK. The problem appears to be increasing (Cuffel, 1992) probably because most psychiatric patients now live in the community and have easy access to alcohol and drugs (Smith & Hucker, 1994). It has been postulated that schizophrenics use alcohol to cope with stress associated with their illness. Schizophrenics with an alcohol problem may be more prone to violence. Alcohol use may be an added risk factor for the development of tardive dyskinesia in some schizophrenics (Duke et al., 1994).

Mental illness: the general implications

The account that has been given in this chapter of the many types of mental illness that can be associated with excessive drinking, and of the nature of those possible relationships, must not be interpreted as meaning that only the psychiatrist can treat the problem drinker. The fact that psychiatric treatment or admission to a psychiatric hospital may be indicated for some of these patients does not mean that the treatment of alcohol problems is a psychiatric preserve. However, what must be evident is that psychiatry may quite often have a part to play, and that a working liaison with psychiatric services should be available to anyone helping with drinking problems. An awareness of this psychiatric dimension must, moreover, be important, whatever the therapist's professional discipline.

References

Allan, C. A. (1995). Alcohol problems and anxiety disorders – a critical review. *Alcohol and Alcoholism* 30, 145–51.

American Psychiatric Association (1994). *Diagnostic and Statistical Manual of Mental Disorders*, 4th edn. Washington D.C.: American Psychiatric Association.

Babor, T. F., Hofmann, M., Del Boca, F. K., Hesselbrock, V., Meyer, R. E., Dolinsky, S. & Rounsaville, B. (1992). Types of alcoholics, I: Evidence for an empirically derived typology based on indicators of vulnerability and severity. *Archives of General Psychiatry* 49, 599–608.

Bates, M. E. (1993). Social and cultural perspectives: psychology. In *Recent Developments in Alcoholism*, ed. Galanter, M., vol. 11, *Ten Years of Progress*, pp. 45–72. New York: Plenum Press.

Brennan, F. N. & Lyttle, J. A. (1987). Alcohol and seizures: a review. *Journal of the Royal Society of Medicine* 80, 571–3.

Brown, S. A. & Schuckit, M. A. (1988). Changes in depression amongst abstinent alcoholics. *Journal of Studies on Alcohol* 49, 412–17.

Brown, S. A., Irwin, M. & Schukit, M. A. (1991). Changes in anxiety among abstinent male alcoholics. *Journal of Studies on Alcohol* 52, 55–61.

Chick, J. (1989). Delirium tremens. *British Medical Journal* 298, 3–4.

Cloninger, C. R. (1987). Neurogenetic adaptive mechanisms in alcoholism. *Science* 236, 410–16.

Coid, J. (1979). 'Mania a potu': a critical review of pathological intoxication. *Psychological Medicine* 9, 709–19.

Cuffel, B. (1992). Prevalence estimates of substance abuse in schizophrenia and their correlates. *Journal of Nervous and Mental Disease* 180, 589–92.

Cushman, P. (1987). Delirium tremens – update on an old disorder. *Postgraduate Medicine* 82, 117–22.

Davidson, K. M. (1995). Diagnosis of depression in alcohol dependence: changes in prevalence with drinking status. *British Journal of Psychiatry* 166, 199–204.

Duke, P., Pantelis, C. & Barnes, T. R. E. (1994). South Westminster Schizophrenia Survey. Alcohol use and its relationship to symptoms, tardive dyskinesia and illness onset. *British Journal of Psychiatry* 164, 630–6.

Earnest, M. P., Feldman, H., Marx, J. A., *et al.* (1988). Intracranial lesions shown by CT scans in 259 cases of first alcohol-related seizures. *Neurology* **38**, 1561–5.

Eckert, E. D., Goldberg, S. C., Halmi, K. A., Casper, R. C. & Davis, J. M. (1979). Alcoholism in anorexia nervosa. In *Psychiatric Factors in Drug Abuse*, ed. Pickens, R. W., Heston, L. L. New York: Grieve and Stratton.

George, G. T., Nutt, D. J. & Dwyer, B. A. (1990). Alcoholism and panic disorders: is the comorbidity more than coincidence? *Acta Psychiatrica Scandinavica* **81**, 97–107.

Glass, I. B. (1989a). Alcoholic hallucinosis: a psychiatric enigma – I. The development of an idea. *British Journal of Addiction* **84**, 29–41.

Glass, I. B. (1989b). Alcoholic hallucinosis: a psychiatric enigma – 2. Follow-up studies. *British Journal of Addiction* **84**, 151–64.

Goldbloom, D. S. (1993). Alcohol misuse and eating disorders: aspects of an association. *Alcohol and Alcoholism* **28**, 375–81.

Goodwin, D. W., Crane, B. J. & Guze, S. B. (1969a). Phenomenological aspects of the alcoholic 'blackout'. *British Journal of Psychiatry* **115**, 1033–8.

Goodwin, D. W., Crane, B. J. & Guze, S. B. (1969b). Alcoholic 'blackouts': a review and clinical study of 100 alcoholics. *American Journal of Psychiatry* **126**, 191–8.

Halmi, K. A., Eckert, E., Marchi, P., Sampugnaro, V., Apple, R. & Cohen, J. (1991). Comorbidity of psychiatric diagnosis in anorexia nervosa. *Archives of General Psychiatry* **48**, 712–18.

Helzer, J. E. & Pryzbeck, T. R. (1988). The co-occurrence of alcoholism with other psychiatric disorders in the general population and its impact on treatment. *Journal of Studies on Alcohol* 49, 219–24.

Hemmingsen, R. & Kramp, P. (1988). Delirium tremens and related clinical states. *Acta Psychiatrica Scandinavica Supplement* **345**, 94–107.

Higuchi, S., Suzuki, K., Yamada, K., Parrish & K., Kono, H. (1993). Alcoholics with eating disorders: prevalence and clinical course. A study from Japan. *British Journal of Psychiatry* **162**, 403–6.

Johnston, A. L., Thevos, A. K., Randall, C. L. & Anton, R. F. (1991). Increased severity of alcohol withdrawal in in-patient alcoholics with a co-existing anxiety diagnosis. *British Journal of Addiction* **86**, 719–25.

Kendler, K. S., Heath, A. C., Neale, M. C., Kessler, R. C. & Eaves, L. J. (1993). Alcoholism and major depression in women: a twin study of the causes of comorbidity. *Archives of General Psychiatry* **50**, 690–8.

Kopelman, M. D. (1991). Alcoholic brain damage. In *The International Handbook of Addictive Behaviour*, ed. Glass, I. B., pp 141–51. London: Routledge.

Kushner, M. G., Sherk & Beitman, B. (1990). The relation between alcohol problems and anxiety disorders. *American Journal of Psychiatry* **147**, 685–95.

Lacey, J. H. (1993). Self-damaging and addictive behaviour in bulimia nervosa. *British Journal of Psychiatry* **163**, 190–4.

Lacey, J. H. & Moureli, E. (1986). Bulimic alcoholics: some features of a clinical sub-group. *British Journal of Addiction* **81**, 389–93.

Lishman, W. A. (1987). *Organic Psychiatry*, 2nd edn. Oxford: Blackwell Scientific Publications.

Maier, W., Lichtermann, D. & Minges, J. (1994). The relationship between alcoholism and unipolar depression – a controlled family study. *Journal of Psychiatric Research* **3**, 303–17.

Maletzky, B. M. (1976). The diagnosis of pathological intoxication. *Journal of Studies on Alcohol* **37**, 1215–28.

Menezes, P., Johnson, S., Thornicroft, G., Marshall, J., Prosser, D., Bebbington, P. & Kuipers, E. (1996). Drug and alcohol problems among individuals with severe mental illness in South London. *British Journal of Psychiatry* **168**, 612–19.

Merikangas, K. R., Leckman, J. F., Prusoff, B. A., Pauls, D. L. & Weissman, M. M. (1985). Familial transmission of depression and alcoholism. *Archives of General Psychiatry* **42**, 367–71.

Mueller, T. I., Lavori, P. W., Keller, M. B., Swartz, A., Warshaw, M., Hasin, D., Coryell, W., Endicott, J., Rice, J. & Akiskal, H. (1994). Prognostic effect of the variable course of alcoholism on the 10-year course of depression. *American Journal of Psychiatry* **151**, 701–6.

Mullaney, J. A. & Trippett, C. J. (1979). Alcohol dependence and phobias: a clinical description and relevance. *British Journal of Psychiatry* **135**, 565–73.

Murphy, G. G. & Wetzel, R. D. (1990). The lifetime risk of suicide in alcoholism. *Archives of General Psychiatry* **47**, 383–92.

Naranjo, C. A. & Sellers, E. M. (1986). Clinical assessment and pharmacotherapy of the alcohol withdrawal syndrome. In *Recent Developments in Alcoholism*, ed. M. Galanter, pp. 265–81. vol. 4. New York: Plenum Press.

O'Sullivan, K., Whillans, P., Daly, M., Carroll, B., Clare, A. & Cooney, J. (1983). A comparison of alcoholics with and without co-existing affective disorder. *British Journal of Psychiatry* **143**, 133–8.

Peveler, R. & Fairburn, C. (1990). Eating disorders in women who abuse alcohol. *British Journal of Addiction* **85**, 1633–8.

Regier, D. A., Farmer, M. E., Rae, D. S., Locke, B. Z., Keith, S. J., Judd, L. L. & Goodwin, F. K. (1990). Comorbidity of mental disorders with alcohol and other drug abuse. *JAMA* **264**, 2511–18.

Ross, H. E., Glaser, F. B. & Germanson, T. (1988). The prevalence of psychiatric disorders in patients with alcohol and other drug related problems. *Archives of General Psychiatry* **45**, 1023–31.

Roy, A., DeJong, J., Lamparski, D., George, T. & Linnoila, M. (1991). Depression among alcoholics. *Archives of General Psychiatry* **48**, 428–32.

Schuckit, M. A., Irwin, M. & Brown, S. A. (1990). The history of anxiety symptoms among 171 primary alcoholics. *Journal of Studies on Alcohol* **51**, 34–41.

Schuckit, M. A., Smith, T. L., Anthenelli, R. M. & Irwin, M. (1993). The clinical course of alcoholism in 636 male inpatients. *American Journal of Psychiatry* **150**, 786–792.

Smith, J. & Hucker, S. (1994). Schizophrenia and substance abuse. *British Journal of Psychiatry* **165**, 13–21.

Soyka, M. (1995). Pathophysiological mechanisms possibly involved in the development of alcohol hallucinosis. *Addiction* **90**, 289–94.

Stockwell, T. & Bolderston, H. (1987). Alcohol and phobias. *British Journal of Addiction* **82**, 971–9.

Stockwell, T., Smail, P., Hodgson, R. *et al.* (1984). Alcohol dependence and phobic anxiety states. II: a retrospective study. *British Journal of Psychiatry* **144**, 58–63.

Tarter, R. E. (1991). Developmental behaviour – genetic perspective of alcoholism etiology. In *Recent Developments in Alcoholism*, ed. Galanter, M. vol. 9, pp. 69–85. New York: Plenum Press.

Tsuang, J. W., Irwin, M. R., Smith, T. L. & Schuckit, M. A. (1994). Characteristics of men with alcoholic hallucinosis. *Addiction* **89**, 73–8.

World Health Organisation (1992). *The ICD-10 Classification of Mental and Behavioural Disorders*. Geneva: World Health Organisation.

Zuckerman, M. (1991). Sensation seeking: the balance between risk and reward. In *Self-Regulatory Behaviour and Risk Taking: Causes and Consequences*, ed. Lipsitt, L. P., Muttnick, L. L., pp 143–52. Norwood: Ablex.

7

Drug problems and alcohol problems

'Chemical dependence'

In many countries the contemporary pattern of substance misuse, particularly in individuals under the age of 40, is of multiple substances. Drug and alcohol problems may occur either concurrently or as problems that develop in sequence. The patterns of relationship, which can exist between the use of different types of mind-acting chemical, are many and the following case-extract illustrates one variation on this theme.

The patient was a successful and wealthy entrepreneur aged 35. His working day was lived at a great pitch of tension and every evening he would go out to restaurants and night clubs and get through a lot of alcohol. He would on average drink a couple of bottles of wine and up to a dozen double vodkas before becoming, in his terms, 'pretty incoherent'. He was beginning to feel 'dreadful, sick, sweaty' on most mornings and would often be unable to remember how he had reached his bed. Cocaine then began to be available in his social circle and before long he discovered that this drug appeared to provide an antidote to some of the unwanted effects of alcohol. For instance, if he snorted (sniffed) cocaine a few times during the evening 'it lifted me up, I could go on drinking, it stopped me passing-out with the alcohol'. He also found that a snort or two of cocaine helped to alleviate the unpleasant early-morning symptoms caused by the previous night's drinking. Within a few months he progressed from snorting to free-basing (inhaling) cocaine, and his cocaine use rapidly and disastrously went out of control. His problem came to attention when a club was raided and he was arrested for possession of cocaine. Seen by a doctor at the request of the defence solicitor this man said, 'OK, I'm addicted to cocaine but let's not keep on about the alcohol.

What this patient's history illustrates is that another type of chemical often lies behind the immediately presenting drug. It would be unprofitable in such circumstances to debate whether alcohol or cocaine was the 'real' problem. This man's problem was his tendency to misuse chemicals. Both the alcohol and cocaine aspects of his history have to be taken seriously but what the patient himself and those who are seeking to help him need to realise is that dependence can often resemble the many headed Hydra of mythology: one head can be lopped off and another grows. Unless with such a patient there is a focus on the central issue of their tendency to develop dependence on chemicals, the story will all too probably progress in terms of a further switching or mixing of different substances – in terms perhaps of tranquillisers or sleeping tablets then being added to alcohol. Nicotine is an almost inevitable part of the mix.

The most common reason for concurrent drug use is to enhance effects (Clayton, 1986). For instance, alcohol can enhance the effects of stimulants such as cocaine and amphetamines, and also the effects of benzodiazepines and volatile solvents. Alcohol is also commonly used to counteract the effects of other drugs. It reduces jittery feelings associated with stimulant use and may help in the withdrawal phase. A heroin user may substitute with alcohol, cannabis or benzodiazepines, either alone or in combination to tide them over until heroin is again available. A further reason for poly-drug use is peer influence. The combined use of alcohol, cannabis, and nicotine is commonplace.

This chapter describes some of the more commonly encountered connections between alcohol and other drug problems. The characteristics of benzodiazepine dependence is described in some detail and guidelines for the treatment of this condition are given. Lastly the general implications both for prevention and for clinical practice which stem from the realisation that alcohol and other drug problems potentially constitute one continuous domain rather than two distinct problem areas are fully discussed. Box 7.1 summarises some of the main points which this chapter will emphasise.

Poly-drug problems

Poly-drug use has become increasingly prevalent over recent decades and shows no sign of abating. It occurs in the general population and is not confined to individuals heavily involved in the 'drug scene' or in contact with treatment services. Nevertheless, the number of poly-drug users in contact with treatment services is increasing and is a cause of serious worry.

Box 7.1. Drug problems and alcohol problems: key issues

- Poly-drug use is the contemporary pattern of substance misuse
- Alcohol is almost always implicated in poly-drug use
- Poly-drug use is associated with significant physical and psychosocial morbidity
- Therapists and treatment services need the skills to meet mixed problems

Young people who experiment with drugs appear to be particularly at risk. Often there is a primary drug of choice, but a variety of other drugs can also be used, depending on availability, price, the social situation, peer group usage, and fashion (Clayton, 1986). Heroin may, for a time, be the prime focus, or alternatively some other drug such as cocaine. Drug fashions switch and combine with great rapidity and although one particular drug may, for a few years, constitute the major cause for concern, the drug problem can never be defined satisfactorily in terms of one substance. Alcohol is almost always implicated in the shifting picture of poly-drug use, together with various combinations of cannabis, opioids, cocaine, amphetamines, hallucinogens and benzodiazepines, and more recently MDMA (ecstasy). Poly-drug use is associated with significant medical and psychosocial complications. The drug-using career of the young person who later turns to injecting heroin or to other forms of illicit addiction, is often marked at an early stage by the heavy use of 'gateway' drugs, namely tobacco, cannabis, and alcohol. Multiple drug use can develop in stages, with individuals moving from licit to illicit drugs, and from less to more serious drugs. Drug users also tend to carry forward the substances used at earlier stages in their career, often at levels of increasing severity.

History taking may need to incorporate a set of questions for each drug class, in order to define the sequencing and pattern of drug use, and the combinations of drugs used (alcohol and cannabis; alcohol and cigarettes; alcohol and cocaine, and so on).

Specific combinations

Alcohol and cocaine

The combination of alcohol and cocaine is an increasingly familiar pattern of poly-drug use and in the USA, alcohol is more likely to be used in conjunction with cocaine than with any other type of drug (Helzer & Pryzbeck, 1988). Alcohol is typically used during a cocaine binge in order to prolong the euphoriant effects of cocaine and, as already mentioned, to diminish unpleasant experiences associated with cocaine use, such as agitation and paranoia, and to ameliorate the dysphoria associated with acute abstinence from cocaine (the 'crash'). The mechanism underlying these effects is not known, but cocaethylene, a pharmacologically active metabolite formed after ingestion of both cocaine and alcohol, has been implicated (McCance *et al.*, 1995).

For many people, treatment of the cocaine problem may lead to an improvement in the alcohol problem (Kosten, 1989). However, the presence of alcohol problems and dependence in treated cocaine users is associated with poor outcome (Walsh *et al.*, 1991; Carroll *et al.*, 1993), and more needs to be learnt about how to treat this difficult combination (Brower *et al.*, 1994)

Alcohol and opioids

Problematic use of alcohol is common among opioid users. Alcohol consumption typically precedes first use of heroin in the early career of heroin addicts, but levels of alcohol use tend to drop off when regular opioid use is established (Rounsaville *et al.*, 1982). However, the impact of treatment of opiod dependence on alcohol use is uncertain, some studies finding that rates of alcohol misuse remain constant or decline, and others reporting that treatment entry is associated with increased alcohol use. The theme that emerges from these studies is that alcohol problems frequently predate opioid use, and that when one dependence has developed, a variety of drugs will be misused.

Two general patterns of drinking have been recognised in heroin dependent subjects during and following treatment – concurrent use while on licit or illicit opioids and use of alcohol as a substitute for opioids. Methadone treatment, in particular, is associated with alcohol problems, because methadone blocks the intoxicating effect of opioids, thus causing addicts to look for another intoxicating substance. Prevalence rates of problem drinking in patients undergoing methadone treatment programmes have varied from 20–50% in the majority of (mainly North American) studies (Liebson *et al.*, 1973). A

113

British study of patients enrolled in a methadone treatment programme in a London teaching hospital, reported that 32% had actual or potential drinking problems (Stastny & Potter, 1991). Those with alcohol problems were also likely to use benzodiazepines. Here is a case example:

> A 32-year-old woman was referred from a Methadone Maintenance Clinic. She had been attending daily for one year, and was stabilised on a script of 50 mg methadone daily. Her alcohol consumption had increased dramatically over this period and at the time of referral she was drinking four to six cans of strong lager daily and experiencing marked symptoms of alcohol withdrawal. Her history revealed a period of heavy alcohol consumption earlier in life and before her first involvement in heroin at age 23.

Alcohol problems may substitute for opioids, when heroin users attempt to detoxify on their own, in a treatment programme or during prolonged periods of abstinence. A typical story may be of a young man or woman who stops using heroin, who spends a few months in a therapeutic community where no alcohol is allowed, and who then moves into lodgings and starts to drink rather heavily in the evenings. One or two years later, that individual may have to accept the fact that alcohol dependence has begun to consitute a problem as was heroin at an earlier stage. A seemingly promising recovery from a drug problem is being brought down because the danger of contracting a later cross-dependence on alcohol was not foreseen. A long-term national study in the USA found that substitution of alcohol for heroin occurred in about 10% of the clients followed up, and was strongly associated with cannabis use (Sells & Simpson, 1987). Treated opioid users who go on to develop alcohol problems are more likely to have had disrupted childhoods, more legal problems and poly-drug use, more problems with social functioning, and higher rates of psychiatric disorders than 'non-alcoholic addicts' (Rounsaville et al., 1982). Here is a typical story of early heavy drinking in a setting of poly-drug use, this youthful pattern of mixed use may lead to a dominant use of heroin, and recovery from heroin dependence being followed a few years later by a plunge into alcohol.

> A 34-year-old unemployed man was referred for assessment of his heavy drinking and depression. He had experienced extreme emotional deprivation in childhood and had been in care. At 14 years of age he began to drink beer and to smoke cannabis 'for comfort'. He soon began to use amphetamines and diazepam, and his daily alcohol consumption gradually increased to three to four cans of strong lager. He first smoked heroin in his early 20s and very soon switched to intravenous use, sharing needles. He also snorted cocaine on a regular basis, injecting it on occasion. Other drug use included LSD intermittently, 'mushrooms', and ecstasy. When he was 30 he entered a residential rehabilitation unit and gave up all illicit drug use. However, his alcohol consumption escalated

and four years later, at the time of referral, his drinking was out of control. He was also experiencing marked craving for heroin and cocaine and was worried that he would begin to use them again.

Drinking problems and benzodiazepines

At various points in this book, reference will be made to the dangers which can arise from patients with drinking problems being introduced to heavy use of sedatives or tranquillisers as a result of unwise medical prescribing. Such occurrences are far from rare. The result may be that pills come to be mixed with concurrent drinking in a haphazard fashion or alternatively dependence on benzodiazepines or chlormethiazole may substitute for the drinking and at least for a time become the dominant problem. Barbiturates are still, on occasion, responsible for a cross-dependence but are much less widely prescribed than previously.

> A 39-year-old man was admitted for in-patient treatment. He had well-established alcohol dependence. Throughout his 20s he had regularly used cannabis, cocaine, and amphetamines. In his mid-30s he had developed marked anxiety for which his GP prescribed small doses of diazepam. When his GP refused to increase the dose he threatened self-harm. He regularly forged prescriptions. The GP made arrangements for him to pick up his diazepam on a daily basis at a local chemist. However, he also obtained benzodiazepines from several hospitals, both general and psychiatric. In total he was probably taking 60–80 mg of diazepam daily, mixed with alcohol. On admission he refused to consider a reduction in his benzodiazepines and therefore was only withdrawn from alcohol. He relapsed on the day of discharge and continued to drink and to use benzodiazepines.

Dependence on benzodiazepines has become such a frequently encountered complication among patients who present with alcohol problems that it is appropriate to give special attention to this issue in a book which takes the treatment of drinking problems as its central concern. Therapists working in this field today need as a basic skill to be able to recognise and treat benzodiazepine dependence. They should also be constantly aware of the dangers that so easily result from lax prescribing of this class of drugs.

The benzodiazepine group of drugs

Benzodiazepines were introduced to clinical practice in 1960 and have since become widely used in the treatment of anxiety and insomnia.

They are also accepted as the treatment of choice for alcohol withdrawal symptoms. A wide variety of benzodiazepines has been marketed and Box 7.2 lists the commoner substances giving both their official and trade names.

Box 7.2. Some common benzodiazepines

Non-proprietary name	Proprietary name	Active Metabolites	Approx. duration of action	Approximate equivalent dose (mg)
Diazepam	Valium	Several	2–4 days	10
Chlordiazepoxide	Librium	Several	2–4 days	20
Nitrazepam	Mogadon	None	12–24 hours	10
Clonazepam		Several	1–2 days	1
Lorazepam	Ativan	None	8–12 hours	1
Temazepam	Normison	None	8 hours	20
Oxazepam	Oxanid	None	8–12 hours	30

Drugs within this group have many properties in common. Important differences exist, however, in relation to duration of action either of the drug itself or of its active metabolite. Lorazepam, oxazepam, and temazepam are all relatively short acting; chlordiazepoxide and diazepam are long acting, while the other substances listed in Box 7.2 produce an action of intermediate duration.

Dependence potential

Most benzodiazepine prescribing is appropriate (Woods *et al.*, 1988). Nevertheless long-term, continuous use of benzodiazepines carries a risk of dependence. This is most evident for high doses, but dependence can develop in patients who take therapeutic doses for prolonged periods. The relatively short-acting compounds have a greater dependence potential than the long-acting compounds. The proportion of patients taking therapeutic doses of benzodiazepines at risk of developing dependence is not known. Neither is there enough information other than in broad terms to identify the level of exposure (dose and duration) associated with an increased risk of dependence. New prescriptions of benzodiazepines should be restricted to approximately two weeks, and certainly no longer than four weeks, and lorazepam should be avoided. Patients with alcohol problems should not generally be given benzodiazepines, except for treatment of acute alcohol withdrawal, and then only on a careful and time-limited basis.

Clinical characteristics of benzodiazepine dependence

Benzodiazepine dependence can, like alcohol dependence, exist with any degree of severity. It typically develops within weeks or months. Difficulty in withdrawing the drug after regular use of as little as a few weeks is not uncommon.

The more gross symptoms of benzodiazepine withdrawal at the extreme end of the spectrum include seizures or a state resembling delirium tremens. Milder symptoms include insomnia, anxiety, agitation, hypersensitivity to light and sound, giddiness, tremor, perspiration, and headache. Withdrawal symptoms usually develop two to three days after stopping or reducing a short- or medium-acting benzodiazepine and after 7–10 days with longer acting drugs (Lader, 1987). Symptoms may also be present during dose reduction. Withdrawal symptoms usually subside within one to six weeks, but can persist for many months with risks of further drug taking or alcohol consumption. Rebound of the original and underlying symptoms can also contribute to the picture.

Treatment of benzodiazepine dependence

The first step in the treatment of this condition must be sympathetically but firmly to convey to the patient the nature of the problem which has to be met. Treatment should, if possible, be accomplished on an out-patient or doctor's surgery (office) basis, but in-patient admission may sometimes be needed. Assistance may be locally available from a self-help organisation which deals with tranquilliser problems.

The basic treatment is then a matter of gradual stepwise withdrawal at a rate that does not produce symptoms which the patient finds intolerable. Abrupt withdrawal should never be attempted because of the risk of seizures, toxic psychosis, and other severe symptoms. Benzodiazepine withdrawal should be a joint effort between doctor and patient, based on a trusting relationship and a schedule of reductions negotiated with the patient. Every case sets individual problems and different drugs will require different regimes. Patients with fluctuating intake should have their dose stabilised before starting withdrawal. It may be helpful to transfer patients from their existing benzodiazepine to an equivalent daily dose of diazepam. This is particularly necessary for the shorter acting compounds such as lorazepam. Diazepam should be given in small tablet sizes (2 mg) in order to segment the volume of drugs being taken, and to facilitate reduction. It may be helpful to agree a written timetable with the patient and to allow them responsibility to control their own rate of withdrawal. Schedules should not usually last less than six to eight weeks; many patients will need longer. If the rate of reduction leads to the recurrence of unacceptable symptoms, the pace must be slowed, temporarily stopped or reversed. As a rough guide it might generally be acceptable to aim at a reduction in total daily dose of about 2 mg of diazepam each fortnight, but initial reductions can be greater where the starting dose is high. Complete withdrawal may take several weeks or months. Very slow withdrawal (six months or longer) may herald poor outcome and should be avoided if possible. Throughout the withdrawal period the patient should have regular support sessions and telephone access to a member of the team. It may be helpful to keep a diary of symptoms. Some patients will reach an impasse and it may be better to leave them on a low dose rather than withdrawing completely. Other drugs such as clonidine or beta blockers may be of some assistance in suppressing withdrawal symptoms and antidepressant treatment may sometimes be indicated (Lader & Morton, 1991; Russell & Lader, 1992).

Nicotine

Individuals with drinking problems are two to three times more likely to smoke than those without such problems. They are often heavy smokers and when they stop drinking may compensate by even heavier use of cigarettes. Problem drinkers have high rates of tobacco-related disease and their all-cause mortality rates are twice as high as 'non-alcoholic' smokers (Rosengren *et al.*, 1993).

Drugs and alcohol as one domain: the practical implications

Several of the most immediate implications of this perspective have already been discussed in earlier sections of this chapter. At this point it may, however, be useful to bring together the core implications and in Box 7.3 we draw attention to some matters of special clinical relevance.

Implications for training and service organisation

Anyone taking professional responsibility for treatment of alcohol problems should recognise that multiple drug use is pervasive and should possess a good working knowledge of drug problems (and vice versa). There may be a continuing place for specialised drug or specialised alcohol treatment services, but the intensity of specialisation must not be of such a degree as to be out of tune with clinical realities. The problems with which patients present often do not respect the specialists' demarcations. Inadequate training may mean that individuals with joint drug and alcohol problems find it difficult to obtain treatment, are incompletely evaluated and treated, and often rejected. If treatment services are to face the challenge of poly-drug use successfully they must have a capacity to integrate alcohol and drug treatment.

Box 7.3. Tips for therapists

- Have a good working knowledge of alcohol and drugs

- Always take a complete alcohol and drug history

- Update substance use history appropriately

- Organise spot urine drug screens where indicated

A prime responsibility for prevention

Therapists who are treating patients with drinking problems have a special responsibility not to do their patients damage by careless prescription of sedatives or minor tranquillisers. It is similarly important that anyone who is treating opioid dependent patients should offer counselling on the use of alcohol and the dangers of alcohol dependence.

Diagnosis and screening

With a patient whose presenting problem is with one type of substance, an open eye should be kept on the possible existence of problems with other types of chemical. It is, for instance, less than useful to concentrate exclusively on a patient's drinking while failing to detect the fact that massive quantities of benzodiazepines are being consumed. A complete alcohol and drug history should be obtained. This means charting, as necessary, the evolution of use and dependence for every drug taken, as well as for alcohol. In this way the sequence of drug use can be mapped out, for example, solvents as a child, alcohol and later amphetamines in the teenage years, heroin as an adult. Many clients presenting to alcohol services may have a past history of intravenous drug use and will need assessment of hepatitis and human immunodeficiency virus (HIV) status. Routine urine testing should be more widely employed. The history may need to be updated at regular intervals.

Treatment goals

Therapists working within treatment programmes that take the concept of chemical dependence as a central tenet would probably advise a patient who has encountered difficulties with either alcohol or other drugs to avoid all mood-altering chemicals for ever after. For many patients this is the best advice and although it is unlikely to be acceptable for all patients (some former heroin addicts may for instance later use alcohol moderately and safely), the insistence that patients should be made aware of the dangers of crossing over from one substance to another is generally appropriate.

A constant two-way vigilance

This heading cross-cuts with all the other entities in this section. When seeing a patient or client for the first time, when planning and carrying through a treatment programme, and when assessing success, patient and therapist should be thinking in terms of drugs and alcohol and not just alcohol or just drugs. And to turn a blind eye to nicotine is not in the health interest.

References

Brower, K. J., Blow, F. C., Hill, E. M. & Mudd, S. A. (1994). Treatment outcome of alcoholics with and without cocaine disorders. *Alcoholism: Clinical and Experimental Research* **18**, 734–9.

Carroll, K. M., Power, M.-E. D., Bryant, K. & Rounsaville, B. J. (1993). One-year follow-up status of treatment-seeking cocaine abusers. *Journal of Nervous and Mental Disease* **181**, 71–9.

Clayton, R. (1986). Multiple drug use: epidemiology, correlates and consequences. In *Recent Developments in Alcoholism*, ed. Galanter, M., vol. 4, pp. 7–38. New York: Plenum Press.

Helzer, J. E. & Pryzbeck, T. R. (1988). The co-occurrence of alcoholism with other psychiatric disorders in the general population and its impact on treatment. *Journal of Studies on Alcohol* **49**, 219–24.

Kosten, T. R. (1989). Pharmacotherapeutic interventions for cocaine abuse. *Journal of Nervous and Mental Disease* **177**, 379–89.

Lader, M. (1987). Long-term anxiolytic therapy: the issue of drug withdrawal. *Journal of Clinical Psychiatry* **48** (suppl. 12), 12–16.

Lader, M. & Morton, S. (1991). Benzodiazepine problems. *British Journal of Addiction* **86**, 823–8.

Liebson, I., Bieglow, G. & Flamer, R. (1973). Alcoholism amongst methadone patients. A special treatment method. *American Journal of Psychiatry* **130**, 483–5.

McCance, E. F., Price, L. H., Kosten, T. R. & Jatlow, P. I. (1995). Cocaethylene: pharmacology, physiology and behavioural effects in humans. *Journal of Pharmacology and Experimental Therapeutics* **274**, 215–23.

Rounsaville, B. J., Weissman, M. M. & Kleber, H. D. (1982). The significance of alcoholism in treated opiate addicts. *Journal of Nervous and Mental Disease* **170**, 479–88.

Rosengren, A., Wilhelmsen, L. & Wedel, H. (1993). Separate and combined effects of smoking and alcohol abuse in middle-aged men. *Acta Medica Scandinavia* **223**, 111–18.

Russell, J. & Lader, M. (1992). *Guidelines for the Prevention and Treatment of Benzodiazepine Dependence*. Substance Abuse Committee of the Mental Health Foundation. London: The Mental Health Foundation.

Sells, S. B. & Simpson, D. D. (1987). Role of alcohol use by narcotic addicts as revealed in the DARP research on evaluation of treatment for drug abuse. *Alcoholism: Clinical and Experimental Research* **11**, 437–9.

Stastny, D., Potter, M. (1991). Alcohol abuse by patients undergoing methadone treatment programmes. *British Journal of Addiction* **86**, 307–10.

Walsh, D. C., Hingson, R. W., Merrigan, D. M., Levenson, S. M., Cupples, A., Heeren, T. *et al.* (1991). A randomised trial of treatment options for alcohol abusing workers. *New England Journal of Medicine* **325**, 775–82.

Woods, J. H., Katz, J. L., Winger, G. (1988). Use and abuse of benzodiazepines: issues relevant to prescribing. *Journal of the American Medical Association* **260**, 3476–80.

8

Physical complications of excessive drinking

Within a total and balanced approach to drinking problems the physical element must be seen as often very important. Helping services must be so organised as to cope effectively with diagnosis and treatment in the physical domain, and whatever the particular professional affiliation of the person who is working with the drinker, there is need for an alertness towards possible physical pathologies. For instance, the voluntary worker in a lay counselling centre is, of course, practising their own special types of skill, and no one would suggest that they should also cultivate a highly specialised knowledge of liver pathology. It is, though, a reasonable expectation that they should know enough about the liver to understand the significance to their client of a diagnosis of cirrhosis, rather than themselves being mystified by this term and consequently deflecting that client from talking about something of vital importance. A polite conspiracy can be set up which pretends that the body does not exist.

Why physical complications matter

Alcohol consumption is a significant cause of physical morbidity. In Great Britain, approximately 15–30% of male and 8–15% of female admissions to general hospitals in urban areas have alcohol-related problems (Chick, 1994). The equivalent figure in the United States is 20–40% (Lieber, 1995).

Although, on the one hand, physical complications are common in any population of heavy drinkers, early detection and cessation of drinking can often lead to recovery. Continued drinking, on the other hand, is likely to exacerbate the alcohol-related problem and may seriously threaten life. Physical complications impinge upon all aspects of the patient's life and it is unrealistic to compartmentalise psychological, social, and physical disability.

Often physical complications are the main reason for seeking help. If information about the physical symptoms is imparted clearly, so that the patient can understand their significance, this information can be used to appraise their position. Thus an understanding of the physical symptoms may have the potential to influence drinking behaviour. As ever, the therapist is the informant, the person who brings up the issue, and who shares and reflects the patient's feelings and concerns, rather than the disembodied pronouncer of facts. The way in which information on physical problems is presented to the patient can be part of the therapy. Here are two dialogues that illustrate different ways in which the patient's concern over their physical health can be met at interview. Firstly, and very briefly, a dialogue which is not to be dismissed as caricature:

PATIENT: What did the doctor mean when he said my liver had been hit by the drinking?
COUNSELLOR: You will have to ask the doctor to explain.
PATIENT: But he never explains anything.
COUNSELLOR: Well, he's the person to ask.

Secondly, and more constructively:

PATIENT: What did the doctor mean when he said my liver had been hit by the drinking?
COUNSELLOR: That's something pretty important to talk about. What did you think he meant?
PATIENT: I suppose I was dead scared. Not sure I believe him, though. He may just be trying to put the frighteners under me. But if what he's really saying is that I'm going to die of cirrhosis I'll go out in the crest of the all-time greatest booze-up.
COUNSELLOR: I don't think anyone is wanting to scare you in a horror-story sort of way, but it's your own liver and you have a right to know about it.
PATIENT: So what's the score?
COUNSELLOR: I spoke to your doctor on the phone. You have undoubtedly done your liver some harm, and if you go on drinking you would be risking cirrhosis, and that's a miserable way to die. If you stop drinking, your liver's going to heal. You've a right to know all the facts. It's reasonable to be anxious, but at least there is something positive you can do towards repairing the damage – stop drinking.
PATIENT: When I was getting that pain, I guessed it must be my liver,

123

but I suppose I have been shutting my eyes, doing the 'it can't happen to me' trick.

The vital question is what any information on physical consequences means to the patient. Too often the results of the physical examination and laboratory tests are left in the case notes, and no one thinks to ask whether these findings have been shared with the person most intimately affected. Patients and their families are concerned about their physical health and deserve to be given the facts. Explaining and talking through this information is an opportunity for the therapist to strengthen the quality of the relationship with the patient.

Some patients stop drinking abruptly when persuaded that alcohol is posing a tangible threat to their physical health. One may suspect, however, that even if the news of physical damage constitutes the turning point, in reality this is only the final event to tip a decision where the moment for change has been set up by many previous happenings. But using the results of the physical examination or the laboratory tests for crude scare tactics is likely to be counter-productive. The patient may dismiss what they are being told simply because the information is too frightening to be accepted, or they may decide that all is lost and that they may as well drink themselves to death.

Causes of physical complications

Heavy alcohol consumption causes physical damage by many direct and indirect effects on the body. Alcohol is a source of calories and therefore displaces normal nutrients, causing malnutrition, in particular deficiencies of folate, thiamine, and other vitamins. Pancreatic insufficiency and impaired liver metabolism cause malabsorption and secondary malnutrition. Alcohol and its metabolite acetaldehyde are toxic substances that have the potential to cause tissue damage. Cytochrome P450, the key enzyme in the microsomal ethanol-oxidising system (MEOS), produces a toxic variety of active oxygen which can cause liver damage (Lieber, 1995). In some conditions, both the toxic element and disturbance of nutritional status may be implicated as a cause of damage at the same time.

What level of alcohol intake constitutes a threshold for physical dangers? The answer must vary according to the particular condition, but in general the evidence points to the probability that risk for many varieties of damage increases in proportion to alcohol intake, even within the ranges of what passes as 'social drinking'. This is probably true, for instance, in relation to alcohol-related brain damage, cirrhosis, the foetal alcohol syndrome, and certain other alcohol-related problems. In particular, a pattern of heavy weekend or binge drinking, even an amount equivalent to an average of two or three drinks a day, carries risks for physical health. Paradoxically, light or moderate drinking of one or two drinks per day is likely to reduce the risk of coronary heart disease in some populations (see p. 134). As we have argued earlier, the issue of level of consumption and risk of physical harm is complex and does not allow for an easy calculation of a 'safe' level.

But whatever the risks at the relatively lower ranges of intake, by the time someone is drinking in the fashion dictated by the dependence syndrome, the question of whether their level of intake carries dangers hardly needs to be asked. The answer is resoundingly 'yes' for nearly every tissue of the body. And quite apart from any specific tissue damage discussed in this chapter, it should be remembered that as a consequence of heavy drinking and dietary neglect, almost every aspect

---

Box 8.1. Patients presenting to the GP or general hospital with the following should be assessed for an alcohol problem

- Hepatitis/cirrhosis

- Hypertension

- Stroke

- Cardiomyopathy

- Pneumonia and TB

- Myopathy

- Osteoporosis

- Seizures

- Wernicke-Korsakoff syndrome

- Accidents

- Resistant psoriasis and eczema

- Anaemia/raised mean corpuscular volume (MCV)

All patients, whatever their presentation, should on first contact be *asked about their drinking*

---

of the body's chemistry may in some circumstances be put out of balance; even such seemingly obscure aspects as serum zinc or magnesium levels may be disturbed.

In the ensuing sections of this chapter, a range of physical complications that can result from excessive drinking will be described. This list is comprehensive but does not claim to be exhaustive. As far as possible technical language is explained, but as noted in the 'Introduction' this is a chapter where the non-medical reader will have to show some forbearance.

In Box 8.1 are listed physical conditions where particular alertness is appropriate as to the possibility of an underlying drinking problem, while stressing that basic enquiry into the patient's drinking history should be absolutely routine in medical practice.

Acute alcohol intoxication and coma

A life-threatening overdose with alcohol is unlikely to occur with the alcohol dependent person both because of their experience with handling their drinking and their raised tolerance: that is not to deny the possibility of such a patient at times getting very drunk, or drinking to unconsciousness. Drinking to the point of collapse and 'passing out' is more likely to be the result of a casual drinking spree, or a Saturday night celebration, and it is this type of patient who is the familiar late-night visitor to the hospital's Accident and Emergency Department. The tablets which are taken with suicidal intention are sometimes washed down with a quantity of alcohol and a mixed sedative/alcohol overdose then results. Occasionally a child will overdose accidentally with alcohol and this is discussed in relation to hypoglycaemia (pp. 135–6).

Intoxication can usually be dealt with on a sensibly conservative basis and the patient left to sleep off their binge, with due care taken to ensure that they do not inhale their vomit – examination must of course also ensure that there is no other cause for the unconsciousness. A stomach wash-out may sometimes be indicated. But with a higher level of intoxication there is a risk of respiratory depression and death. The BAC likely to be associated with such a tragedy must vary with the individual but a BAC of 400 mg per 100 ml is usually quoted as the threshold for very serious danger (Peters, 1996). Because of the occasional risk of death from respiratory paralysis, the more common danger from inhaled vomit and the many possibilities of being unwarily caught out by some underlying or complicating condition (for example, head injury, hypoglycaemia, ketoacidosis, systemic infection, overdose of other licit or illicit drugs), the problem set by alcoholic overdose and by the often rather unwelcome visitor to the Emergency Room should not be too casually dismissed as 'routine'. When coma is thought to be caused by alcohol, it is important that a high alcohol concentration is shown by measurements of breath or blood alcohol. Skull radiography and urine toxicology are other fundamental investigations (Quaghebeur & Richards, 1989). Alcoholic coma has a mortality rate of approximately 5%.

Acute poisoning with methyl alcohol (methanol) is both a rarer and a much more threatening condition than intoxication with ordinary beverage alcohol (ethanol). There are substantial risks of blindness or death and intensive emergency medical care will be required, possibly with dialysis.

Gastroenterological disorders

Alcoholic liver disease

Alcohol misuse is the commonest cause of liver damage in the UK, Europe, the United States, and Australia. Three types of alcoholic liver disease have been described – fatty liver, alcoholic hepatitis, and alcoholic cirrhosis. All three may coexist. Fatty liver is present in up to 90% of persistent heavy drinkers at some time. Alcoholic hepatitis is seen in approximately 40% of individuals with a history of persistent heavy drinking. Between 8–30% of heavy drinkers will develop alcoholic cirrhosis, typically after a 10–20 year history of daily heavy drinking. However, not all heavy drinkers develop cirrhosis; some individuals appear to be genetically more susceptible (see p. 23). For instance, genetic factors that increase the oxidation of alcohol or reduce the rate of acetaldehyde clearance will increase acetaldehyde levels in the liver and cause greater injury. In women, a reduced 'first pass' metabolism of alcohol in the stomach by gastric ADH leads to increased blood alcohol levels. This further exacerbates the higher blood alcohol levels in women compared with men, due to their lower body water content and weight. Environmental factors such as hepatitis B and C (HBV and HCV) may contribute to the development of alcoholic liver disease and continuing heavy alcohol consumption may worsen liver disease associated with HBV or HCV infection (Sherman & Williams, 1994; James, 1996). The main features of alcoholic liver disease are summarised in Box 8.2.

Box 8.2. Alcohol and the liver

- Fatty liver rarely causes illness and is reversible with abstinence
- Alcoholic hepatitis may be fatal but can be reversible with abstinence
- Alcoholic cirrhosis is often progressive and fatal but can stabilise with abstinence
- Abstinence is the single most important component of treatment for alcoholic liver disease

---

Fatty liver

The first histological change seen in persistent heavy drinkers is deposition of fat. While this is usually asymptomatic, patients may present with non-specific symptoms such as malaise, tiredness, nausea, an enlarged tender liver, or abnormal liver function tests. Occasionally very severe fatty liver can lead to obstructive jaundice, liver failure, or death due to a fat embolism (globules of fat getting into the circulation and obstructing arteries to the brain). Fatty liver is reversible with abstinence.

Alcoholic hepatitis

Minor degrees of alcoholic hepatitis may be asymptomatic and clinically indistinguishable from fatty liver. More severe episodes reflect liver inflammation and are characterised by loss of appetite, abdominal pain, nausea, weight loss, jaundice, and fever. Severe alcoholic hepatitis has a mortality of about 60% during the first six weeks after hospital admission. Corticosteroids may improve survival in the early stages, but abstinence is the best 'treatment', and is essential for long-term survival. Abstinence leads to reversal of the histological changes but alcoholic hepatitis almost always progresses to cirrhosis in women, even following abstinence.

Alcoholic cirrhosis

Cirrhosis may arise *de novo* in some cases, without passing through the intermediate state of hepatitis. Here liver tissue becomes scarred with the development of fibrous tissue. This scarring, together with the regeneration of liver tissue, disturbs the normal liver architecture, and the consequences are two-fold. Firstly, the actual loss of functioning liver tissue causes a range of metabolic disturbances and ultimately liver failure may occur. Secondly, and very importantly, the scarring and disorganisation lead to the squeezing and blocking off of blood vessels. This physical damming causes a build-up of pressure in the portal venous system (the veins that carry blood from the alimentary tract to the liver), called portal hypertension. This can, in turn, cause bleeding from veins at the lower end of the oesophagus (oesophageal varices), and this bleeding can be severe or fatal.

Cirrhosis can exist in degrees. If the condition is not too advanced, abstinence may lead to stabilisation and enhance life expectancy. From the patient's point of view, they may know nothing of this insidious condition until they suddenly becomes jaundiced, find their abdomen swelling up with fluid (ascites), or have a massive bleed. More often, the diagnosis is picked up at an earlier stage, with confirmation coming from various special investigations. Liver transplantation is now an option for some individuals with alcoholic liver disease (Lucey *et al.*, 1994).

Patients with alcoholic liver disease may develop Zieve's Syndrome, characterised by a combination of cholestasis (blocking of bile channels in the liver), haemolysis (breakdown of red cells) and gross hyperlipidaemia (rise in blood fats).

Acute pancreatitis

Alcohol misuse and biliary disease are the two main causative factors in acute pancreatitis. Individuals with acute alcoholic pancreatitis are likely to be young men, drinking in excess of 80 g of alcohol per day. The most common form of presentation is a sudden onset of severe upper abdominal pain, typically penetrating through to the back, associated with vomiting. The pain lessens in severity over the first 72 hours after onset. Patients with severe acute pancreatitis may be feverish, hypotensive, have rapid breathing and suffer with acute ascites, pleural effusions, and paralytic ileus (paralysis of the intestines). The diagnosis is usually made from the clinical presentation and confirmed by gross elevations of amylase and lipase in the blood. The mortality rate is between 10 and 40% (Imrie, 1996).

Chronic pancreatitis

Heavy drinking is the most frequent cause of chronic pancreatitis in adults, particularly the calcifying form. The main presenting symptom is chronic abdominal pain which is often associated with steatorrhoea (fat in the faeces), diarrhoea, and weight loss. All this is indicative of reduced pancreatic exocrine tissue which secretes digestive enzymes. Damage to the Islets of Langerhans within the pancreas occurs more slowly, with consequent failure of insulin secretion and diabetes mellitus. Severe and chronic pain may lead to opioid dependence (Toskes, 1996). Further acute attacks of pancreatitis may occur against the background of the chronic condition.

> A businessman aged 52 years had a long history of alcohol dependence. On occasion he would stop drinking for a few months, but was never willing to consider long-term abstinence as the goal. One weekend he relapsed once more into drinking with a very heavy binge. On the Sunday night he was admitted as an emergency to his local hospital with appalling abdominal pain radiating through to the back. A raised serum amylase confirmed the diagnosis of acute pancreatitis. Despite the hospital's best efforts he died in shock 36 hours later. Post-mortem showed extensive necrosis of the pancreas and some old scarring. There was also evidence of early liver cirrhosis.

Peptic ulceration and gastritis

Alcohol has long been thought to be associated with the development of peptic ulceration, but recent research suggests that *Helicobacter pylori* infection is the major causative factor, particularly in duodenal ulceration and in chronic gastritis. However, acute erosive ulcers can develop in patients whose upper gastro-intestinal mucosa is damaged by alcohol (Misiewicz & Pounder, 1996).

Mallory-Weiss syndrome

This is a tear of the lower end of the oesophagus caused by severe retching, with a consequent vomiting of blood. It is common after a heavy bout of drinking.

Musculoskeletal disorders

Gout

Gout is a constitutional metabolic disorder characterised by episodic painful swelling of peripheral joints, especially the fingers and toes. Individuals with gout have high uric acid levels, and the joint inflamation is produced by the deposition of uric acid in the joints (Doherty, 1996). Most gout occurs in middle-aged men, who often have a family history of the disorder and drink heavily. Beer is particularly liable to produce hyperuricacidaemia, because of its high purine content (Scott, 1989). Other conditions predisposing to gout include obesity, hyper-lipidaemia, and hypertension, all of which are independently associ-ated with heavy drinking. Heavy drinking can bring out a latent tendency towards gout or make established gout worse.

Osteoporosis

Chronic alcohol misuse is associated with a reduced bone mass and osteoporosis (reduction in the amount of bone per unit volume without a change in its composition), an increased frequency of skeletal bone fractures, and avascular necrosis (Diamond et al., 1989; Moniz, 1994). Disorders, such as nutritional deficiencies of calcium and Vitamin D, pancreatic or liver disease and endocrine dysfunction, arising as a result of heavy drinking could account for the reduced bone mass. However, heavy alcohol consumption causes impaired bone formation (reduced osteoblastic activity) and may increase bone degradation. These effects of alcohol on bone metabolism appear to be reversible with abstinence. Heavy drinkers are therefore at risk of fractures, even after minimal trauma. Symptoms of back pain indicative of osteoporosis and possible vertebral collapse should not be overlooked, particularly as these patients are also likely to develop dependence on opioid-based anal-gesics. Post-menopausal women may be particularly susceptible to the effects of alcohol on bone.

Myopathy

Acute myopathy produced by alcohol poisoning is characterised by severe pain, tenderness, swelling and weakness of the skeletal muscles. In its severe form, acute rhabdomyolysis (breakdown of muscle tissue) is associated with myoglobinuria, renal damage, and hyperkalaemia (raised potassium levels). Alcohol consumption reduces the normal metabolic responses of skeletal muscle to the action of insulin by causing an acute insulin resistance (Xu et al., 1996).

Chronic alcoholic myopathy is a relatively common complication of long-standing alcohol problems and is easily overlooked or misattrib-uted to poor nutrition. As is the case with alcoholic liver disease and brain damage, women are more susceptible than men. Individuals typ-ically present with proximal muscle weakness, pain and abnormal gait, and show evidence of atrophy and loss of muscle fibre in the shoulder and pelvic girdle region (Preedy & Peters, 1990). Histology reveals a selective myopathy of type II skeletal muscle fibres. This weakness and atrophy tends to improve with abstinence (Urbano-Marquez et al., 1995).

The following is a case abstract illustrating a fairly typical picture:

A 45-year-old storekeeper who was severely alcohol dependent came along to complain that he had developed 'terrible rheumatics'. There was severe pain and some tenderness and swelling of both upper arms and he could no longer lift his stock down from the shelves. It took about two months for him to make a reasonable recovery.

Endocrine disorders

Alcohol-induced pseudo-Cushing's syndrome

Alcohol-induced pseudo-Cushing's syndrome is a term used to describe heavy drinkers who present with a clinical picture similar to that seen in Cushing's Syndrome – truncal obesity with thin extremities, plethoric appearance, 'moon-face', bruising, striae, muscle wasting and hypertension (Jeffcoate, 1993). Biochemical abnormalities include elevated urinary and plasma cortisol levels (the latter failing to suppress with dexamethasone) and reduced circadian rhythm of plasma cortisol, and normal or suppressed ACTH (adrenocorticotrophic hormone). The biochemical abnormalities rapidly revert to normal with abstinence from alcohol. The mechanism of this disorder is poorly understood.

Male hypogonadism

Alcohol causes a lowering of plasma testosterone concentrations through a direct toxic effect on the Leydig cells in the testis where testosterone is synthesised.

Cancers

Heavy alcohol consumption is associated with an increased risk for cancers of the oropharynx, larynx and oesophagus (gullet), and liver in men and women, and possibly with breast cancer in women (Longnecker, 1992; Arria & van Thiel, 1992). Most studies show a dose response relationship. Alcohol is not thought to increase the risk of cancers of the stomach, pancreas, or lung. Its role in colorectal cancer is equivocal.

The risk for cancer of the oropharynx is related to the number of drinks consumed per day, even after adjustment for smoking. For cancers of the larynx, the effect of alcohol consumption is exacerbated by smoking (Tuyns, 1991). Alcohol misuse is an important co-factor in the development of primary liver cancer and liver cancer may arise consequent on alcoholic cirrhosis.

Cardiovascular disease

Alcohol-related arrythmias

Arrythmias, or disturbances of the normal heart rhythm, may occur as a result of acute alcohol intoxication, or during withdrawal. Binge drinking may be particularly involved. The mildest presentation is that of palpitations, caused by a few extra and irregular beats (extrasystoles). Atrial fibrillation (irregular twitching of the atrial muscle) is the most common arrythmia associated with alcohol use (Koskinen & Kupari, 1992). Ventricular arrythmia has also been reported.

Hypertension

Over the past 20 years epidemiological findings have suggested an association between alcohol consumption and blood pressure (Saunders, 1987; Kaplan, 1995). Chronic excessive alcohol consumption is associated with increased blood pressure in both men and women, independent of age, body weight, and cigarette smoking, and is thought to be the second most important non-genetic risk factor for hypertension. Binge-drinking may be particularly implicated. Approximately 7–11% of hypertension in men can be attributed to alcohol consumption of over 40 g per day. The figure is nearer 1% in women because of their lower consumption. Intervention studies indicate that persistent heavy drinkers who cut down on their alcohol consumption, or abstain, lower their blood pressures. Individuals presenting with hypertension to a GP or physician should always have an alcohol history taken, together with appropriate laboratory investigations.

Cerebral vascular disease or stroke

There are two broad categories of stroke – ischaemic and haemorrhagic. In ischaemic stroke, thromboembolism causes cerebral infarction. Haemorrhagic stroke is due to either intracranial haemorrhage or sub-arachnoid haemorrhage. Alcohol may interact with a variety of risk factors for stroke, including hypertension, cigarette smoking, diabetes, and obesity. However, there appears to be an independent, dose-dependent relationship between the level of alcohol consumption and the risk of intracerebral and sub-arachnoid haemorrhage (Stampfer et al., 1988;

Anderson, 1995). This risk is present even at levels of 20 g per day. A two to threefold increase in risk is seen at levels of consumption of over 30 g daily. In contrast there is no association between alcohol consumption and ischaemic stroke, although there is some suggestion that low levels of consumption reduce the relative risk.

Coronary heart disease

Population-based epidemiological studies indicate a 'J-shaped' relationship between alcohol consumption and the risk for coronary heart disease (Edwards *et al.*, 1994). This means that non-drinkers and perhaps very light drinkers have a higher rate of morbidity and mortality resulting from coronary heart disease than light or moderate drinkers, and that heavy drinkers have an elevated risk. These studies have controlled for cigarette smoking, obesity and hypertension. This 'protective' effect is present in men and women and appears stronger in men over 40 and in post-menopausal women. The reduced risk for coronary heart disease occurs at levels as little as 10 g per day and remains similar up to 30–40 g per day (beyond about 20–30 g for men and 15–20 g for women, advantages for the heart will be outweighed by other risks). Individuals drinking over this level have an increased incidence of coronary heart disease which is dose-related (Edwards *et al.*, 1994). The protective effect appears to derive from ethanol itself rather than any specific beverage type.

The mechanisms underlying the 'protective effect' are not fully understood. Alcohol may have a partial inhibitory effect on atherosclerosis by increasing levels of high density lipoproteins (HDLs) which carry cholesterol to different parts of the body. HDLs are associated with a reduced risk of coronary heart disease and are thought to protect the arteries from a build-up of cholesterol. Alcohol also reduces platelet stickiness and aggregation, reduces fibrinogen, and increases fibrinolysis.

Alcoholic cardiomyopathy (alcohol-induced heart muscle disease)

Alcoholic cardiomyopathy is associated with excessive alcohol consumption and is thought to arise as a result of the toxic action of alcohol on heart muscle (Preedy & Richardson, 1994; Rubin & Urbano-Marquez, 1994). A genetic predisposition may also be an important factor. Previously, alcoholic cardiomyopathy was attributed to thiamine deficiency but this is probably not the case because it occurs in heavy drinkers who are well nourished. The disorder usually manifests itself between the ages of 30 and 60 years. Although commoner in men, due to their heavier consumption, women seem to be particularly vulnerable (Urbano-Marquez *et al.*, 1995).

Alcoholic cardiomyopathy is characterised by an enlarged, hypertrophied heart. The left ventricle is dilated and there is dysfunction in cardiac contractility, leading to a depressed output (ejection fraction). In the early stages of hypertrophy and dilatation, there may be few symptoms. However, as the disorder progresses, patients develop arrythmias, including atrial and ventricular tachyarrythmias and atrioventricular conduction defects. Congestive cardiac failure is another typical form of presentation (breathlessness on exertion, breathlessness at night, and peripheral oedema).

Sub-clinical forms of alcoholic cardiomyopathy are evident in problem drinkers, as revealed by echocardiography. Early detection and abstinence may arrest or reverse the progress of this disorder.

Respiratory disease

Heavy alcohol consumption is associated with defects in the body's immune responses and clinically this is reflected in an excess of lower respiratory tract infections with *Streptococcus pneumoniae*, *Mycobacterium tuberculosis* and *Klebsiella pneumoniae*. Self-neglect and the associated way of life, particularly among Skid Row drinkers, are also important factors predisposing to infections. Because heavy drinkers may both vomit and become stuporose, they are prone to inhale material into their lungs and hence develop lung abscesses or bronchietasis (dilation and infection of the smaller bronchi).

Many problem drinkers also smoke heavily. A carcinoma of the lung is not, therefore, an uncommon coincidental finding, sometimes confusing the diagnostic picture. What is thought to be an alcoholic 'dementia' turns out, for instance, to be a secondary cancer of the brain or a severe 'alcoholic' peripheral neuropathy is found to be a cancer-related (carcinomatous) neuropathy. The simple message is that if a patient with a drinking problem presents for an assessment and has not had a recent chest X-ray, such an examination should be arranged.

Metabolic disorders

Hypoglycaemia

Alcohol-induced hypoglycaemia (lowering of blood sugar) can occur as a result of alcohol intoxication or after a modest intake of alcohol in individuals who are malnourished or fasting (Turner, 1996). Clinically the patient may present as flushed and sweaty with a rapid pulse and the appearance of being 'drunk' and inco-ordinated. An alternative presentation is of a patient who is in coma and hypothermic, without obvious features of hypoglycaemia. Children and adolescents are particularly susceptible to alcohol-induced hypoglycaemia and the condition for them is much more dangerous than in the adult (Lamminpaa, 1995).

Alcoholic ketoacidosis

This is a rare condition and usually arises after an episode of heavy drinking which has been followed by cessation in eating or by vomiting. Thus the patient can present drowsy and collapsed, and have a blood alcohol level of zero. Typically the patient presents with a metabolic acidosis, which responds to rehydration and glucose. A metabolic alkalosis may also be evident if there has been vomiting.

Hyperlipidaemia

Heavy drinking is associated with a rise in circulatory blood fats (serum triglycerides). This will only be picked up by laboratory tests, but probably carries implications for enhanced risk of arteriosclerosis.

Haematological effects

Heavy drinking gives rise to anaemia, macrocytosis, simple iron deficiency, neutropaenia, and thrombocytopaenia (Weatherall, 1996).

Anaemia

Anaemia is common among heavy drinkers and can be caused by a variety of factors including malnutrition, chronic blood loss, liver disease, malabsorption, chronic infections, and the direct toxic effect of alcohol on the bone marrow.

Macrocytosis

Macrocytosis (enlarged red blood cells) is also common among such patients and an unexplained macrocytosis should always alert clinicians to the possibility of an alcohol problem. If nutrition is adequate, macrocytosis is probably caused by the direct toxic action of alcohol on the bone marrow. Folate deficiency in malnourished problem drinkers can give rise to a megaloblastic anaemia. However, alcohol may interfere directly with folate metabolism.

Iron deficiency

Iron deficiency among heavy drinkers will probably reflect a poor diet or chronic blood loss due to gastritis or bleeding varices. It may be associated with folate deficiency.

Neutropaenia and thrombocytopaenia

Heavy drinking may cause a neutropaenia (lowering of white cells), either by a toxic effect on the bone marrow, or as a result of folate deficiency, and thereby render patients susceptible to infections. Alcohol may also interfere with neutrophil locomotion. Thrombocytopaenia (decrease in platelets) is frequent in heavy drinkers. The platelet count usually returns to normal with abstinence.

Neuropsychiatric disorders

The mechanisms underlying alcohol-related brain damage are complex. Poor nutrition and diminished vitamin reserves predispose to thiamine and nicotinic acid depletion. Alcohol is neurotoxic and acetaldehyde, its main metabolite, may have a similar action. Metabolic factors, resulting from acute and chronic intoxication and withdrawal, such as hypoxia, electrolyte imbalance, and hypoglycaemia, are also important as are alcohol withdrawal seizures, hepatic encephalopathy, subarachnoid haemorrhage, haemorrhagic stroke, and head injury.

Disorders of the central and peripheral nervous system

Seizures

Withdrawal seizures have been fully discussed on p. 85, but a number of other possible reasons for seizures in patients with drinking problems must be borne in mind, as well as the fact that seizures may be entirely coincidental. Heavy drinking may, for example, lower the threshold of seizures in a person with an underlying epileptic tendency of any origin. An epileptic patient who is being treated with anti-convulsants may forget to take their tablets when they go on a drinking binge. Heavy drinking can as a result of liver enzyme induction lead to increased metabolic clearance of such medication.

Heavy drinkers are often heavy cigarette smokers and a seizure may on occasion be the first and tragic signal of the secondary spread to the brain (metastases), from a carcinoma of the lung (see p. 135). Problem drinkers are prone to accidents and a seizure may be symptomatic of an old or more recent head injury. Alcoholic 'dementia' may sometimes be accompanied by seizures. A rather common cause of seizures is coincidental withdrawal of sedative or hypnotic drugs, particularly chlormethiazole. Rarer causes include alcohol-related hypoglycaemia (lowered blood sugar, pp. 135–6), and fatty emboli lodging in the brain (p. 128).

Alcoholic cerebellar degeneration

The cerebellum is a part of the brain concerned with balance and motor integration, and it is sometimes the focus for alcohol-related brain damage (Charness, 1993). Alcoholic cerebellar degeneration usually develops insidiously and is characterised by ataxia of gait and incoordination of the legs. It is thought to be due to thiamine deficiency but alcohol neurotoxicity may also be an important factor. Abstinence and treatment with thiamine (vitamin B1) may halt the progress of the disorder but the patient may still be left with a disabling condition.

Alcohol amblyopia

This uncommon condition presents as a gradual blurring of vision, accompanied perhaps by difficulty in distinguishing red from green. Testing reveals a central blind spot (scotoma), with the peripheral field of vision intact. The most likely cause is a deficiency of both thiamine and vitamin B12. The same picture sometimes occurs as 'tobacco amblyopia'.

The Wernicke-Korsakoff syndrome

Although Wernicke's encephalopathy and Korsakoff's psychosis were originally described as different entities, both are caused by thiamine (vitamin B1) deficiency and show the same underlying pathological lesions in the periventricular and periaqueductal grey matter (Lishman, 1987). Cortical abnormalities have also been reported in a proportion of cases.

Wernicke's encephalopathy, the acute component, consists of the triad of ophthalmoplegia (paralysis of eye muscles), ataxia, and confusion. However, the diagnosis is often missed in life because clinical signs are atypical or absent. The Korsakoff syndrome, the chronic component, is characterised by a profound anterograde and retrograde amnesia, disorientation in time and place, and lack of insight. Polyneuropathy, nystagmus, and ataxia may also be present, the latter two signs being related to earlier Wernicke episodes. The Korsakoff syndrome, however, can develop insidiously, with no clear prior history of a Wernicke episode.

Recent evidence suggests that the circuit involving the hippocampus, the mammillary bodies, the mammillo-thalamic tract, and the anterior (rather than the medial dorsal) nucleus of the thalamus, is particularly critical in the formation of new memories (Kopelman, 1995). Neuroimaging studies have reported a range of subcortical lesions and cortical atrophy. Functional imaging studies report impaired frontal cortical blood flow (Joyce, 1994).

Wernicke's encephalopathy responds to treatment with parenteral thiamine, but the amnesia of the Korsakoff syndrome does not generally respond. Alcohol problems are not the only cause of the disorder, but autopsy studies suggest that the Wernicke-Korsakoff syndrome occurs in about 2–3 % of 'alcoholics'.

These rather strange-sounding eponyms should not deflect the non-specialist from trying to understand what is being talked about and the following case abstract illustrates both how the acute element can present very suddenly and the type of chronic disorder that may occur when the Wernicke-Korsakoff syndrome supervenes.

A woman aged 48 years who had been drinking a bottle of whisky each day for 10 or more years was admitted to a psychiatric hospital for detoxification. It was noted that she was suffering from severe peripheral neuropathy (weakness, tingling, and pain in the legs). On the evening of admission, she was found to be rather confused, to be complaining of double vision, and to be staggering. By the next evening, she was stuporose, and her eye movements were unco-ordinated (external ocular palsies). At this stage, and much too late, she was started on massive doses of thiamine – the classical picture of confusion, staggering gait, and ocular palsies should have alerted the staff to the dangerous onset of Wernicke's encephalopathy. After five days of the acute illness, the confusion cleared and the patient was then found to have a grossly impaired memory for recent events, a tendency to make things up to fill her gaps in memory (confabulation), and very little ability to remember new information, as witnessed by her difficulty in finding her way around the ward. This amnesic syndrome (Korsakoff syndrome), showed little recovery over the ensuing months, and arrangements had to be made for the patient's transfer to long-term residential care.

This is a story of a tragedy that might have been averted, and there is a good argument for giving thiamine prophylactically to any patient who is in danger of this sort of complication.

Alcoholic pellagra encephalopathy

This is caused by a deficiency of nicotinic acid and its precursor trypto-phan. It is rarely reported in the British and US literature, perhaps because of the routine use of parenteral multi-vitamin therapy (Lishman, 1987). However, it is still evident in other countries, such as Japan. Clinical features include a fluctuating confusional state with global memory loss, visual hallucinations, restlessness alternating with apathy, and other neurological signs including myoclonic jerks and hyper-reflexia.

Alcoholic 'dementia'

Many individuals with a history of chronic alcohol misuse have mild to moderate impairment in short- and long-term memory, learning, visuo-spatial organisation, visuo-perceptual abstraction, maintenance of cognitive set, and impulse control (Oscar-Berman, 1990). Neuro-psychological tests improve with abstinence but some impairments may still be evident even five years later. With the advent of computer-ised tomographic (CT) scanning, cortical shrinkage (particularly in the frontal area) and ventricular enlargement have been confirmed in about two-thirds of 'alcoholics', compared with age-matched controls (Lishman, 1987). Abstinence was shown to lead to reversal of brain shrinkage, particular in younger individuals and in women. Neuropathological studies have shown that in comparison with controls, brain weight is significantly reduced in heavy drinkers at autopsy, with selective neuronal loss.

Magnetic Resonance Imaging (MRI) confirms cortical atrophy and mild ventricular enlargement, also volume reductions in various parts of the brain (Jernigan et al., 1991; Pfefferbaum, 1992). Functional imaging studies suggest a reduced cerebral blood flow within the medial frontal cortex. Implications of alcohol-related brain damage for the treatment of alcohol dependence are discussed on p. 100.

Central pontine myelinolysis

This is a rare disorder of cerebral white matter in the brain stem, which is seen in alcohol dependent individuals, but can also occur in malig-nancy, non-alcoholic liver disease, chronic renal disease, rapid correction of hyponatraemia, and other debilitating diseases (Charness, 1993). Clinical features include a pseudobulbar palsy and spastic or flaccid quadraplegia which evolves over a few days or weeks, often resulting in coma or death. Lesions can be visualised on scanning.

Marchiafava-Bignami disease

This rare disorder of the corpus callosum and adjacent white matter is again not confined to problem drinkers (Charness, 1993). A nutritional deficiency or a contaminent of alcohol have been postulated as cause. Presentation can either be acute with agitation, apathy, hallucinations, epilepsy, and coma, or insidious with dementia, spasticity, dysarthria, and inability to walk. Lesions can be visualised on scanning, but the diagnosis is usually made only at post-mortem.

Hepatic encephalopathy

In heavy drinkers with alcoholic liver disease the presenting and predominant clinical picture can be that of hepatic encephalopathy. This is a chronic organic reaction with psychiatric and neurological abnormalities that come and go and are extremely variable. Psychiatric features include impaired consciousness (ranging from hypersomnia to coma), delirium, impaired recent memory and mood swings. Liver function tests are usually abnormal and the EEG (electroencephalogram) shows a typical picture that can be extremely helpful in diagnosis.

Peripheral neuropathy

Alcoholic peripheral neuropathy is a sensorimotor neuropathy detectable in some degree among approximately 10% of chronic heavy drinkers. The main aetiological factors are thought to be vitamin B deficiency and the toxic effect of alcohol. The lower limbs are more frequently affected than the upper limbs and the typical presentation is with an insidious onset of weakness, pain, parasthesiae, and numbness in the feet, which progresses proximally and symmetrically in a 'glove and stocking' distribution. Bilateral foot drop and weakness of the small hand muscles and finger extensors may occur. Distal reflexes are usually absent. Treatment includes B group vitamins and abstinence. Recovery is usually slow and sometimes incomplete, with residual sensory loss.

Foetal alcohol syndrome

That the mother's drinking can cause foetal damage was widely believed in the nineteenth century, but was later to be forgotten or dismissed as temperance scaremongering. It is only over the last two decades or so that firm evidence has accumulated for the reality of the danger, and even so there are questions remaining as to the level of maternal drinking which carries risk. The distinctive syndrome is much more widely prevalent in the United States than in the UK, and it is unclear whether this reflects differing levels of awareness or a real difference in occurrence rate. Estimates even within the United States do, however, vary and the incidence of foetal alcohol syndrome (FAS) has been put as low as 0.33 cases per 1000 live births (Abel & Sokol 1991), or as high as 1.7 to 5.9 (Phillips *et al.*, 1989). Rates of FAS vary with ethnicity, socio-economic, and medical status.

The fully developed picture of FAS includes reduced growth and morphological abnormalities of the face and head (a small head, shortened eyelids, under-developed upper lip and flattened wide nose). Associated abnormalities include limb deformities and congenital heart disease. As they grow up these children remain small for their age and often have significant cognitive impairment. Cognitive deficits, together with concentration, attention, and behavioural problems, may handicap education or employment.

Alcohol-related birth defects which do not meet criteria for the full foetal alcohol syndrome are referred to as a foetal alcohol effect (FAE). Women who drink heavily during pregnancy also have increased rates of complications of pregnancy and delivery, of spontaneous abortion and stillbirth. The greatest risk to the foetus from the mother's drinking is probably within the first few weeks of conception.

The crucial public health question relates to what is meant by 'heavy drinking' in this context. It is not known what levels of pre-natal alcohol exposure produce what intensity of developmental problems. However, there is no doubt that a woman who is drinking at a level which implies her having developed alcohol dependence is at risk of damaging her baby. For any alcohol treatment service the practical message must be that a woman of child-bearing age who has a serious drinking problem requires very special counselling, and should be discouraged from having a baby until the drinking has been dealt with successfully. One has to think not only of the potential damage to an unborn child, but also of the lifetime guilt of the mother should a deformed child be born.

When one is seeking to advise as to what is the safe upper limit of drinking for a pregnant woman or a woman intending to have a child, the evidence from different studies is conflicting. It seems best at present to advise such women not to drink.

Skin disease

Heavy drinkers and individuals misusing alcohol are prone to a variety of skin disorders including psoriasis, discoid eczema, and superficial cutaneous fungal infections such as tinea pedis and pityriasis versicolor (Higgins & du Vivier, 1994). Rosacea and acne may be exacerbated by alcohol.

Psoriasis is a potentially alcohol-related skin condition which deserves special note. The daily alcohol consumption of men with psoriasis is higher than in men with other skin diseases and heavy drinking appears to be related to the severity of the disease (Poikolainen *et al.*, 1990). Two patterns of psoriasis are seen in heavy drinkers (Higgins & du Vivier, 1994). Alcohol-induced psoriasis will respond poorly to treatment unless the patient stops drinking.

The immune system

The immune system may be suppressed in heavy drinkers as a result of alcoholic liver damage, malnutrition, or as a direct effect of the action of alcohol (Dunne, 1988). Heavy drinkers are therefore prone to respiratory infections, including TB (see p. 135) but may also be at risk of both hepatitis and HIV infection. Alcohol-induced skin disorders, particularly fungal infections (see above) are also possibly mediated in part by the action of alcohol on the immune system.

Accidents

Alcohol is an underlying and frequently overlooked risk factor for accidents in the general population, not just in individuals with alcohol problems or alcohol dependence (Glucksman, 1994). Ingestion of alcohol causes diminished co-ordination and balance, increased reaction time, and impaired attention, perception, and judgement, all of which increase accidental injury (Cherpitel, 1993). Road traffic accidents in which alcohol is implicated are more serious than accidents in which it is not, and the risk of being involved in an accident rises as a function of the increased BAC. Approximately one-third of pedestrians killed in road traffic accidents by day have measurable BACs; the figure rises to approximately 70% for those killed at night. The literature on alcohol-related accidents has historically focused largely on road traffic accidents and drink-driving, but accidents in the home, work-place and civil aviation, and also leisure accidents such as drownings, now receive more prominence.

Studies from various countries suggest that drinking is involved in 26–54% of home and leisure injuries (Edwards *et al.*, 1994). It is particularly associated with violent family incidents (see p. 63) and is implicated in child abuse. Positive blood alcohol levels have been obtained in 40% of fatal industrial accidents and 35% of non-fatal work-related accidents.

Anaesthesia

It is worth entering a brief general reminder as to the potential importance of the patient's heavy drinking to the work of the anaesthetist both operatively and post-operatively (Payne, 1986). Emergency surgery may in particular run into difficulties if intoxication is overlooked and recovery complicated by a seizure or by other unexpected withdrawal symptoms. Tolerance to alcohol may result in cross-tolerance to certain anaesthetics, notably thiopentone.

The need for two kinds of alertness

This chapter started with the plea that everyone working with problem drinkers should be more aware of the physical element within the assessment and treatment plan. It should similarly be pleaded that everyone who works in the medical field should be vigilant as to the possibility of undeclared problem drinking being behind any one of a host of clinical presentations.

References

Abel, E. L. & Sokol, R. J. (1991). A revised conservative estimate of the incidence of FAS and its economic impact. *Alcoholism: Clinical and Experimental Research* **15**, 514–24.

Arria, A. M. & Van Thiel, D. H. (1992). The epidemiology of alcohol-related chronic disease. *Alcohol, Health and Research World* **16**, 209–16.

Anderson, P. (1995). Alcohol and risk of physical harm. In *Alcohol and Public Policy: Evidence and Issues*, ed. Holder, H. D. & Edwards, G., pp. 82–113. Oxford: Oxford University Press, Oxford.

Charness, M. E. (1993). Brain lesions in alcoholics. *Alcoholism: Clinical and Experimental Research* **17**, 2–11.

Cherpitel, C. (1993). Alcohol and injuries: a review of international emergency room studies. *Addiction* **88**, 923–37.

Chick, J. (1994). Alcohol problems in the general hospital. In *Alcohol and Alcohol Problems*, ed. Edwards, G. & Peters, T. J., pp. 200–10. British Medical Bulletin **50**. London: Churchill Livingstone.

Diamond, T., Stiel, D., Lunzer, M., Wilkinson, M. & Posen, S. (1989). Ethanol reduces bone formation and may cause osteoporosis. *The American Journal of Medicine*, **86**, 282–8.

Doherty, M. (1996). In *Oxford Textbook of Medicine*, ed. Weatherall, D. J., Ledingham, J. G. G. & Warrell, D. A., 3rd edn, vol. 3, pp. 2983–92. Oxford: Oxford University Press.

Dunne, F. (1989) Alcohol and the immune system. *British Medical Journal* **298**, 543–4.

Edwards, G., Anderson, P., Babor, T. F., Casswell, S., Ferrence, R., Giesbrecht, N. *et al.* (1994). *Alcohol Policy and the Public Good*. Oxford: Oxford University Press.

Glucksman, E. (1994). Alcohol and accidents. In *Alcohol and Alcohol Problems*, ed. Edwards, G. & Peters, T. J., pp. 76–84. British Medical Bulletin **50**. London: Churchill Livingstone.

Higgins, E. M. & du Vivier, A. W. P. (1994). Cutaneous disease and alcohol misuse. In *Alcohol and Alcohol Problems*, ed. Edwards, G. & Peters, T. J., pp. 85–98. *British Medical Bulletin*, **50**. London: Churchill Livingstone.

Imrie, C. W. (1996). Diseases of the pancreas: acute pancreatitis. In *Oxford Textbook of Medicine*, ed. Weatherall, D. J., Ledingham, J. G. G. & Warrell, D. A., 3rd edn, vol. 2, pp. 2027–34. Oxford: Oxford University Press.

James, O. F. W. (1996). Alcoholic liver disease. In *Oxford Textbook of Medicine*, ed. Weatherall, D. J., Ledingham, J. G. G. & Warrell, D. A., 3rd edn, vol 2, pp. 2080–5. Oxford: Oxford University Press.

Jeffcoate, W. (1993). Alcohol-induced pseudo-Cushing's syndrome. *Lancet* **341**, 676–7.

Jernigan, T. L., Butters, N., Di Traglia, G., Schafer, K., Smith, T., Irwin, M., Grant, I., Schuckit, M. & Cermak, L. S. (1991). Reduced cerebral gray matter observed in alcoholics using magnetic resonance imaging. *Alcoholism: Clinical and Experimental Research* **15**, 418–27.

Joyce, E. M. (1994). Aetiology of alcoholic brain damage: alcoholic neurotoxicity or thiamine malnutrition? In *Alcohol and Alcohol Problems*, ed. Edwards, G. & Peters, T. J., pp. 99–114. British Medical Bulletin **50**. London: Churchill Livingstone.

Kaplan, N. M. (1995). Alcohol and hypertension. *Lancet* **345**, 1588–9.

Kopelman, M. D. (1995). The Korsakoff Syndrome. *British Journal of Psychiatry* **166**, 154–73.

Koskinen, P. & Kupari, M. (1992). Alcohol and cardiac arrythmias. *British Medical Journal* **304**, 1394.

Lamminpaa, A. (1995). Alcohol intoxication in childhood and adolescence. *Alcohol and Alcoholism* **30**, 5–12.

Lieber, C. S. (1995). Medical disorders of alcoholism. *The New England Journal of Medicine* **333**, 1058–65.

Lishman, W. A. (1987). *Organic Psychiatry*, 2nd edn. Oxford: Blackwell Scientific Publications.

Longnecker, M. (1992). Alcohol consumption in relation to risk of cancers of the breast and large bowel. *Alcohol, Health and Research World* **16**, 223–9.

Lucey, M. R., Merion, R. M. & Beresford, T. P. (1994). *Liver Transplantation and the Alcoholic Patient: Medical, Surgical and Psychosocial Issues.* Cambridge: Cambridge University Press.

Misiewicz, J. J. & Pounder, R. E. (1996). Peptic ulceration. In *Oxford Textbook of Medicine*, ed. Weatherall, D. J., Ledingham, J. G. G. & Warrell, D. A., 3rd edn, vol. 2, pp. 1877–91. Oxford: Oxford University Press.

Moniz, C. (1994). Alcohol and bone. In *Alcohol and Alcohol Problems*, ed. Edwards, G. & Peters, T. J., pp. 67–75. *British Medical Bulletin* **50**, 67–75. London: Churchill Livingstone.

Oscar-Berman, M. (1990). Learning and memory deficits in detoxified alcoholics. *NIDA Research Monograph* **101**, 136–55.

Pfefferbaum, A., Lim, K. O., Zipursky, R. B., Mathalon, D. H., Rosenbloom, M. J., Lane, B., Ha, C. N. & Sullivan, E. V. (1992). Brain gray and white matter volume loss accelerates with aging in chronic alcoholics: a quantitative MRI study. *Alcoholism: Clinical and Experimental Research* **16**, 1078–89.

Poikolainen, K., Reunala, T., Karvonen, J., Lauharanta, J. & Karkkainen, P. (1990). Alcohol intake: a risk factor for psoriasis in young and middle aged men? *British Medical Journal* **300**, 780–3.

Payne, J. P. (1986). Anaesthesia and the problem drinker. *Hospital Update* **12**, 287–96.

Peters, T. J. (1996). Physical complications of alcohol misuse. In *Oxford Textbook of Medicine*, ed. Weatherall, D., Ledingham, J. G. G. & Warrell, D. A., 3rd edn, vol. 3, pp. 4276–8. Oxford: Oxford University Press.

Phillips, D. K., Henderson, G. I. & Schenker, S. (1989). Pathogensis of foetal alcohol syndrome. *Alcohol, Health and Research World* **13**, 219–27.

Preedy, V. R. & Richardson, P. J. (1994). Ethanol-induced cardiovascular disease. In *Alcohol and Alcohol Problems*, ed. Edwards, G. & Peters, T. J., pp. 152–163. British Medical Bulletin **50**. London: Churchill Livingstone.

Preedy, V. R. & Peters, T. J. (1990). Alcohol and skeletal muscle disease. *Alcohol and Alcoholism* **25**, 177–87.

Quaghebeur, G. & Richards, P. (1989). Comatose patients smelling of alcohol. *British Medical Journal* **299**, 410.

Rubin, E. & Urbano-Marquez, A. (1994). Alcoholic Cardiomyopathy. *Alcoholism: Clinical and Experimental Research* **18**, 111–14.

Saunders, J. B. (1987). Alcohol and hypertension. *British Medical Journal* **294**, 1045–6.

Scott, J. T. (1989). Alcohol and gout. *British Medical Journal* **298**, 1054.

Sherman, D. I. N. & Williams, R. (1994). Liver damage: mechanisms and management. In *Alcohol and Alcohol Problems*, ed. Edwards, G. & Peters, T. J., pp. 124–38. British Medical Bulletin **50**. London: Churchill Livingstone.

Stampfer, M. J., Colditz, G. A., Willett, W. C., Speizer, F. E. & Hennekens, C. H.

(1988). A prospective study of moderate alcohol consumption and the risk of coronary disease and stroke in women. *New England Journal of Medicine* **319**, 267–73.

Toskes, P. P. (1996). Diseases of the pancreas: chronic pancreatitis. In *Oxford Textbook of Medicine*, ed. Weatherall, D. J., Ledingham, J. G. G. & Warrell, D. A., 3rd edn, vol. 2, pp. 2034–9. Oxford: Oxford University Press.

Turner, R. C. (1996). Hypoglycaemia. In *Oxford Textbook of Medicine*, ed. Weatherall, D. J., Ledingham, J. G. G. & Warrell, D. A., 3rd edn, vol. 2, pp. 1505–12. Oxford: Oxford University Press.

Tuyns, A. J. (1991). Alcohol and cancer. An instructive association. *British Journal of Cancer* **64**, 415–16.

Urbano-Marquez, A., Estruch, R., Fernandez-Sola, J., Nicolas, J. M., Pare, J. C. & Rubin, E. (1995). The greater risk of alcoholic cardiomyopathy and myopathy in women compared with men. *JAMA* **274**, 149–54.

Weatherall, D. J. (1996). The blood in systemic disease. In *Oxford Textbook of Medicine*, ed. Weatherall, D. J., Ledingham, J. G. G. & Warrell, D. A., 3rd edn, vol. 3, pp. 3676–87. Oxford: Oxford University Press.

Xu, D., Dhillon, A. S. & Palmer, T. N. (1996). Metabolic effects of alcohol on skeletal muscle. *Addiction Biology* **1**, 143–55.

9

Women with drinking problems

Drinking patterns of women

In most cultures, women are less likely than men either to drink or to drink heavily. Those who do drink, consume alcohol less frequently than men and drink smaller amounts per drinking occasion. Social and cultural factors still exert a powerful influence on the pattern and degree of drinking in women, altering their vulnerability to the development of alcohol problems. Despite social and cultural changes there is still less social pressure on women to begin drinking and more pressure for them to stop.

However, society is harsh in its judgement of women with drinking problems. They are held in low-esteem, are perceived as having deserted the roles of wife and mother, and as being vulnerable to sexual promiscuity. Such misperceptions are often mirrored in the attitude of health professionals who view women with drinking problems in a negative light, as deviant personalities who are particularly untreatable. These attitudes have no place in the treatment setting.

We believe that the role of this chapter is rather especially to sensitise as well as inform, and thus to challenge the still too prevalent stereotyping of the woman who has a drinking problem. As for structure, we firstly provide a note on basic epidemiological findings. In the following section a range of factors that can be correlated with drinking problems among women is identified and risk factors across the life course are discussed. Attention is then given, in turn, to physical complications, psychosocial comorbidity and social complications. The treatment inferences emerging from this factual background are considered. Physiological factors that may predispose women to alcohol-related tissue vulnerability have already been discussed (pp. 22 and 127).

Epidemiology of alcohol problems in women

The five site Epidemiologic Catchment Area (ECA) study in the United States reported a 4.6% lifetime prevalence of DSM-III alcohol abuse or dependence in women (Helzer *et al.*, 1991). The corresponding figure for men was 23.8%, and rates were highest in the 18–29 and 30–44 year age groups for both sexes. In Great Britain, the Office of Population Censuses and Surveys (OPCS) estimates that 11% of women drink more than the recommended 'sensible' level of 14 units per week, of whom 2% are drinking very heavily, that is more than 35 units per week (OPCS, 1995). There is evidence of a modest decline in drinking amongst women in the United States throughout the 1980s – although the overall drinking rate has changed little, the proportion of heavy drinkers has decreased, and there has been a reduction in heavy episodic drinking.

Correlates of women with alcohol problems – a heterogeneous group

Women with alcohol problems are a heterogeneous population. Drinking behaviour in women is influenced by a number of demographic factors such as age, marital status, employment status, and ethnicity. These factors interact with other risk factors such as genetic predisposition (Kendler *et al.*, 1995) and environmental factors to determine the onset and course of drinking problems (Wilsnack *et al.*, 1994). Risk factors are summarised in Box 9.1.

Box 9.1. Some risk factors for problem drinking in women

- Positive family history

- Childhood problem behaviours related to impulse control

- Early use of nicotine, alcohol, and other drugs

- Poor coping responses in the face of stressful life events

- Depression

- Divorced/separated/cohabiting

- Heavy drinking partner

- Working in a male-dominated environment

- Sexual dysfunction

Age

Younger women have higher rates of heavy drinking and drinking problems than older women.

Marital Status

Never married, divorced, and separated women have the highest rates of heavy drinking and drinking problems. Married women have inter-mediate rates and widowed women the lowest. Divorce appears to put women without a drinking problem at greater risk for increased drink-ing but it may also provide a 'remedy' for women with established drinking problems, who appear to reduce their alcohol consumption following divorce (Wilsnack et al., 1994). Many surveys of women's drinking classify individuals who cohabit in the 'married' category but when analysed separately, cohabitation is strongly associated with problem drinking.

Employment

Contrary to expectation, there appears to be little relationship between full-time employment and alcohol problems in women (Wilsnack et al., 1994). Multiple roles (family, marriage, employment) appear to have a beneficial effect on women, reducing their risk for problem drinking. However, women working in male-dominated environments are more likely to drink heavily and to have drinking problems. Peer influence, increased drinking opportunities, and the stress of working in a male-dominated culture have been invoked as reasons for this (Wilsnack & Wilsnack, 1993).

Race and ethnicity

In the USA white women are most likely to drink, African-American the least, and Hispanic women are intermediate. Little is known about the cultural and ethnic differences in drinking amongst women in the UK.

Drinking partner

Women appear to be more influenced by the drinking habits of their male partners than vice versa (Wilsnack & Wilsnack, 1993).

Childhood sexual abuse and relationship violence

Women with drinking problems have higher rates of childhood sexual abuse and are more likely than other women to have experienced physical violence, either as children or adults. Women are often in violent relationships with men when they enter treatment. Distressing and vivid memories of childhood sexual abuse and rape may resurface during abstinence. Post-traumatic stress disorder (PTSD) resulting from childhood sexual abuse is best treated at the same time as the alcohol problem.

Sexual experience

Sexual dysfunction may contribute to the chronicity of excessive drinking in women. Problem drinking amongst women may be associated with risky sexual behaviour, putting them at high risk for HIV/AIDS. This is particularly true of women with poly-drug use who may share injecting equipment with their partners and engage in high rates of unprotected sex.

Depression

Depression is more likely to be associated with chronicity of problem drinking amongst women than as a risk factor for the onset of problem drinking (Wilsnack *et al.*, 1991). However, depression may also precede problem drinking (Helzer *et al.*, 1991).

Stressful life events

Negative life events during childhood and adolescence (death of a parent, economic deprivation, illness in the family) may predispose to drinking as a coping style to relieve stress. The way in which women respond to such events in early life may be the critical factor in determining whether they go on to develop an alcohol problem (Gomberg & Nirenberg, 1993).

Poly-drug use

Many women with alcohol problems also have significant drug problems and dependence. In the 1970s and 1980s prescription drugs such as minor tranquillisers and sedatives were typically used, but illicit drugs such as cannabis, cocaine, other stimulants, and hallucinogens are becoming increasingly common, particularly in women under the age of 30 years (see also Chapter 7).

Risk factors across the life-span

Although most risk factors are relevant to all age groups, some are more specific to certain stages in the life cycle. Peer influence plays a greater role amongst female adolescents than amongst their male counterparts (Wilsnack *et al.*, 1994). During their 20s and 30s, the time of career, marriage, and child bearing, women frequently alter their drinking patterns. Infertility, post-natal depression, marital or other relationship breakdown, bereavement, and physical illness are all factors which may influence drinking behaviour at this stage. Different stresses in the 40s and 50s may also influence drinking behaviour, including marital or relationship break-up, lack of employment, departure of children, and loss of attractiveness.

Physical complications

Women are at greater risk of certain physical complications associated with heavy drinking than are men and complications develop earlier in their drinking careers (Dunne, 1988). These include liver disease, cardiomyopathy, myopathy, and brain damage (see chapters 2 and 8). Chronic heavy drinking is also associated with inhibition of ovulation, infertility, and a wide variety of gynaecological and obstetric problems (Blume, 1992). Heavy alcohol consumption during pregnancy is associated with spontaneous abortion, intrauterine growth retardation, FAS and FAE (see chapter 8). Treatment programmes must therefore pay special attention to the physical health and pregnancy status of women. Women with alcohol problems have a considerable excess mortality when compared with their male counterparts and the general population.

Psychological comorbidity

Both men and women with drinking problems have high rates of associated psychiatric disturbance (see Chapter 6). A consistent finding of clinical studies is that depression is more commonly diagnosed in women with alcohol problems. Women also have higher rates of anxiety disorder, psychosexual dysfunction, and bulimia (Ross *et al.*, 1988). Even socially intact women with drinking problems, early in their treatment careers, have high levels of mood and anxiety disorders (Haver & Dahlgren, 1995).

Social complications

Women with alcohol problems often drink alone at home, thus reducing the likelihood that their problem will be uncovered, and increasing the risk of social isolation. Women drinkers report more marital problems than their male counterparts. Children are more likely to be taken into care, particularly if the mother is a single parent, or her partner is also a heavy drinker.

More women now live independently and own their own cars and drive, and recent studies report an increased crash risk for women who drink and drive. This may be due in part to the fact that women metabolise alcohol differently from men and have higher BACs for a given volume of alcohol consumed (see Chapter 2). It is also possible that women are more sensitive than men to the effects of alcohol on driving performance.

Three clinical vignettes

The illustrations given below point to just three among a host of different ways in which a woman may present with a drinking problem.

Early onset and progression to physical disaster

Ms A was a shy woman from a privileged background. Her father and paternal grandmother were both problem drinkers. She began to drink and smoke when she was aged 15 at her parents' cocktail parties and found that she could tolerate alcohol well and that it gave her confidence. After school she did an Arts degree, and lived a student life to the full, drinking most evenings and bingeing at weekends. She married in her mid-twenties, but by this time early signs of alcohol dependence were evident. She had a successful career as a media consultant, but following a series of miscarriages and the breakdown of her marriage, she became depressed and her drinking escalated. She lost her job when she was 35 because of absenteeism and going to work intoxicated. She did not present to the treatment services until she was 40, but by this time she had alcoholic cirrhosis and alcohol-related brain damage, and was living in a squat with a partner who also had an alcohol problem. She died of liver failure shortly after.

An alcohol problem following sexual abuse

Ms B, a 32-year-old woman, was referred for treatment by her GP. She was one of nine children and her early life was one of poverty and deprivation. Her mother was an invalid, and her father, a labourer, sexually abused her and her two sisters when they were between the ages of 5 and 16 years. She began to drink whisky at the age of 13 years and soon found that it anaesthetised her 'raw emotional pain' and made life bearable. She left school at 15 and worked as a waitress in a restaurant. She enjoyed her work and was well-liked by patrons. Her drinking, however, increased and by the time she was 25-years-old she was drinking every day, both at lunch time and in the evening. She lost her job and began to drink in local parks. Two attempts at in-patient treatment failed because horrific and unbearable memories of her childhood sexual abuse emerged with abstinence.

A problem of later onset

Mrs C, a 56-year-old woman, was referred for treatment by her GP who reported in the referral letter that her husband, 'a good man', could no longer cope with her drinking and was threatening to leave her. Mrs C was a quiet person who worked as a cleaner. She had been a devoted mother to her three sons and was proud that they were doing well in life. However, their leaving home had left an emptiness and loneliness and she realised that she had little in common with her husband, who was himself a heavy drinker. She had always been close to her mother who, until her death five years previously, had lived near-by. Following her mother's death she became depressed and began to drink sherry. Her consumption had increased slowly over the years and she was now consuming about one bottle per day.

Treatment issues

Barriers to help-seeking and detection

Although the numbers of women presenting to alcohol treatment services has increased over recent years, they still under-use such resources (Blume, 1992). The failure to seek help may reflect barriers, either real or perceived, which are specific to women. Moralistic societal attitudes and the social stigma associated with drinking problems are important. Often women do not see drinking as their primary problem and present with associated health and psychosocial problems, such as depression (Thom, 1986). The fear of stigma and social disapproval may prevent them from approaching a GP or local community alcohol team. Drinking partners may discourage or actively prevent help-seeking. Low self-esteem may lead women with drinking problems to believe that they are not worthwhile. Sometimes their needs are so basic (housing, money, clothing, food) that more specific help is deferred.

Lack of resources to arrange child care or fear of removal of their children are very potent barriers. All too often children have been removed already and life is so bleak that treatment seems worthless. Opposition from friends and family and negative professional attitudes can also play a part.

Barriers to engaging in and remaining in treatment

Women with alcohol problems are often regarded as more deviant and personality disordered, more difficult to help and less motivated than their male counterparts. Confrontational techniques may be harmful and compound feelings of anxiety, low self-esteem, and depression (Beckman, 1994). They are likely to receive less support from their partners and families and lack of adequate child care facilities. Often the treatment is not tailored sufficiently to their needs. For instance a woman with a history of childhood sexual abuse will find it difficult to cope on an in-patient unit where she is the only woman. There is considerable debate as to whether women are better served in a women-only treatment programme or a 'mixed' facility (Dahlgren & Willander, 1989). It is possible that women-only services have a role in attracting women of particular backgrounds into treatment, possibly women with dependent children, lesbians, women with a maternal history of a drug or alcohol problem, and those who have suffered childhood sexual abuse.

Treatment outcomes

There is a prevailing assumption that women with alcohol problems have poorer outcomes than men. However, closer scrutiny of the literature reveals that women are under-represented in treatment outcome research (Vannicelli & Nash, 1984) and that outcomes are often similar. There is a suggestion that women do better in the first year after treatment, whereas men have better results at follow-up after 12 months. Women may be better than men at using self-help material to reduce heavy or problem drinking (Sanchez-Craig et al., 1989).

Very few studies have examined the factors that predict outcome in women with drinking problems. Factors from women-only samples associated with poor outcome include marital problems prior to treatment, a dysfunctional relationship with an important person, few primary relationships prior to treatment and multiple life problems (MacDonald, 1987), a history of delirium tremens, early onset of the drink problem, unemployment, antisocial personality disorder, and not living with a husband (Smith & Cloninger, 1984). These matters are summarised in Box 9.2. Paradoxically women with major depressive disorders and alcohol dependence have better outcomes than women with no other psychiatric diagnosis (Rounsaville *et al.*, 1987).

Box 9.2. Factors predicting poor outcomes in women with drinking problems

- Early onset

- Few primary relationships prior to treatment

- Multiple life problems

- Dysfunctional relationship with an important person

- Unemployment

- A history of delirium tremens

Fundamental commonalities

Whatever the differences that men and women bring to the origins and presentations of their drinking problems, whatever the special sensitivities needed to analyse and appreciate the position of the woman with a drinking problem, and whatever the special issues which the treatment of the woman with the drinking problem may raise, there is fundamentally much in common between the male and female drinker. Men and women equally need individual understanding and individual help unhampered by stereotypes.

References

Beckman, J. L. (1994). Treatment needs of women with alcohol problems. *Alcohol Health and Research World* **18**, 206–11.

Blume, S. B. (1992). Alcohol and other drug problems in women. In *Substance Abuse, a Comprehensive Textbook*, ed. Lowinson, J. H., Ruiz, P. & Millman, R. B., 2nd edn. Baltimore: Williams and Wilkins.

Dahlgren, L. & Willander, A. (1989). Are special treatment facilities for female alcoholics needed? A controlled 2-year follow-up study from a specialized female unit (EWA) versus a mixed male/female treatment facility. *Alcoholism: Clinical and Experimental Research* **13**, 499–505.

Dunne, F. (1988). Are women more easily damaged by alcohol than men? *British Journal of Addiction* **83**, 1135–6.

Gomberg, E. S. L. & Nirenberg, T. D. (1993). Antecedents and consequences. In *Women and Substance Abuse*, ed. Gomberg, E. S. L. & Nirenberg, T. D., pp. 118–41. New Jersey: Ablex Publishing.

Haver, B. & Dahlgren, L. (1995). Early treatment of women with alcohol addiction (EWA): a comprehensive evaluation and outcome study. I. Patterns of psychiatric comorbidity at intake. *Addiction* **90**, 101–9.

Helzer, J. E., Burnam, A. & McEvoy, L. (1991.) Alcohol abuse and dependence. In *Psychiatric Disorders in America: The Epidemiological Catchment Area Study*, ed. Robins, L. N. & Regier, D. A., pp. 81–115. New York: Free Press.

Kendler, K. S., Walters, E. E., Neale, M. C., Kessler, R. C., Heath, A. C. & Eaves, L. J. (1995). The structure of the genetic and environmental risk factors for six major psychiatric disorders in women. *Archives of General Psychiatry* **52**, 374–83.

MacDonald, J. G. (1987). Predictors of treatment outcome for alcoholic women. *International Journal of the Addictions* **22**, 235–48.

Office of Population Censuses and Surveys (1995). *General Household Survey 1992*. Series GHS No.23. London: OPCS.

Ross, H. E., Glaser, F. B. & Stiasny, S. (1988). Sex differences in the prevalence of psychiatric disorders in patients with alcohol and drug problems. *British Journal of Addiction* **83**, 1179–92.

Rounsaville, B. J., Dolinsky, Z. S., Babor, T. F. & Meyer, R. E. (1987). Psychopathology as a predictor of treatment outcome in alcoholics. *Archives of General Psychiatry* **44**, 505–13.

Sanchez-Craig, M., Leigh, G., Spivak, K. & Lei, H. (1989). Superior outcome of females over males after brief treatment for the reduction of heavy drinking. *British Journal of Addiction* **84**, 395–404.

Smith, E. M. & Cloninger, C. R. (1984). A prospective twelve-year follow-up of alcoholic women: a prognostic scale for long-term outcome. *National Institute of Drug Abuse Research Monograph Issues* **55**, 245–51.

Thom, B. (1986). Sex differences in help-seeking for alcohol problems. I. The barriers to help seeking. *British Journal of Addiction* **81**, 777–88.

Vannicelli, M. & Nash, L. (1984). Effect of sex bias on women's studies on alcoholism. *Alcoholism: Clinical and Experimental Research* **8**, 334–6.

Wilsnack, S. C., Wilsnack, R. W. & Hiller-Sturmhofel (1994). How women drink. Epidemiology of women's drinking and problem drinking. *Alcohol Health and Research World* **18**, 173–84.

Wilsnack, S. C. & Wilsnack, R. W. (1993). Epidemiological research on women's drinking: recent progress and directions for the 1990s. In *Women and Substance Abuse*, ed. Gomberg, E. S. L. & Nirenberg, T. D., pp. 62–99. New Jersey: Ablex Publishing.

Wilsnack, S. C., Klassen, A. D., Schur, B. E. & Wilsnack, R. W. (1991). Predicting onset and chronicity of women's problem drinking: a five year longitudinal analysis. *American Journal of Public Health* **81**, 305–18.

10

Some special presentations

This chapter gives nine special clinical presentations: the patient with impaired brain function; the person who is drunk and violent; the situation where a child is at risk; the younger person with a drinking problem; a drinking problem in later life; the patient who comes from a culture other than the therapist's; the situation where it is a concerned family member rather than the patient who is making contact; a presentation on a general hospital ward; and, finally, what may be called 'the very important patient'. These pictures are selected arbitrarily from a much wider gallery, and anyone who practises in this field will themselves soon begin to identify additional headings. To keep a mental card index which allows one to see patterns of presentation and use the last such case to illuminate understanding of the next, will add to the reward and interest of therapeutic work. The only proviso to be borne in mind is the latent danger of forcing people into pigeonholes; management of the next elderly patient will be helped by thinking through one's previous case experience with individuals in this age group, but each new patient is different.

The patient with impaired brain function

A description of the brain pathologies that can result from excessive use of alcohol has been given in Chapter 8. Here discussion will focus on the everyday clinical implications of the fact that brain damage will in some patients compromise their ability to respond to and engage in the usually available treatment programmes. The following passage gives a nurse's report on a 50-year-old man with a long history of alcohol dependence.

He gets everyone else irritated in the group. He doesn't seem to listen to what other people say and then butts in with his own views, saying exactly the same as he said yesterday and the day before. Things like, 'If you keep yourself tidy and clean you've got no problem'. I don't think that after three weeks he even knows anyone else's name.

That observation might be evidence of a particular patient's habitual conversational style but it must also raise a warning flag as to the possibility of brain damage. Subsequent psychological testing with this patient and a scan confirmed this suspicion.

Gross brain damage is not likely to set difficulties in recognition (see p. 140). What has to be cultivated is an alertness to lesser but still clinically important degrees of brain impairment. The problem can present with various severities, but the picture given by the patient who was identified as having difficulties in functioning in the group is fairly typical. There is often some mild sense of the patient's social awareness being blunted, of their not being good at taking in new ideas or information, of their memory for newly learnt material being impaired (hence that patient's difficulty with remembering names), and there may also be difficulty in sustaining concentration.

Ward observation and watching the patient's behaviour in groups can be helpful diagnostically as can a report from an occupational therapist. In many instances recovery in functioning can take place over weeks or months and serial assessments are therefore needed – testing carried out immediately after detoxification can give misleadingly pessimistic results. Beyond the ward observation and routine mental state examination (simple tests of memory and concentration), a full assessment will involve skilled psychological testing and brain imaging.

If testing and a brain scan confirm the presence of significant impairment and damage (the two assessment approaches are complimentary), and if repeated assessment demonstrates that recovery is likely to be incomplete, the implications for clinical management must be considered. A patient who is experiencing cognitive difficulties will become frustrated by a demanding therapeutic regime. The best therapeutic programmes involve a great deal of new learning, emotional awareness, and social interaction, and it is in exactly the skills needed to engage successfully in those types of experience in which the brain-damaged patient may be deficient. If sympathetic note is not taken of their special needs and handicaps they will either go through the programme without benefit or more probably they will break therapeutic contact.

A programme that acknowledges the needs of this type of patient cannot be formulated on a one-off basis but must be designed by interaction with the patient concerned. Would it be helpful for them to have individual discussions which identify the core simplicities of their personal recovery programme? Would they be helped by written material or by making out checklists?

On return to their own home from the ward, thought must be given to the special after-care needs of such a patient and their family. The programme should put therapeutic emphasis on management of external and situational factors such as arranging how money is to be controlled, how time is to be spent, how work or sheltered employment is to be found, and how the local liquor stores are to be persuaded to be proscriptively helpful.

The patient who is drunk and violent

The general issue of the relation between drinking and violence is discussed elsewhere in this book (p. 74). Every now and then a therapist will be faced by the worrying problem set by the patient who repeatedly turns up drunk and violent and demanding to be seen. The safety of staff and other patients may be at risk, and an enormous amount of anxiety can be engendered. If an alcohol treatment service is coexisting closely with other facilities, it will acquire a bad name if disruption is allowed to get out of hand.

> A 40-year-old man after a long drinking history had been thrown out of his own home, and was now drifting around temporary accommodation or sleeping rough. Over a period of six months he was twice admitted to hospital but on each occasion came back drunk onto the ward, assaulted the nurses, and smashed the furniture. A few days after his last discharge he came up to the hospital late at night and got into a fight with a porter. He then arrived at out-patients drunk and demanding admission, with threats of further violence if admission was not granted.

In such circumstances there are two courses of action that are anti-therapeutic and should not be followed. The first of these is to tolerate further violence or threat of violence. The patient will not be helped, the morale of the treatment service will be torn apart, and staff may indeed be hurt. The second non-answer is to ban the patient from the hospital. Even if the banning is successful, it will only transfer the problem of violence onto someone else's doorstep, and things will not look too good if a week later the man is on an assault charge with the court told that a hospital has abrogated its responsibilities.

Such a problem is dealt with more easily by a treatment service than by anyone working in isolation. A hospital, for instance, ought to be able to meet this type of problem and the GP and other local services will not be grateful if the hospital seeks to pass the buck. What is needed is a firm treatment policy drawn up for this individual, and one which sets explicit limits but which is none the less a treatment rather than a mere containment policy. It must reward constructive behaviour and in no way reinforce unacceptable behaviour, and it must be communicated fairly and openly to the patient themselves, put at the front of the case-notes, and a copy given to all staff who may be involved. It is useful to hold a staff meeting for formulation of the plan so that things go forward by agreement, and with everyone fully in the picture. It may be wise to ensure that the organisation's administrative staff are consulted, with a legal opinion obtained if necessary.

On the basis of consultation a memo such as the following might be put into the case-notes of the man whose story has just been sketched.

Mr Smith: agreed treatment plan
So that we can go on helping this patient within a treatment programme the following guidelines have been agreed by the treatment team, and we would be grateful if everyone will give this plan support.
(1) Mr Smith will only be seen by appointment, and if he comes up without an appointment he should be asked to leave.
(2) He will then only be seen at appointment if he is not intoxicated. If there is any suspicion of intoxication he will be asked to leave without being seen further.
(3) If Mr Smith refuses to leave when asked, or if he threatens or offers violence, help should be summoned through the hospital's usual emergency system and the police should be telephoned. The number is . . . and the police station has been alerted. On no account should an individual staff member attempt to argue with this patient.
(4) Mr Smith has been told that if he commits any chargeable offence on the hospital premises, the hospital will not hesitate to press charges.
(5) These ground rules have been explained to Mr Smith personally, and they have been set up not only to protect the staff but also so as to make it possible for us to go on working with this patient within a constructive treatment plan.

Contained within those seemingly harsh guidelines is a plan designed to enable the team to go on offering help to a man who would probably be rejected by many centres as unhelpable. In practice this drawing of limits is reassuring to the patient. A disorganised and inconsistent response, which may even involve a sort of complicity with his violence, is likely to exacerbate anxiety and violence, whereas a firm policy often results in the patient showing a capacity to go along with constructive expectations. They are able to come to appointments sober, and make a new and positive therapeutic engagement. Things do not, however, always run smoothly, and if the patient does turn up drunk and tries to hit someone, a charge may have to be brought, for otherwise no learning can take place. To be able to use the police therapeutically requires careful liaison with the local police force.

With the immediate threat of violence contained, it should be possible to get down to an individually planned and positive treatment programme. Violence is then no longer the central issue, and the patient's reputation should not be allowed to overshadow therapeutic dealings. There will be need to talk about the violence, and the patient has to come to terms with the full implications of the fact that alcohol for them releases violent feelings.

The problem has also to be met as to how flexibly the stated rules are to be interpreted in certain difficult circumstances. For instance, if there is anxiety about the possibility of head injury, a deterioration in the patient's physical condition, or concern as to whether underlying mental illness is now hidden within the picture, appropriate help should be obtained. There has therefore to be an understanding that individual clinical judgement allows a flexible response to emergency, but the team should whenever possible be brought into the decision or promptly informed as to what has been done. There are some patients who pose extreme threats of violence and staff safety and public safety should then be the paramount consideration without prevarication or apology.

A child at risk

There has over recent years been a sharp increase in public anxiety about the risks to which children may be subjected as a result of parental violence or sexual abuse. Such anxieties provide the context within which Social Service departments will deal with the sensitive problems that arise when a parent's drinking appears to put a young child's safety at risk (see also pp. 62–4).

> Mr and Mrs B had met when they were both patients in an Alcoholism Treatment Unit. He was aged 35, she 30 and they had both experienced deprived childhoods and chaotic adult life histories. In their recovery they gave each other a great deal of mutual understanding, and they started to live together. Seen three years later they reported much improvement but they would still periodically relapse into short bouts of drinking. At these times they were sometimes violent to each other, the furniture was apt to be broken and the police had been called on several occasions. They now had an 18-month-old daughter and the neighbours had reported their concern about the safety of this child to the authorities.

The issues that are being dealt with in this section overlap with the previous discussion of the patient who was drunk and violent, but a new and worrying element is introduced when a child is at risk (Sherr, 1991). Every such case must be approached differently, but guidelines can be helpful.

The child's safety and welfare must come first

In any decision-making around this case, that simple rule of priority must never be lost from sight.

Do not panic, but err on the side of caution

No one would wish reflexly to put every child into care where there is a history of parental drinking or drunken violence, but at the same time it would be culpable to engage in an extended process of leisurely assessment rather than taking firm emergency action in those instances where the safety of the child requires immediate placement in care.

Try to work with, rather than against, the parents

This advice will seem obvious to the experienced case-worker. The parents may feel guilty about and frightened by their own behaviour and their failure adequately to care for a child who is precious to them. Any threat of having that child taken away is likely to cause a reaction not only in terms of self-blame but of angry projected blame of other people. The parents need therefore so far as possible to be helped into a position where they can accept that everyone is working constructively together for a resolution of the problem.

Assess the total background family situation and interactions rather than focus only on the drinking

In the case which has been outlined above there was evidence that when both parents were sober they cared for their child lovingly and competently. When sober the relationship between the parents was also a happy one and whenever they could obtain a baby-sitter they went to AA meetings together. There was no suggestion of violence other than in the setting of drunkenness.

Assess the parental drinking history and the likely consequences of the drinking for the child

Drinking bouts in this family tended to last about three to five days, with one parent's drinking sparking off drinking in the other partner, although sometimes one would drink and the other stay sober. There was evidence that several months (sometimes as long as six months), could elapse without a bout occurring. There had never been any indication of intentional violence to the child, but she had on one occasion been accidentally knocked to the floor. She had also been left neglected and crying in a bedroom when both parents were drinking and rowing. Drunken driving may also cause concern when the child is at risk as a passenger.

Examination of the child

Assessment is not complete without a physical and developmental assessment of the child. This is usually best conducted by a child psychiatrist or a paediatrician. A social worker will also usually be involved in assessing the child. In the case we are describing the little girl showed no abnormalities.

Setting up an appropriate level of safeguard and monitoring

The appropriate level of safeguard must depend on the individual situation and can range from the emergency decision to take a child into care to putting that child on the 'at risk' register, or even some lesser level of intervention. In the present circumstances it was felt that there was a small but real danger of the child coming to accidental harm if the parents continued to drink and fight in this explosive fashion. They agreed to strict supervision, and each decided to take disulfiram and attend a hospital out-patient group. It was agreed that their ability to look after their child would have to be viewed as dependent on their continued sobriety. Twelve months later they had remained abstinent and made good therapeutic progress.

Not every such story has a happy outcome. Circumstances may arise when a child has to be taken into care, but the hope may then still be that a constructive and monitored programme can be set up which allows the parents to work towards getting their child back.

This discussion has been in terms of a situation where both parents have a drinking problem. Situations also of course arise when only one parent is drinking or where there is drinking and a single-parent family.

The young drinker

In many countries a common experience over recent years has been the increasingly frequent presentation of young people (including young women) with drinking problems. 'Young' may in extreme instances mean the early teens, but the particular focus of this discussion will be on patients in the late teens or early twenties. More significant than the exact boundaries of chronological age is the fact that these are people who in an important sense see themselves as *not adult*, and who have not made the social transition from adolescent to adult self-image. The therapist is encountering a person who is still finding a way through adolescent conflicts, and who has not resolved fundamental questions about the balance between dependence on others and independence. For the anxiety, anger, and despair which may be generated by these frustrations, alcohol can be a panacea. It temporarily relieves a painful confusion of feelings, provides at the same time a 'high' of optimism and excitement, while in a state of intoxication the aggressive feelings can be liberated and acted out, and with the natural energy and physicality of this age adding intensity to all this chaos. Moreover, drinking can give companionship and the approbation of peers.

As for the pattern of alcohol use itself, in most instances the young person will not have had a drinking history of sufficient duration for established alcohol dependence. The picture is of repeated drinking to the point of intoxication, often with experience of amnesias.

Possibilities for growth

There is a common belief that severe personality disorder is likely to be associated with a drinking problem of early onset, and a diagnosis of underlying psychopathy is readily pinned on to the patient. But it is important to realise that the immaturity of the behaviour often speaks to the *possibility* of change. There is the paradox with this type of disturbance that the very unformedness of personality can itself bear witness to potential for growth. A uniformly pessimistic attitude towards the prognosis of the young drinker is therefore unjustified, even when their behaviour is flagrantly disturbed. A brief case history on one such young person whose story typifies this kind of presentation follows.

> A 22-year-old man was referred to a counselling centre by the court. He had been charged with assault after a pub fight, and he had also broken a few windows. There had been several suicide gestures. He had been working in a garage but had been sacked. His drinking involved his becoming explosively and obstreperously drunk whenever he had money in his pocket. He had been forced to leave his parental home at the age of 19 because of his rowdy drunkenness, and his respectable parents did not want him back. Five years after being seen at this centre he had a steady job in the Post Office and was happily married. He now drank occasionally and moderately. He looked back on his past as distant, and saw it in terms of 'I was all messed up at that time'.

What needs to be emphasised is that while pessimism is often self-fulfilling, a treatment approach which responds hopefully to the needs for growth may catch a moment of possibility. There is no one recipe for treatment in this type of case, and the basic approach will have much in common with what is done to help the patient of any age. This young man discovered a capacity to talk about his problems and was helped by a counsellor who was able to arrange her schedule so that she had time to see him whenever he dropped in for an hour's talk – he needed to do a lot of talking. He also benefited from a six-month residence in a therapeutic hostel and from a set of friendships which developed from that stay. Later, he was lucky to meet the right partner. In essence what these various relationships offered, each in their own way, was a series of experiments in facets of growing up. If there are common ingredients in such stories of therapeutic success they lie in the qualities of the therapist – someone who is specially and evidently warm, who will be able to tolerate projection of unworked-out feelings towards parents, but who will not be manoeuvred into treating the patient as a child. There is also often a need to find a way of helping this type of young person pull out of a pattern of living (or pattern of drifting) which is a series of makeshifts rather than one which offers either real demands or real rewards.

Special difficulties

Having taken as an illustration a case with a happy outcome, it is necessary also to look at reasons why the story may on other occasions be turbulent or marked by nothing but defeat. One reason may be that the personal handicaps are already more fixed, a matter of psychological damage rather than of frustrated growth. The young man or woman who is profoundly anxious, restless and irritable, who cannot easily use or tolerate a relationship of any kind, who will not stay in a job and who is likely to disappear to another town or go off to sea, is going to be difficult to help. Even so, it is worthwhile holding out the availability of friendship, with the modest expectation of working for small immediate gains and taking a very long-term view.

Another reason for special difficulty, grossly evident or only revealed by assessment, is when excessive drinking in someone of this age is symptomatic of brain damage (see pp. 98–9). A further common diagnostic perplexity is the interpretation to be made when a client in this age group reports 'being depressed'. Most often this complaint is to be understood in terms of the general lability of mood which so often accompanies problems in development. On the one hand, it is a mistake to over diagnose depressive illness or inappropriately to prescribe antidepressant drugs. On the other hand, there are cases where recurrent depressive illness may first declare itself at this age, and where this distress leads to use of alcohol as self-medication.

Yet another type of story is that of the young man or woman who is referred to an alcohol clinic because drinking has been seen as the problem. It then becomes apparent that one is dealing with a major psychiatric illness, the exact nature of which is perplexingly difficult to diagnose. The picture shifts perhaps from that of depression to a presentation that looks worryingly like schizophrenia. The excessive use of alcohol is no more than a confounding factor in a very complex disturbance.

Drinking problems at this age may be accompanied by drug problems, with alcohol being but one substance in a pattern of multiple drug use. The story may, for instance, be of the lad who was drinking heavily at 14 years of age and who later turned to injected drugs, returning once more to heavy alcohol use after giving up injected heroin. Enquiry into the history of drug taking is therefore particularly important in this age group (see Chapter 7).

Taking the problems of the young drinker very seriously

With these young patients there are a number of reasons for arguing with special force the general position that earlier rather than later intervention is to be preferred. They should be helped before dependence supervenes. The young drinker who is left to run deeper into trouble is in danger of becoming increasingly unemployable. It must also be remembered that it is particularly among young drinkers that mortality rates are elevated, often as a consequence of accident or violence (see p. 177). There are therefore good reasons for taking the young drinker seriously.

Alcohol problems in later life

A long-standing history of excessive drinking continuing into old age may often be marked by brain damage, and other physical complications and nutritional neglect are common. The drinking pattern may have become fragmented compared with previous years, and loss of tolerance to alcohol is a frequent manifestation (see pp. 45–6).

In contrast is the elderly patient who has taken to excessive drinking as a response to a problem or cluster of difficulties which he or she has encountered only recently. Widowhood, retirement, and a general loss of purpose in life are often important factors in the onset of a drinking problem at this age. The possible significance of underlying brain disease or of depressive illness should also be considered as cause of a late onset problem.

The division of the drinking problems that occur in this epoch of life into those of early and late onset is clinically useful and carries implications for management of the problem. A not unusual story is of the seemingly late onset condition being found to have a much longer background history on closer enquiry. Many of the basic features can, however, be the same whether the onset of the problem was remote or recent, and one should be aware of elements that can very generally colour the presentation at this age. For instance, there is often the likelihood of social isolation. The psychiatric picture may give rise to diagnostic confusion – delirious states are common in the elderly and at this time of life depression and a degree of brain impairment often go together. There are often multiple physical pathologies.

Help for the older patient

Basic principles have to be borne in mind, but for patients in this age group special skills will be needed to design a treatment plan that effectively responds to their situation in life (Janik & Dunham, 1983; Hinrichsen, 1984; Koford et al., 1987; Fitzgerald & Mulford, 1992). This implies a knowledge of the local resources that are available to help the elderly, including clubs, day centres, home helps, community nurses, and so on. Mobilising whatever family support is available can also be important. The patient may be ambivalent about surrendering independence, but sheltered accommodation can provide companionship and enable better adjustment than continued isolation. Initial hospital admission may be needed for diagnosis, but it should not be too prolonged. The sensitivity of the ageing nervous system to drugs should be borne in mind with tranquillisers or sedatives used only in the short-term and with caution. Disulfiran is too dangerous at this age. Some older people will join AA, but that kind of group experience is usually difficult to utilise at that age.

Whatever the specifics of therapy, the non-specifics are again important, including the warmth, the hopefulness, and the goal-setting. An elderly person may need things explained slowly, positions explored, and solutions negotiated at an acceptable pace. Abrupt and clumsy interference will be met deservedly with tetchiness, and there will be no therapeutic gain.

The approach to old-age drinking problems still tends sometimes to be negatively influenced by a gulf in understanding, 'Well, drink is all she's got, and if she drinks herself to death . . .'. Such attitudes are unjustified. Elderly people with drinking problems can be helped, with large benefit in terms of health, enjoyment of life, and dignity.

The patient from a cultural background other than the therapist's

'I don't understand him at all,' said the community psychiatric nurse who was reporting on a visit to her patient's home. 'He is a Pakistani who owns a fruit shop, aged about 60, very much the head of the family, two grown-up sons who help in the business and take orders from their father. He only speaks poor English, and his wife doesn't speak one word of our language. He has a bottle of whisky at the back of the shop, and swigs at it steadily throughout the day. When I went round I was treated with deference, loaded with presents of fruit, and met with massive denial. He says that he uses a little whisky for medicine.'

The community psychiatric nurse had the openness to admit that she did not understand this patient, and no doubt the shopkeeper was equally puzzled as to the role, credentials, and purpose of this person whom his doctor had asked to call. To admit bafflement can be the necessary preliminary to forward movement.

The cultural meaning of the drinking itself may be puzzling. What does 'normal' drinking mean within a particular culture, and how are religious prohibitions in practice interpreted? What are the legitimate functions of alcohol and its symbolism? What are the culturally determined ideas which define 'drinking too much', and if there is a concept equivalent to 'alcohol dependence' with what adverse connotations is that idea loaded? These questions, which relate to difficulties in understanding the drinking itself, constitute only a small part of the total cross-cultural puzzle. The essential background problems relate to such issues as understanding of personality, family and family roles, religion, social class and status, and who has a right to say what to whom (Blane, 1993; Heath, 1993). Different cultures will carry different assumptions as to what constitutes 'treatment', the primacy given to the prescription of medicines, or the degree of directiveness which is expected (Edwards & Arif, 1980).

The case of that shopkeeper is one example of the many and varied cross-cultural problems in understanding that can be met whatever the country in which one is practising (Brisbane & Womble, 1985; Collins, 1993). The presentation may be the recently immigrated family, the postgraduate student from Africa, the immigrant labourer who is today part of the work-force in many parts of the world, or the patient of the therapist's own culture but with regional or social class identity different from the therapist's. The problems set by the extreme cases of cultural difference can in fact serve as a useful reminder of the need for a more general awareness of the culture-clash which is often present in many 'ordinary' therapeutic encounters.

There can be no one formula for dealing with such situations. It is important to be alert to the need for understanding, and hence to avoid those clumsy errors which come from assuming that everyone else is like us, or that there is something funny about others if they do not comply with our own, parochial expectations. Over time, and with continued work in a particular locality, there will probably be a growing familiarity with cultures other than one's own, with the last case teaching something about the next. Treatment services are still often too ethnically insensitive

Every such case has to be seen as an exercise in building bridges. With the fruit-shop owner it may for instance be possible to find a second generation member of the family who can be a broker in understanding. The patient's son may be subservient to his father and unable to talk in the shop, but eager to talk and a helpful informant when he comes to the nurse's office. He may identify the key figures within the extended family network who have a right to advise and intervene. It may also be possible to find someone within the local agencies or hospitals who speaks the language and understands the culture, and who can help with an assessment interview.

The family member as intermediary

Anyone working in this field will from time to time receive the following type of letter or a phone call of similar nature.

> I wonder whether you can possibly help. It is not about myself but it's my daughter who needs assistance. She will not take any notice of me, but I know she is an alcoholic.

The letter may be from a mother about her son or daughter, a husband about his wife, a divorced wife about her ex-husband, or reflect any one of a wide range of other possible combinations. The common theme is that a concerned family member is seeking help on behalf of someone who is not themselves at that moment of a mind to do so.

Helping agencies ought to have the capacity to meet such requests, at least by offering a preliminary evaluation session. The principal, which guides response to this type of proxy consultation, is that there may be fruitful possibilities of working with the person who is actually in the room (the intermediary), rather than the therapist being lured into the impossible position of trying to find instant solutions for the person who is absent (the problem drinker).

For instance, the mother who has come to talk about her daughter's drinking may in fact be wanting to talk about her own sense of guilt, anger or frustration, or about her need to control, or her difficulty in 'letting go'. More than one session may be required. Information about Al-Anon can be timely.

Secondly, there are possibilities of the encounter with the intermediary leading to help for the individual who is drinking. Information can be passed on about treatment services and AA, or an open and unthreatening invitation can be offered for the drinker to come along to discuss whether there is anything to talk about. Beyond that level of information-giving there may also be indirect ways of working with the drinker through changing the behaviour, attitudes, and level of confidence of a key family member. In terms of family systems theory, one is introducing movement into a system which is otherwise going to maintain the drinking. One should also be aware that this kind of approach can at times be manipulative and an attempt to establish blame, and one does well not to be lured into secret contracts.

A presentation on a general hospital ward

This is an account of a late-night happening on a surgical ward.

> A woman had been admitted three days earlier with an abdominal emergency. A diagnosis of acute pancreatitis had been made and the patient had spent the first two days in intensive care. With her physical condition stabilised she was back in a surgical bed. That evening at about midnight she pulled out her intravenous line, made for the door of the ward and said she was going home in a taxi. She drifted into the belief that she was in a hotel, but then suggested that her husband was hiding in a gas cylinder.

Delirium tremens (see Chapter 6) is not infrequently precipitated by a medical or surgical event with consequent admission to hospital and abrupt withdrawal of alcohol. The condition is often satisfactorily treated in that kind of general ward setting, but sometimes there are difficulties. Here is a case history that reflects the real-life eventuality of the thoroughly competent surgical team suddenly being faced by a dangerous alcohol-related emergency. It is the danger that needs to be emphasised. If that patient is allowed to run off the ward she may get lost in the hospital grounds and die of exposure, or walk into traffic and be killed. If the patient is brought back onto the ward without a safe nursing environment established and appropriate medication given, there is a danger of a fall from a window or other accident.

When a surgical or medical team is confronted by this kind of presentation there are some golden rules. Firstly, the patient must by all means possible be kept on the ward and their physical safely ensured. Secondly, psychiatric advice should immediately be obtained. Thirdly, adequate and appropriate medication should be given to bring the disturbance under control as quickly as possible, but with care taken not to induce overdose (pp. 237–8). The fourth stage of response may need to be a review of staff training and procedures.

The 'very important patient'

Frequently, and despite every supposed personal advantage, the man or woman with a large public reputation is the person whose alcohol problem is likely to be mishandled. Because of the aura of prestige no one quite dares make the diagnosis or take a firm line. Phone calls are made in the middle of the night, a quick visit is demanded to a hotel room, and instead of a full history there is a superficial and interrupted conversation, and everything is a whispering game. The therapist may need considerable confidence to stand their ground when dealing with the demands and expectations of the tycoon, the politician, the famous actress, the judge, or the distinguished surgeon, but unless they are willing to hold to a therapeutic position their patient will not be well served. Paradoxically, the rich and famous may be as much at hazard of receiving inadequate treatment as the drinker on Skid Row.

The key to dealing with such problems is to act with an awareness that this person, as much as the vagrant or any other patient who comes one's way, is indeed to an extent a 'special case'. But at the same time one has to hold to the commonalities and the basic working rules of the therapeutic approach. These two ideas need to be discussed briefly and separately.

Firstly, as regards the 'specialness' of this type of patient, the situation may be clouded by fear of public revelation. For instance, the politician will be concerned about the damage to their reputation and electoral chances from any rumour that they are an 'alcoholic'. Advice that they should attend Alcoholics Anonymous where their face will be recognised may in these circumstances be impractical, and anxiety about the dangers of 'the newspaper getting hold of things' may consequently so dominate their thinking as to block every effort to help them. The truth of the matter can be that their drinking habits are already public knowledge and a known embarrassment to their Party – and a rumour that they are getting help can only do good, not harm. The extent to which it is possible for someone in this position to admit publicly that they have had to deal with a drinking problem must vary from country to country and across professions. In the United States, for example, such openness is increasingly and beneficially possible (Hughes, 1997).

There are certain other rather typical features. The pressure under which such people are living and working can be extreme and engender a great deal of tension, with alcohol used as self-medication. Fear of failure may be potently linked to this stress with an uncertain personal sense of worth and security despite every public success. The life-style may involve frequent entertaining and thus pressures to drink. Marriages are often under strain.

With this kind of patient there may sometimes be difficulty in initiating effective therapy because the patient claims that they are too important to waste their time on treatment – there is a film to make, a business meeting to be attended on the other side of the world, an invitation to Downing Street which must take priority.

So much for a brief consideration of what may be 'special'. It must, however, be obvious that what has been instanced as special could be turned around and argued the other way. There is nothing unique about fear of public exposure, and it may affect the driver of the company car as well as the company president, while stress and fear of failure are common themes whatever the stratum from which patients are drawn. Although it is necessary to be alert to the intensity and clustering of certain factors that affect the 'special' patient, one is soon brought back to the need to hold onto the basics of the therapeutic approach. A full assessment must, for instance, be carried out, rather than the argument accepted that the patient is too busy for proper time to be given this task. The formulation has to be discussed, the diagnosis agreed, and goals appropriately set. And, as always, the quality of the relationship is fundamental. At one level the encounter may be between public figure and psychiatrist or counsellor, but more fundamentally it is between a patient or client with a drinking problem and a person seeking to offer help.

References

Blane, H. T. (1993). Ethnicity. In *Recent Advances in Alcoholism 11. Ten Years of Progress*, ed. Galanter, M., pp. 109–23. New York: Plenum Press.

Brisbane, F. L. & Womble, M. (1985). *Treatment of Black Alcoholics*. New York: Haworth Press.

Collins, R. C. (1993). Sociocultural aspects of alcohol use and abuse: ethnicity and gender. In *Innovations in Alcoholism Treatment: State of the Art Reviews and their Implications for Clinical Practice*, ed. Connors, G. J., pp. 89–116. New York: Haworth Press.

Edwards, G. & Arif, A. (Eds.) (1980). *Drug Problems in Socio-Cultural Perspective*. Geneva, World Health Organisation.

Fitzgerald, J. L. & Mulford, H.A. (1992). Elderly vs younger problem drinkers 'treatment' and recovery experience. *British Journal of Addiction* **87**, 1281–91.

Heath, D. (1993). Anthropology. In *Recent Advances in Alcoholism 11. Ten Years of Progress*, ed. Galanter, M., pp. 29–45. New York: Plenum Press.

Hinrichsen, J. J. (1984). Toward improving treatment services for alcoholics of advanced age. *Alcohol Health and Research World* **8**, 31–9.

Hughes, J. (1997). Journal Interview. *Addiction*, **92**, 137–50.

Janik, S. W. & Dunham, R. G. (1983). A nationwide examination of the need for specific alcoholism treatment programs for the elderly. *Journal of Studies on Alcohol* **44**, 307–17.

Koford, L. L., Tolson, R. L., Atkinson, R. M., Toth, R. L. & Turner, J. A. (1987). Treatment compliance of older alcoholics: an elder-specific approach is superior to a mainstreaming. *Journal of Studies on Alcohol* **48**, 47–51.

Sherr, K. H. (1991). Psychological characteristics of children of alcoholics: overview of research methods and findings. In *Recent Advances in Alcoholism*, vol. 9, *Children of Alcoholics*, ed. Galanter, M., pp. 301–26. New York: Plenum Press.

11

Drinking problems and the life course

Meaning can be given to the phrase 'longitudinal perspective' through a presentation made at a postgraduate teaching forum. At this session it was decided first to review a bundle of case notes from 20 years previously and to use this material for discussion around issues of prognosis. A psychiatric registrar (resident) had gone through these notes and summarised the patient's case history as follows:

> Mr A was aged 42 years at the time of his admission to this hospital 20 years previously. His father had been an army officer, his mother had died young, and his childhood had been loveless and arid. After boarding school he had been commissioned into his father's regiment and had for a time done well and been decorated for bravery. However, by his mid-30s his drinking was becoming notorious and he was faced with the choice of forced discharge or resignation. Back into civilian life and with a wife and two children to support, he went into a security business which was soon insolvent. By the time of the hospital admission he had severe alcohol dependence and most aspects of his life were in ruin – he was separated from his family, heavily in debt, and facing prosecution for financial irregularities. It was unclear whether he had a depressive illness, but he confessed to having at times strong suicidal ruminations and said 'I wonder if I've always been depressed'. The last entry in the notes read 'Removed from ward today by police on charge of fraud'.

The consultant chairing this clinical conference next invited a short presentation from another registrar on the literature dealing with prognosis in alcohol dependence (Lindquist, 1973; Gibbs and Flanagan, 1977; Edwards *et al.*, 1988; Monahan & Finney, 1996), and it was agreed that Mr A's life expectation would probably have been severely curtailed by his drinking (Marshall *et al.*, 1994) – it was all too likely that in a drunken state he would have acted out his suicidal fantasies. If, however, he had survived it was probable that he would have

175

continued to drink (Edwards *et al.*, 1983). One of the nurses present offered the image of 'a shabby and maudlin habitué of a Chelsea pub cadging drinks off other people and still wearing his regimental tie'.

At 11 a.m. precisely, a well-dressed man entered the conference room and was introduced by the consultant chairing the meeting as his former patient, Mr A, who had recently got in touch by letter and who wanted to express his personal thanks for the help and kindness he had received all those years back. He had not drunk since the day he left the ward and he gave a detailed, insightful account of recovery in terms not only of abstinence but of changes within himself, changed relationships and a new marriage and the ability to love, and business success as creative fulfilment. He remembered acutely certain things that had been said to him on admission to hospital by the psychiatric registrar who was at that time on the firm, 'She said that I had a right to be depressed, don't know why, that was some kind of turning point'.

An abstract discussion of case notes transmuted into empathetic reality by a patient walking into a room is a special kind of event which in acute and theatrical form makes a general point. The therapist working with drinking problems needs to cultivate a sense of the longitudinal play, to see their patients' lives not just in terms of the immediate clinical encounter and the immediate problems and anxieties – the snapshot – but in terms also of the moving picture show (Vaillant, 1983, 1995; Edwards, 1984, 1989; Ludwig 1988). Whatever the statistics may say at the aggregate level, it is extraordinarily difficult to foretell at baseline what will have happened 20 years later to the individual person.

Research exists, however, that can support our understanding of the drinker's life course. There are literatures dealing with change and stability in drinking behaviour and problem experience within general populations (Cahalan *et al.*, 1969; Cahalan, 1970; Cahalan & Room, 1974; Fillmore & Midanik 1984; Fillmore, 1987 a, b). Valuable insights have come from follow-up studies on cohorts of subjects recruited not for their drinking but for some other purpose, but with the ensuing drinking behaviour then prospectively explored (McCord & McCord, 1960; Vaillant, 1983; Vaillant, 1995). Another type of study has dealt with the long-term follow-up of patients treated for their drinking problems (Taylor, 1994). Other work has focused specifically on mortality (Sundby, 1967; Marshall *et al.*, 1994). This chapter will give an account of the core conclusions to be drawn from this research background in a statement that is necessarily selective rather than all-inclusive. With the research picture thus sketched the final section of the chapter will return to questions of how linkage is to be made between research findings and clinical insights.

Stability and change in drinking behaviour: the significance of general population surveys

Population surveys of drinking behaviour provide a context within which to understand what happens to clinical populations over time. There are likely to be differences between cultures and the sexes, but the general finding is that young people in their 20s are the section of the population who do a lot of drinking, frequently get drunk, and notch up a tally of often drunkenness-related drinking problems (Cahalan & Room, 1974). Their drinking patterns reflect the life-style, exuberance and irresponsibility of youth, and much which at the time looks like 'drinking pathology' will 10 years later be found to have ameliorated or faded away (Room, 1977). What is remarkable about this kind of behaviour is its flux rather than its fixity, but the dangers that can attach to youthful heavy drinking should not be ignored – what for the most part may appear to be no more than innocent experimentation and transient excess can carry enhanced risk of accident, trauma, and death (Andréasson *et al.*, 1988). Thus a balance should be struck between, on the one hand, an awareness that much drinking in the 20s can be seen as a stage of evolution toward more restricted and sensible drinking, and on the other, the realisation that excessive drinking at this age can carry significant and age-related risk of accident (especially motor vehicle accident) and death by violence. What needs to be emphasised is that the drinking itself can carry risks rather than the problem being defined solely in terms of detecting early signs of alcohol dependence.

While this body of research tends to show that in middle age the prevalence and incidence of heavy drinking or drinking problems is less than in earlier decades, the chronicity of problematic drinking at this age is greater (Fillmore, 1987a). Fewer people are now drinking heavily, but those who do so are more likely to go on doing so rather than moving casually in and out of the problem drinking sector of experience. The explanation is no doubt in part that at this phase in the life course the significance of alcohol's dependence potential is becoming manifest.

The question has also been examined as to whether surrounding changes in society will influence evolution in drinking, so that cohorts recruited and followed over different time periods might show different patterns of change. By and large the age effect appears to be dominant and generalisable whatever the population studied (Fillmore, 1987a).

Alcohol dependence: the long-term outcome

Percentage achieving abstinence and the stability of abstinence

Here different samples recruited at different times and followed up for different periods show widely varying outcomes. Much must depend on sample characteristics and the outcome definition which is employed, and completeness of follow-up (Vaillant, 1995). Less is known about female than male drinkers. Reported rates of abstinence have varied from a high of 64% in a Norwegian sample at 20–35 year follow-up (Sundby *et al.*, 1967), to 13% in a Norwegian 10-year study (Bratfos, 1974). Most but not all reports describe an intermediate category of 'social' or 'asymptomatic' drinking lying between abstinence and continued problemtatic drinking. These subjects are probably a mix of patients who were never severely dependent, those who are sliding toward relapse, and those drinking with lowered tolerance to alcohol (Edwards *et al.*, 1983, 1986). That drinkers interviewed at follow-up do not necessarily tell the truth is a fact that has sometimes been overlooked (Edwards, 1985), with consequently inflated estimates of 'return to normal drinking'.

Research suggests that over the course of any one follow-up year there will be considerable movement of subjects between abstinence and troubled drinking, with individual patterns gradually becoming more stable over time (Taylor, 1994). Two or three years after initial treatment contact it will be possible to identify a sub-group of patients whose abstinence is likely to remain stable in the long-term while there will also be a group of patients whose troubled drinking is relentlessly continuous.

> First seen 25 years previously on an alcohol treatment unit, a doctor saw this now 70-year-old patient again for a consultation on a general hospital ward. The original notes had described him as 'blaming everyone but himself'. A quarter of a century later he complained about 'everyone letting him down'. His alcohol intake was now restricted because of physical illness and lack of resources, but after a stroke he still continued to drink to staggering incapacity as often as his welfare payments would allow.

Alcohol dependent patients do not necessarily 'mature out of dependence', even after many years (Vaillant, 1995).

Recovery from the drinking problem is generally but not universally associated with consequent improvement in health, social functioning and quality of life (Duckitt *et al.*, 1985; Vaillant 1995). There is, however, evidence to suggest that 'good outcome' among more severely dependent drinkers more often involves a degree of dysjunction between stopping drinking and in improvement in health and adjustment (Taylor et al., 1986), but there are many subjects who have dealt with severe dependence and have gone on to establish a resoundingly positive life adjustment.

Within all this human variation, any statement on 'average' outcome expectations must be guarded. With that proviso underlined it is likely that if 100 patients treated for alcohol dependence who were aged 45 years at the intake point were followed for 20 years, about 40% would have died by the 20-year anniversary: alcohol dependent subjects have over a 3.6 fold excess mortality compared with age-matched controls, and excess mortality is probably greater among more dependent drinkers (Finney & Moos, 1991, 1992; Marshall et al., 1994). Of the remaining subjects over 30% will still be experiencing continued or intermittent trouble with their drinking and rather less than 30% will be abstinent or engaging in trouble-free drinking.

Alcohol dependence: what aids recovery in the long-term?

Researchers have found it difficult to identify any strong and consistent baseline pointers to favourable long-term outcome (Lindquist, 1973; Gibbs & Flanagan, 1977; Edwards et al., 1988). Conventional wisdom has it that the patient with better initial social support, less severe dependence and more stable personality will do better than the subject who is not so favoured, but it would be difficult to find conclusive research support for that assertion. There may well be different significant baseline pointers for different sub-groups, and in particular for the more and less dependent subjects. In some circumstances severe baseline dependence and severe problems may actually constitute a favourable prognostic pointer because continued drinking for that person is becoming too punishing (Edwards et al., 1988).

Besides the none too fruitful attempt to identify prognostic indicators, investigators have also examined the change processes, which over the long-term are associated with achievement and maintenance of sobriety – at attempt, as it were, to understand the dynamics of recovery. The strongest conclusion must be that there is no one single pathway to recovery and that people find many different individual paths out of drinking. With the crucial fact of variation stressed (one hundred different drinkers will have one hundred unique life stories), certain recurrent findings can be seen as emerging from research (Vaillant, 1983; Edwards et al., 1987, 1992), and these findings will be summarised below under subheadings (see also Box 11.1).

Box 11.1. Alcohol dependence: what influences recovery in the long-term

- *Baseline patient characteristics*. It is difficult to identify consistent baseline pointers significant for recovery in the longer term.

- *Accepting an appropriate treatment goal*. For severe dependence abstinence is likely to be the appropriate goal, but not always or necessarily so for lesser degrees of dependence.

- *Treatment and AA involvement* can significantly help recovery in terms of pointing up, nurturing, and nudging along the potential for self-determined change.

- *'Natural processes of recovery'* are of vital importance to initiation and support of sobriety. Treatment must work in sensible alliance with these processes

---

Acceptance of the abstinence goal

Recovery from severe alcohol dependence almost inevitably involves personal acceptance of an abstinence goal. Without that crucial cognitive shift the individual will struggle on and on and self-defeatingly against the odds. Insight may come from the buffeting of experience, from what is heard at an AA meeting or from professional advice. The importance of goals and goal-setting is obvious but easily forgotten.

Trigger or 'Damascus' events

A frequent story given by recovered drinkers is that they owe their sobriety to a memorable and emotionally-laden event which for them constituted a turning point (Tuchfield, 1981). Such an instance as reported in a 10-year follow-up study (Edwards *et al.*, 1992) is given below:

> a place in Ireland called Knock where the Virgin appeared . . . I visited the place, atmosphere, and I knew I would never drink again or smoke

Events so trivial, such as being teased in the street for a dishevelled appearance, or so major as drunken carelessness causing the death of a child, illustrate a spectrum of happenings which the drinker may see as responsible for their abrupt and permanent switch toward sobriety. Both negative and positive life events may be precursors to achievement of sobriety (Edwards *et al.*, 1992). Many other similar events occurring over time will be without impact or produce only a brief false dawn. Furthermore, attribution should not be confused with cause and although a 'Damascus' event may stand out in an individual's memory as the unique and immediate cause of a radical change in drinking behaviour, it is more likely that such an event will have triggered or supported cognitive processes that were the preparatory background to a change finally precipitated by the acute event. The personal reality of this kind of event and the potential significance of such phenomena for processes of recovery does, however, suggest that the therapist should be aware of their possible occurrence and be ready, therapeutically, to capitalise on these events when they occur.

The consolidation of sobriety

As emphasised above, although dramatic events may assist or precipitate change, sobriety is usually best conceived as something built and secured over time rather than as a state achieved on a particular day (Moos *et al.*, 1990). Important questions therefore attach to the understanding of what in the individual's life may most effectively support sobriety. In sum the research here strongly suggests that sobriety is most likely to be held onto in the longer term when the sober state is felt to be rewarding – the negative reinforcement relating to the possible pains of any further drinking are not so potent at the enhancement in quality of life which can stem from what AA calls 'contented sobriety' (Vaillant, 1983; Edwards *et al.*, 1992). A prime example of this kind of positive influence is the reward that can come from a loving relationship and the discovery of a capacity for altruism – an ability to give to other people is often associated with achievement of sobriety. Meaningful employment, energies put into creating a business, hobbies, home-making, house decoration, further educational involvements and enjoyment of holidays provide additional examples of the kinds of activities which can provide substitution for rewards previously found only in drinking (p. 258).

One may suspect that the final arrival of a stable and rewarding sobriety after many years of turmoil may also quite often be related to processes of psychological maturation (Vaillant, 1977), and people who experience drinking problems are likely as the years go by to undergo the same kinds of maturations and life-cycle changes as other people, albeit perhaps delayed or overlaid by the drinking. Maturation may make sobriety more possible and the continuing destructiveness of drinking less bearable. Within this complex lies the intangible reality of what some people will want to call the growth of spiritual awareness. To shut off that aspect of people's lives when trying to understand processes of recovery is unwise, but that does not imply any belief in likely benefits from moralising at the drinker.

What the long-term perspective suggests as to the significance of treatment and of AA involvement

Long-term research gives messages that are by no means nihilistic as to the contribution which treatment can make to recovery from alcohol dependence but within this kind of timeframe treatment takes its place as one kind of interactive influence within the play of many other self-determined, other determined, and accidental forces. As with the case conference example at the beginning of this chapter, there is evidence that many years later, patients or clients will remember 'what a psychiatrist said or did' or the intervention of some other professional as being significantly related to recovery (Edwards *et al.*, 1987). It is the nudging of the person towards a more constructive way of seeing things, the encouragement of self-actualisation and the enhancement of self efficacy, help with choice of appropriate goal, and the alliance between therapeutic intervention and natural processes of change, that research suggests are in the long-term the most potent contributions which treatment can make to recovery. There is no evidence that intensive psychotherapy aids long-term recovery (Vaillant, 1983). Research also again points to the reality of between-person variation – what one person takes from therapy may be different from someone else's gain. Treatment is in general seen as more influential by more dependent drinkers (Edwards *et al.*, 1987).

As regards the long-term significance of AA involvement in the achievement and stabilisation of recovery (Edwards, 1996), the impact of AA on drinking behaviour is notoriously difficult to assess in any controlled sense and even in the short-term (see Chapter 16). Long-term research in this arena not too unexpectedly provides more hints than firm conclusions. Within a British sample at a 10-year follow-up point, about one-third of alcohol-dependent patients spoke positively of some aspect of AA involvement – 'hearing other people's stories at AA' and 'friendship through AA' were for these people particularly favoured elements, while the religious element in AA rated relatively low (Edwards *et al.*, 1987). Again the degree of dependence enters the equation, with evidence that it is the most dependent subjects who will more probably find AA helpful in the long-term.

Research evidence and clinical insight

In the paragraphs above the attempt has been to summarise findings on what happens to drinkers as the years go by and the parallel findings on what explains the observable changes and transitions. The relevances of the perspective which emerges for everyday clinical work and the importance of the clinical feel for things that can be developed from taking the life-course view of dependence will now be brought into focus in this final section of the chapter.

The insights for therapy that can be derived from this long-term view can be ordered under two headings. Firstly, there is the benefit that comes from the pervasive impact on the therapeutic position once we comprehend the significance of the truth that our interventions although often valuable are part of a longer, broader play (Vaillant, 1988; Sobell et al., 1991; Vaillant, 1996). That view is an antidote to therapeutic arrogance and any tendencies towards a belief in our omnipotence – therapy does matter and can contribute, but only insofar as the therapist respects, is intrigued by, and cultivates awareness of how patients themselves effect change in the context of their ongoing lives. Another aspect of this kind of broad perspective-setting that derives from the longitudinal view is the impact that long-term follow-up data may properly be expected to have on the therapist's personal balance of optimism. On the one hand, the data show that alcohol dependence is a potentially destructive condition and awareness of the multiple threats which are posed by this condition should never be staled by familiarity. On the other hand, an equally fair conclusion is that dependence is recoverable and that no one should ever be discarded because of presumed unfavourable baseline prognostic loadings. For patient and therapist alike there is never any reason not to try, and to deny anyone the possibility of help is wrong.

The second summary heading on clinical relevance relates to the more point-by-point application of this perspective to treatment strategies. What may here profitably again be emphasised is the importance of proposing the appropriate drinking goal, willingness to ride with, and therapeutically exploit naturally occurring potential change points, the awareness that recovery is process rather than event, the willingness to encourage and support strategies such as substitution of positive and rewarding activities, the cultivation of open-mindedness and the awareness that rather than there being any one unique pathway to recovery there are different paths for different people. The therapist's job is that of assisting each patient to identify his or her own pathway to recovery and find the means to stay on course.

References

Andréasson, S., Romelsjö, A. & Allebeck, P. (1988). Alcohol and mortality among young men: longitudinal study of Swedish conscripts. British Medical Journal **296**, 1021–5.

Bratfos, O. (1974). *The Course of Alcoholism, Drinking, Social Adjustment and Health.* Oslo: Universitets Forlaget.

Cahalan, D. (1970). *Problem Drinking: a National Survey.* San Francisco: Jossey Bass.

Cahalan, D. & Room, R. (1974). *Problem Drinking Among American Men.* New Brunswick: Rutgers Center for Alcohol Studies.

Cahalan, D., Cisin I. H. & Crossley H. M. (1969). *American Drinking Practices: A National Survey of Behaviour and Attitudes.* Monograph No.6. New Brunswick: Rutgers Center for Alcohol Studies.

Duckitt, A., Brown, D., Edwards, G., Oppenheimer, E., Sheehan, M. & Taylor, C. (1985). Alcoholism and the nature of outcome. *British Journal of Addiction* **80**, 171–83.

Edwards, G. (1984). Drinking in longitudinal perspective: career and natural history. *British Journal of Addiction* **79**, 175–83.

Edwards, G. (1985). A later follow-up of a classic case series: D. L. Davies's 1962 report and its significance for the present. *Journal of Studies on Alcohol* **46**, 181–90.

Edwards, G. (1989). As the years go rolling by. Drinking problems in the time dimension. *British Journal of Psychiatry* **154**, 18–26.

Edwards, G. (1996). Alcoholics Anonymous as mirror held up to nature. *Psychotherapy, Psychological Treatments and the Addictions*, ed. Edwards, G. & Dare, C., pp. 220–39. Cambridge: Cambridge University Press.

Edwards, G., Duckitt, A., Oppenheimer, E., Sheehan, M. & Taylor, C. (1983). What happens to alcoholics in the long-term? *Lancet* **ii**, 269–71.

Edwards, G., Brown, D., Duckitt, A., Oppenheimer, E., Sheehan, M. & Taylor, C. (1986). Normal drinking in a recovered alcohol addict. *British Journal of Addiction* **81**, 127–37.

Edwards, G., Brown, D., Duckitt, A., Oppenheimer, E., Sheehan, M. & Taylor, C. (1987). Outcome of alcoholism: the structure of patient attributions as to what causes change. *British Journal of Addiction* **82**, 533–45.

Edwards, G., Brown, D., Oppenheimer, E., Sheehan, M. & Taylor, C. (1988). Long-term outcome for patients with alcohol problems: the search for predictors. *British Journal of Addiction* **83**, 917–27.

Edwards, G., Oppenheimer, E. & Taylor, T. (1992). Hearing the noise in the system. Exploration of textual analysis as a method for studying change in drinking behaviour. *British Journal of Addiction* **87**, 73–81.

Fillmore, K. M. (1987a). Prevalence, incidence and chronicity of drinking patterns and problems among men as a function of age: a longitudinal and cohort analysis. *British Journal of Addiction* **82**, 77–83.

Fillmore, K. M. (1987b). Women's drinking as compared to men's: a longitudinal analysis. *British Journal of Addiction* **82**, 801–11.

Fillmore, K. M. & Midanik, L. (1984). Chronicity of drinking problems among men: a longitudinal and cohort analysis. *Journal of Studies on Alcohol* **45**, 228–36.

Finney, J. W. & Moos, R. H. (1991). The long-term course of treated alcoholism. I. Mortality, relapse and remission rates and comparisons with community controls. *Journal of Studies on Alcohol* **52**, 44–54.

Finney, J. W. & Moos, R. H. (1992). The long-term course of treated alcoholism. II. Prediction and correlates of 10-year functioning and mortality. *Journal of Studies on Alcohol* **53**, 142–53.

Gibbs, L. & Flanagan, J. (1977). Prognostic indicators of alcoholism treatment outcome. *International Journal of Addiction* **12**, 1097–141.

Lindquist, G. A. R. (1973). Alcohol dependence. *Acta Psychiatrica Scandinavica* **49**, 332–40.

Ludwig, A. M. (1988). *Understanding the Alcoholic's Mind: The Nature of Craving and How to Control It*. New York: Oxford University Press.

Marshall, J., Edwards, G. & Taylor, C. (1994). Mortality in men with drinking problems: a 20-year follow-up. *Addiction* **89**, 1293–8.

McCord, W. & McCord, J. (1960). *Origins of Alcohol*. Stanford: Stanford University Press.

Monahan, S. C. & Finney, J. W. (1996). Explaining abstinence rates following treatment for alcohol abuse: a quantitative synthesis of patient, research design and treatment effects. *Addiction* **91**, 787–805.

Moos, R. H., Finney, J. W. & Cronkite, E. (1990). *Alcoholism Treatment: Context, Process and Outcome*. New York: Oxford University Press.

Room, R. (1977). Measurement and distribution of drinking patterns and problems in general populations. In *Alcohol Related Disabilities*, ed. Edwards, G., Moser, J., Gross M., Keller, M. & Room, R. WHO Offset Publication No.32. Geneva: World Health Organisation.

Sobell, L. L., Sobell, M. B. & Toneatto, T. (1991). Recovery from alcohol problems without treatment. In *Self Control and the Addictive Behaviors*, ed. Heather, N., Miller, W. R. & Greeley, J., pp. 198–242. New York: Pergamon.

Sundby, P. (1967). *Alcoholism and Mortality*. Oslo: Universitets Forlaget.

Taylor, C. (1994). What happens over the long term? In *Alcohol and Alcohol Problems*, ed. Edwards, G. & Peters, T. J., pp. 50–60. British Medical Bulletin vol. 50. Edinburgh: Churchill Livingstone.

Taylor, C., Brown, D., Duckitt, A., Edwards, G., Oppenheimer, E. & Sheehan, M. (1986). Alcoholism and the patterning of outcome: a multivariate analysis. *British Journal of Addiction* **81**, 815–23.

Tuchfield, B. S. (1981). Spontaneous remission in alcoholics: empirical observations and theoretical implication. *Quarterly Journal of Studies on Alcohol* **42**, 626–41.

Vaillant, G. E. (1977). *Adaptation to Life*. Boston: Little Brown.

Vaillant, G. E. (1983). *The Natural History of Alcoholism*. Cambridge, MA: Harvard University Press.

Vaillant, G. E. (1988). What can long-term follow-up teach us about relapse and prevention of relapse in addiction? *British Journal of Addiction* **83**, 1147–57.

Vaillant, G. E. (1995). *The Natural History of Alcoholism Revisited*. Cambridge, Mass: Harvard University Press.

Vaillant, G. E. (1996). Addiction over the life course: therapeutic implications. In *Psychotherapy, Psychological Treatments and the Addictions*, ed. Edwards, G. & Dare, C., pp. 3–18. Cambridge: Cambridge University Press.

II

Screening, assessment, and treatment

12

Case identification and screening

Excessive drinking is frequently and in many settings overlooked. Only about a quarter of 'high risk' or 'excessive' drinkers are correctly identified by primary care physicians (Wallace & Haines, 1985; Reid *et al.*, 1986). Even in the hospital setting, where one might imagine more time was available for enquiry and investigation, the problem often goes unrecognised (Barrison *et al.*, 1980; Rowland *et al.*, 1987; Farrell & David, 1988). The detection rate in the social work setting has not been adequately investigated, but there can be little doubt that the contribution made by drinking to all manner of social presentations is passed by. We all, in fact, need to cultivate a more alert eye, and aim at earlier and more complete diagnosis. If the element of drinking is allowed to remain hidden, it will defeat our plans to help that patient or client. The 'depression' will not respond to the prescribed antidepressant, a stomach ulcer will fail to heal, a family's situation will deteriorate, and we will be left puzzled and frustrated. Treatment which is blind to the drinking problem may indeed do actual harm rather than simply fail in its goal, while early diagnosis which can lead to help before dependence is advanced, or irreversible damage established, is very much in the patient's best interests.

In this chapter we will look at the barriers to detection and diagnosis of drinking problems and we will consider ways in which rates of detection may be enhanced. Special consideration will also be given to the use of laboratory tests and questionnaires in screening and diagnosis.

Why the diagnosis is frequently missed

There are various reasons why drinking problems so often remain under cover, and several of these reasons may conspire together. They can be listed as follows.

Not knowing what we are looking for

The diagnostician may only be attuned to looking for alcohol dependence or the extreme case (with their ideas even on these presentations no more than vaguely formed), but with no real knowledge of the many different types of alcohol-related problems which may be daily impinging on their work. He or she must be familiar with the common diagnostic clues. Neither alcohol dependence nor alcohol-related problems necessarily declare themselves in direct terms, and the shrewd diagnostician has to be familiar with the wide range of signs and symptoms (physical, psychological and social), which can hint at the underlying drinking problem.

Lack of vigilance

The possibility of a drinking problem should always be borne in mind, for otherwise even the person who is armed with all the necessary book-learning is at risk of missing the obvious case (Barrison et al., 1980; Rowland et al., 1987; Farrell & David, 1988).

Embarrassment at asking questions

The therapist may experience a certain degree of social inhibition in asking about drinking problems, which is very much related to society's general difficulty in facing up to such matters (Thom & Téllez, 1986). This may be especially so if the doctor knows the patient socially.

Not knowing what to do if the case is uncovered

If the therapist lacks confidence in his or her ability to respond to a drinking problem, if and when it is uncovered, they may be reluctant to make enquiries that threaten to put them in an uncomfortable position.

The patient's denial or evasion

A patient who is ashamed of their drinking will have difficulty in bringing the problem forward, perhaps especially so if the patient is a woman. That difficulty will only be overcome if the therapist can convey the message that no one is sitting in judgement. It must be safe to talk.

These five subheadings together point to a need for investment in relevant professional training, by educators who are themselves close to the realities of practice.

Enhancing recognition rates

The headings above, which outline common reasons for failure in recognition, point to how the blocks on diagnosis need to be overcome. The practical business of diagnosis will be aided by consideration of the following issues.

The use of disarming questions

It is useful to have as one's personal stock-in-trade a few disarming questions about drinking problems that can be fed into any history-taking in almost throwaway fashion. The scene is often best set by a casual introductory remark, such as, 'I always ask everyone about drinking – it can be important to feel that one can talk about one's drinking without being got at'. The implication is that it is routine to question in this area rather than the patient being singled out as a special case, and this is coupled with an immediate indication that anything the patient reveals will be sympathetically heard. The questions that follow are then usually best phrased in very open terms, for instance, 'Tell me, have you ever been worried about your drinking? Ever? In any way? I mean, has it led to any rows or troubles at home or at work? Health troubles? Ever thought you ought to cut down? Anyone criticised your drinking?'

Questions which thus feel out the possibility of worry or trouble are more likely to provide a way into fruitful dialogue than mechanistic questions along such lines as 'How much do you drink?'. The latter type of interrogation does not immediately reach across barriers towards what the patient is feeling and experiencing. It is too readily deflected by a bland answer, such as 'Just socially'. But if the preliminary questions about worries and troubles suggest that enquiry has to be taken further, it is then essential to construct the outlines of a 'typical drinking day' (see Chapter 13) and go fully into quantity and frequency of drinking.

Remembering who may be specially at risk

To bear in mind a list of who may be especially at risk is useful, provided the therapist does not, as a result, become blinkered to the wider truth that drinking problems can affect both sexes, and, either directly or indirectly, people of any age and every occupation. With that proviso, an awareness of particular occupational hazard is then important (see Chapter 1). The single person and the separated and the recently bereaved also go in this 'at risk' list. Certain ethnic groups are more at risk of drinking problems, with the Irish providing a familiar example. The person who is homeless and drifting might almost be presumed to have a drinking problem until proved otherwise.

Common social presentations

One should always be on the look-out for a hidden drinking problem with the client or patient who is frequently changing house, changing jobs or changing relationships. Family presentations are common – marital disharmony or family violence, the wife presenting with depression or the children with truanting, school failure, antisocial behaviour or neurotic symptoms. Criminal offences also suggest the need to ask about drinking.

Common psychiatric clues

Here the essential background list derives from Chapter 7. In particular one should be alert to the possibility of a drinking problem when the patient or client complains rather non-specifically of 'bad nerves', insomnia, or depression. Phobic symptoms, pathological jealousy, paranoid symptoms, and dementia or delirium may all at times be alcohol-related. A drug problem may also often be associated with a drinking problem. A suicidal attempt or gesture always demands enquiry into drinking.

Common medical clues

An account of the medical complications of heavy drinking is given in Chapter 8. In practical terms one should be particularly on the alert if a patient repeatedly asks for a 'certificate', is a frequent visitor to the doctor's office on a Monday morning, is suffering from malnutrition or obesity, is complaining of any gastro-intestinal disorder or liver problem, has otherwise unexplained heart trouble, or if the patient presents with 'epilepsy' of late onset. Bruising may be a clue, or burns which have resulted from a cigarette being dropped on the skin while the drinker is intoxicated. Accidents of any sort may be alcohol-related, and drink-driving offenders are particularly likely to have other drinking problems, with over 40% being identified as problem drinkers with a score of 5 or more on the MAST (Michigan Alcoholism Screening Test) questionnaire (Lapham *et al.*, 1995).

Not overlooking the obvious

The patient may declare the diagnosis by the smell of alcohol on their breath, by the bottle sticking out of their pocket, by their flushed face and bloodshot eyes, or by their tremor, but even the fact that they are obviously intoxicated can be overlooked if the possibility of drinking is not held in mind. The patient who makes jokes about their drinking should have those jokes taken seriously. Similarly obvious presentations may be seen on a visit to the home: bottles and glasses lying around; decoration neglected and furniture reduced to a few sticks; the home may be a sad parody of a stage-set portraying decay. It would, however, be a mistake to think only in terms of such flagrant presentations and therefore overlook lesser clues.

Having a word with the spouse

If there is any cause to suspect excessive drinking, a word privately with the spouse is essential, and particularly so if the patient says that 'the wife's too busy to come along'. It cannot be automatically assumed that the spouse will be ready and willing to talk about a family drinking problem; loyalty, fear of reprisal, embarrassment, or a determined unwillingness to face up to the painful truth may all stand in the way. Much the same sort of tactful and open questioning may therefore be needed as with the partner who is drinking.

Laboratory tests

A number of laboratory tests are useful in the screening of clinical populations for possible drinking problems – within, for instance, a routine medical examination when staff are recruited or undergo annual health checks. These tests can also be confirmatory in the individual case where excessive drinking is suspected but has not been admitted. No one test by itself is of as much value as a battery of investigations, and it seems likely that a properly chosen array of tests should today detect over 80% of patients with an at least moderately severe drinking problem (see review by Chan, 1990). A negative result does not rule out the possibility that excessive drinking has begun adversely to affect the individual's life, and false positives also occur. Laboratory tests therefore need to be interpreted shrewdly and no test results stand by themselves; they can only be read in the context of all those considerations that have been listed above.

Sensitivity and Specificity

Before listing the individual tests that may be used, it is helpful to identify two characteristics of such tests that provide a guide to their usefulness in making a diagnosis. The *specificity* of a test is a guide to the extent to which a positive result is indicative of the condition of interest – in this case, heavy drinking. A non-specific test for excessive alcohol consumption would show a positive result not just in heavy drinking, but in a range of other unrelated disorders as well. The ideal test would be 100% specific, indicating that it only became positive as a result of heavy drinking. The *sensitivity* of a test indicates the extent to which it reliably detects every case of a disorder. For our present purpose, we would like a 100% sensitive test, which would always be positive, and never negative, in every case of excessive alcohol consumption.

To date, no one has devised a 100% specific and 100% sensitive test for heavy drinking. Different tests are more or less specific and more or less sensitive. The extent to which these tests will serve practical diagnostic needs depends upon the prevalence of heavy drinking in the population in which they are being used. In order to understand this better, let us consider a fictitious illustration:

A new test for heavy drinking, 'alcoholin' has 95% specificity and 60% sensitivity. It is used to screen 1000 apparently healthy employees at their annual medical review. Let us assume that 10% of these employees are actually drinking sufficient amounts of alcohol to be a cause for concern. How useful will the new test be?

Out of 1000 employees, 10% (n=100) are drinking too much, and 60% of these (n=60) will be correctly identified by the test as being 'heavy drinkers'. However, out of the whole group of 1000, 5% (n=50) will be identified as positive due to non-specific (i.e. not alcohol related) results of the test. Therefore, a total of 110 people will be identified by the test, and only 60 of these (55%) will actually be drinking too much. The 'alcoholin' test is therefore of limited usefulness, and must be followed by other tests and by more detailed enquiries, in order to confirm whether or not each of the individuals testing positive actually is drinking too much. Furthermore, 40 people who are drinking excessively will not be identified by the test.

The problems illustrated by this example become more severe the rarer is the disorder. Thus, if the prevalence of heavy drinking were only 1%, only 1 in 9 of those who tested positive with the same test would actually be heavy drinkers. Conversely, if used in a population where almost everyone had a drinking problem (say in an alcohol clinic), then more than 9 out of 10 of those who tested positive would be heavy drinkers.

Screening tests for heavy drinking

Let us now give consideration to the actual tests that are used to screen for heavy drinking. We will not go into the technical detail here at any length, but the most useful tests are as follows.

Mean corpuscular volume (MCV)

This is a measure of the size of red blood cells, which may increase in response to heavy drinking. Sensitivity is 20–50% and specificity 55–100% (Conigrave *et al.*, 1995). MCV, if it has been elevated as a result of heavy drinking, will remain raised for several months after a reduction or cessation of alcohol consumption. This is because of the relatively long life of red blood cells (about 120 days).

Liver function tests

Serum gamma glutamyl transpeptidase (γGT), serum aspartate aminotransferase, and serum glutamate dehydrogenase are all indicators of alcoholic hepatotoxicity, which may be elevated as a result of heavy drinking. Of these, γGT is generally considered to be the most useful as a screening test for heavy drinking. However, with a sensitivity of 20–90% and specificity of 55–100% (Conigrave *et al.*, 1995) it is of debatable value in this role, and its true usefulness has been questioned (Penn & Worthington, 1983). If γGT has been elevated due to drinking, it will fall again after abstinence is established. This is more rapid than the restoration of MCV, but may still take several weeks to return to normal, depending upon the level to which it has been raised. With more serious liver damage other biochemical parameters, such as alkaline phosphatase and bilirubin, will also be altered and in such cases there may be enduring abnormalities of some enzyme levels, even after prolonged abstinence.

Carbohydrate deficient (asialylated) transferrin (CDT)

This is a variant of a serum protein that transports iron. Levels are increased in response to heavy drinking. Its sensitivity as a test of heavy drinking is probably about 60–70%, but may be less, and its specificity is about 95% (Conigrave *et al.*, 1995; Godsell *et al.*, 1995). This is arguably better than most other tests, and it is now considered by some to be the best available screening test for heavy drinking. However, it is probably not much better than γGT.

Blood alcohol level

Blood alcohol concentration (BAC) returns to zero quickly with abstinence: in humans, the average rate of clearance of alcohol from the blood is 15 mg/100 ml per hour. This results in a fairly low sensitivity when used as a screening test. Depending upon the time and context of testing, as well as the threshold alcohol concentration used to define a positive result, moderate social drinkers will also be detected, thus making BAC fairly non-specific as well. Blood alcohol (or breath alcohol as an indirect measure) is therefore not often used as a screening test in the way that γGT or CDT may be used. However, BAC is known to be related to impairment of psychomotor performance and therefore provides a particularly valuable measure in the workplace, or in other safety sensitive contexts, such as driving. BAC may also have an underestimated utility as a screening test in the clinical setting (Wiseman *et al.*, 1982).

Even if not used as a screening test, BAC may be a useful confirmatory investigation. A patient may say, for instance, that he 'only had a few drinks' the previous evening, but at 9 a.m. next morning he still has a blood alcohol level of say 60 mg/100 ml, suggesting much heavier consumption. The finding of a high blood alcohol level in the absence of evident intoxication suggests a high level of tolerance and is therefore important presumptive evidence for habitual heavy drinking.

Other tests

Although rarely used specifically as screening tests for heavy drinking, uric acid, cholesterol, and a variety of other markers all show alterations in response to heavy drinking and may therefore be helpful indicators, particularly in combination with the results of other tests (Chan, 1990).

It will be apparent that none of the tests mentioned above offers improvement over the fictitious 'alcoholin' test. In fact, 'alcoholin' could easily be γGT or CDT. All these tests are limited in their usefulness as screening instruments and in some circumstances medical history and clinical signs will do better (Skinner *et al.*, 1986). However, the sensitivity and specificity of laboratory tests as screening instruments may be improved when they are used in combination. A profile of, for example, MCV, γGT, CDT and other biochemical tests is of considerably more value than any of these tests in isolation.

Laboratory tests may also prove useful in other situations. Comment has already been made regarding the usefulness of a confirmatory BAC in the clinical context. Similarly laboratory tests can be helpful in confirming a diagnosis and where there is clinical suspicion but initial denial from the patient, the feeding of test results into discussion may help the development of insight. Once an abnormal result on one of these tests has been identified, and assuming that this is attributable to heavy drinking, repeat measures over time can also be useful in monitoring clinical progress.

The overall judgement on the value of these tests might therefore be that they are of assistance to therapist and patient if used with discrimination; in this field of practice there are skills to be learnt in using this technology to best advantage.

Screening questionnaires

A number of screening questionnaires have been devised that are intended to aid in the detection of heavy drinking or alcohol related problems. The test which has been most widely researched for its reliability and validity is the 25–item MAST (Selzer, 1971), which has also been published in a shorter 10–item form (Pokorny *et al.*, 1972). The CAGE questionnaire is even briefer, containing only four items (Barrison *et al.*, 1982; King, 1986). These tests generally tend to pick up the more extreme rather than the early case. The MAST, for instance, has among its items delirium tremens and hospital admission for drinking. However, they show remarkably good sensitivity and specificity, for 'excessive drinking' as well as 'alcoholism', and may be superior to laboratory tests when used as screening instruments (Bernadt *et al.*, 1982).

Such instruments are therefore of value for routine screening, for example, in a hospital setting (Barrison *et al.*, 1982; Bernadt *et al.*, 1982), where there is a more or less captive population which is reasonably attuned to the idea of filling in questionnaires. Questionnaires may also be of value in primary care, although usefulness in this setting is more debatable (King, 1986). But these tests in general have found more application as research tools than in the front-line medical and social settings where a paper and pencil test provides no substitute for vigilance, sympathetic questioning, and the very real skills needed for identifying drinking problems of all manner of degree, type, and hiddenness.

In this context, the development of a more recent instrument, the Alcohol Use Disorders Identification Test (AUDIT) is of interest. The AUDIT was developed by an international group of investigators, at the request of the World Health Organisation (Babor & Grant, 1989; Babor *et al.*, 1989). It was designed for use by health care workers in developed and developing countries. It is useful in screening for both currently harmful and potentially hazardous drinking, and shows good sensitivity and specificity, and can identify mild dependence. Potentially, this is the screening questionnaire that should be of most future value to clinicians and researchers in primary care.

Table 12.1. *Advantages and disadvantages of different screening procedures*

Procedure	Advantages	Disadvantages
Clinical interview	Flexibility Potentially high specificity Potential to detect cases that laboratory tests or questionnaires will miss	Subjectivity Dependent upon clinical skill and time/trouble taken Poor sensitivity if the subject is embarrassed or covering up Can be time consuming
Laboratory tests	Objective Quick and convenient for screening large numbers of subjects If positive, useful to monitor subsequent progress Detect heavy use/some tissue toxicity (e.g. liver/blood)	Limited sensitivity and specificity (CDT arguably best, but γGT not much worse) CDT is expensive (γGT much cheaper) Do not detect social/psychological problems
Breath alcohol estimation	Objective Cheap and convenient Good for detecting drinking in safety sensitive context (e.g. drinking and driving) Useful to confirm history/monitor progress	Rapid clearance of alcohol from the blood/breath limits sensitivity Detects alcohol use, not problems *per se* (i.e. poor specificity)
Questionnaires	Standardised and objective Cheap and convenient	Subject to honesty of the respondent Limited sensitivity and specificity (but better than laboratory tests)

Practical conclusions

The relative utility of the various procedures described above, for detection and diagnosis of heavy drinking and drinking problems, is summarised in Table 12.1. To a large extent their utility for detection and screening is determined by their sensitivity, and their utility for diagnosis depends upon their specificity. However, both parameters are important in both contexts. Cost, convenience, and flexibility are also important.

There is no substitute for careful clinical enquiry as a means for detecting heavy drinking, either in specialist practice or in primary care, or other generalist settings. However, information gained in this way may valuably be supported by the discerning use of appropriate laboratory investigations, BAC, and questionnaires.

Where a large, healthy population must be screened, as for example in the occupational setting, even a brief clinical interview may not be possible and questionnaires are therefore advantageous. However, where the follow through of detection includes disciplinary procedures or other adverse consequences, responses to questionnaires may not be reliable. In such circumstances, laboratory tests such as γGT, MCV or CDT can give useful information. Where ensurance of a safety sensitive environment is of concern, such as drinking and driving or certain work settings, BAC estimation may also constitute cost effective technology.

References

Babor, T. F. & Grant, M. (1989). From clinical research to secondary prevention: International collaboration in the development of the Alcohol Use Disorders Identification Test (AUDIT). *Alcohol Health and Research World* **13**, 371–4.

Babor, T. F., de la Fuente, J. R., Saunders, J. & Grant, M. (1989). *AUDIT, The Alcohol Use Disorders Identification Test: Guidelines for Use in Primary Health Care.* Geneva: World Health Organisation.

Barrison, I. G., Viola, L. & Murray-Lyon, I. M. (1980). Do housemen take an adequate drinking history? *British Medical Journal* **281**, 1040.

Barrison, I. G., Viola, L., Mumford, J., Murray, R.M., Gordon, M. & Murray-Lyon, I. M. (1982). Detecting excessive drinking among admissions to a general hospital. *Health Trends* **14**, 80–83.

Bernadt, M. W., Mumford, J., Taylor, C., Smith, B. & Murray, R. M. (1982). Comparison of questionnaire and laboratory tests in the detection of excessive drinking and alcoholism. *Lancet* **1**, 325–8.

Chan, A. W. K. (1990). Biochemical markers for alcoholism. In *Children of Alcoholics*, ed. Windle, M. & Searles, J. S., pp. 39–72. New York: Guilford.

Conigrave, K. M., Saunders, J. B. & Whitfield, J. B. (1995). Diagnostic tests for alcohol consumption. *Alcohol and Alcoholism* **30**, 13–26.

Farrell, M. P. & David, A. S. (1988). Do psychiatric registrars take a proper drinking history? *British Medical Journal* **296**, 395–6.

Godsell, P. A., Whitfield, J. B., Conigrave, K. M., Hanratty, S. J. & Saunders, J. B. (1995). Carbohydrate deficient transferrin levels in hazardous alcohol consumption. *Alcohol and Alcoholism* **30**, 61–6.

King, M. (1986). At risk drinking among general practice attenders: validation of the CAGE questionnaire. *Psychological Medicine* **16**, 213–17.

Lapham, S. G., Skipper, B. J., Owen, J. P. *et al.* (1995). Alcohol abuse screening instruments: normative test data collected from a first DWI offender screening program. *Journal of Studies on Alcohol* **56**, 51–9.

Penn, R. & Worthington, D. J. (1983). Is serum gamma-glutamyltransferase a misleading test? *British Medical Journal* **286**, 531–5.

Pokorny, A. D., Miller, B. A. & Kaplan, H. B. (1972). The brief MAST: a shortened version of the Michingan alcoholism screening test. *American Journal of Psychiatry* **129**, 342–5.

Reid, A. L. A., Webb, G. R., Hennrikus, D., Fahey, P. P. & Sanson-Fisher, R. W. (1986). Detection of patients with high alcohol intake by general practitioners. *British Medical Journal* **293**, 735–8.

Rowland, N., Maynard, A., Beveridge, A., Kennedy, P., Wintersgill, W. & Stone, W. (1987). Doctors have no time for alcohol screening. *British Medical Journal* **295**, 95–6.

Selzer, M. L. (1971). The Michegan alcoholism screening test. *American Journal of Psychiatry* **127**, 1653–8.

Skinner, H. A., Holt, S., Sheu, W .J. & Israel, Y. (1986). Clinical versus laboratory detection of alcohol abuse: the alcohol clinical index. *British Medical Journal* **292**, 1703–8.

Thom, B. & Téllez, C. (1986). A difficult business: detecting and managing alcohol problems in general practice. *British Journal of Addiction* **81**, 405–18.

Wallace, P. & Haines, A. (1985). Use of a questionnaire in general practice to increase the recognition of patients with excessive alcohol consumption. *British Medical Journal* **290**, 1949–53.

Wiseman, S. M., Tomson, P. V., Barnett, J. M., Jenns, M. & Wilton, J. (1982). Use of an alcometer to detect problem drinkers. *British Medical Journal* **285**, 1087–90.

13

Assessment as the beginning of therapy

Case history as initiation of therapy

Taking a history from a patient should not be a matter only of obtaining facts to be written down in the case-notes. It is an interaction between two people, and ought to be as meaningful for the person who answers the questions as for the questioner. The patient should be invited to use the occasion as a personal opportunity to review his or her past and present, and to make sense of what may previously have been a chaotic array of happenings. There is research evidence which demonstrates the potential power of the initial clinical encounter to change the drinker's attitudes, enhance commitment, and clarify goals (Thom *et al.*, 1992).

Assessment is therefore the beginning of therapy (Novey, 1968). The relationship between patient and therapist begins to be determined at this moment, and if the occasion is mishandled, the patient may not attend for a second appointment.

This chapter seeks to cover practical issues related to the art and technique of history-taking. The earlier chapters have sought to lay out the general groundwork of understanding, and we now have to explore how that understanding is to be addressed to practical ends. The present chapter is cast in the form of a series of working guidelines. The framework builds on the general format for the psychiatric history-taking which has for many years been employed at the Maudsley Hospital, London (Departments of Psychiatry *et al.*, 1987). This assessment should be conducted in a carefully created setting which should make open self-appraisal possible.

History-taking is a rewarding aspect of therapeutic work, and the reader should not be daunted by the details of this presentation. Anyone coming to this type of work for the first time should not attempt to absorb everything that is being said here at one sitting. The full meaning of this discussion will only become alive as the therapist's experience of working with drinking problems feeds back and modifies this outline. A seemingly small or theoretical point may then suddenly find its context in what a patient or client has just been saying.

With the format for the patient interview outlined, the chapter will describe a parallel approach to history-taking from spouse or 'significant other'. Tables provide a summary of the key points in history-taking, both for the person presenting with the problem and the spouse. A scheme for the construction of a case formulation is finally given.

Our concern here is with clinical interviewing. Structured approaches to the alcohol research interview are provided by relevant sections of the Diagnostic Interview Schedule or DIS (Griffin *et al.*, 1987; McCrady *et al.*, 1992), and the Structured Clinical Interview for DSM-III-R or SCID (Segal *et al.*, 1994; Kranzler *et al.*, 1996). Another widely used approach is the Comprehensive International Diagnostic Interview or CIDI (Cottler *et al.*, 1989; Cottler & Compton, 1993; Compton *et al.*, 1996). A comparison of five types of diagnostic interview has been given by Hassin (1991).

Setting the tone

Handling the initial contact with someone who has a drinking problem does not stand entirely apart from work with any other type of patient, but it may have been especially difficult for this person to get themselves so far as to recognise that they have a need for help, and then to keep the first appointment. To admit that they are not fully in control of their drinking can be felt by the patient as tantamount to admitting failure or disgrace, and they may be highly ambivalent about walking into that consulting room.

It is therefore worthwhile for the therapist to ensure that they are not taking their own goodwill as self-evident. Special care must be put into showing ordinary courtesies; to walk up the corridor with the patient rather than five paces in front, to take a coat and hang it up, to show that person towards a comfortable chair, are small but telling gestures. It may be useful to say, 'I'm glad you've decided to come, and I hope that this afternoon will be helpful for you'.

Case-notes have to be recorded and a semi-structured approach is useful. There is a way of handling this procedure which makes it informal and unthreatening. The first question should always be something like, 'Tell me what it is that we should talk about'. There should then be a willingness to listen to the answer while looking at the person who is talking. The answer may be discursive or brief, may bear on the drinking or deal with other issues, but the patient is setting the scene in the way that he or she themselves finds useful. It can be useful to explore the circumstances that have led to this appointment being made.

The therapist then has to introduce the fact that they are going to take a history. A statement such as the following can be made.

> I've listened to what you are saying carefully. If you don't mind, it would help if I asked you some questions and made notes. I'm going to assume that all your answers are as honest and open as you can possibly make them. If there's anything too difficult to talk about, let me know, and I'll respect your feelings.

This might seem to be emphasising the ordinary assumption of the therapeutic position in a way that is overdrawn. But against this fear has to be placed the fact that the patient or client may be coming with the expectation that if they admit the reality of their behaviour they are putting themselves at risk. They are having to face the painful consequences of admitting that their behaviour really was their own behaviour. He or she is exposing themselves to the reactions of a person they do not know, and they may be afraid that this stranger will demean them. There are therefore potentially good, apparent reasons for that patient to adopt a defensive posture to protect against these risks. If history-taking is clumsily handled and the initial relationship not sympathetically established, the interview will be interpreted as attack and defences will rapidly be brought into play. The history obtained will then be filtered through these defences and be inaccurate. The stereotype of the drinker as someone who 'never tells the truth' will have been confirmed.

The disadvantages that stem from a neglect of the dynamic interactions of the initial interview are not only that the information obtained will be wrong and the assessment technically unsatisfactory, but also that damage will be done to what should have been the initiation of therapy. Rather than the patient having a good experience, they will have had a bad experience. The self-image as someone who is untrusting and untrustworthy is reinforced, and self-esteem is further lowered.

How much time for history-taking?

The scheme described in this chapter for the patient's history-taking envisages two parts to the reconstruction – the background history and the drinking history. To cover all the matters that lie in either area, and to conduct the interview at a pace that allows useful pauses and human interactions, clearly means that the process cannot be accomplished in a few minutes. The GP may know that five minutes is all that can be allowed for a routine consultation. It might therefore seem impractical to lay out a scheme for history-taking which might on occasion require two hours for completion.

The causes for believing that it is reasonable to set things out in this way are several. There need be no apologies for the worthwhileness of investing time in thorough initial history-taking (especially if this is also seen as the start of therapy and therapeutic time well-spent). The only problem is how that time is to be found. In some settings it may not be out of step with usual practices to expect that considerable time can be found for the initial history – for instance, a hospital in-patient unit. In other settings it may be feasible to take part of the history and then ask the patient to come back so that the work can be completed. It is often possible to find a point at which the history-taking can temporarily be interrupted, and the patient may return for the second session with some reflective working-through accomplished meanwhile, and an enhanced ability to join in the work of historical review.

Another consideration is the usefulness of extended history-taking for training. The process of taking, say, 5–10 histories at full-length and with supervision and feedback, can mean the acquisition of very worthwhile skills. With trained practice an interview may then be conducted more quickly than had previously seemed feasible (and without undue sense of hurry). To acquire skill in handling such an enquiry, and then to design for oneself a shorter approach based on what has been learnt and the needs of a particular setting or agency, is better than to start out with a greatly abbreviated approach. Once familiar, the essential framework of this scheme is, moreover, not overwhelmingly complex.

In the paragraphs that follow (up to p. 219), the discussion will first focus on the meeting with the patient or client, and then turn to the interview with the spouse.

Background history

It is assumed that anyone coming to this work will already have developed their own general style of case-taking, or that the agency in which they operate will have its preferred format. Whatever is useful in this section of the chapter will have therefore to be reconciled and integrated with many different and already established ways of working. No attempt will be made to lay out in detail all the basic aspects of constructing a general medico-social history. Emphasis will be placed on elucidating those features of background history that are likely to be especially relevant to the understanding of drinking problems.

In taking this history a habit that may be useful is to check what is coming in from the questioning by mentally pausing now and then to ask oneself whether one can imagine what the patient was experiencing at the point in their life now reached by the history. What did their parents' house look like and how would it have felt for a small child to be walking in at the front door? In what sort of street did that house stand and what kind of a street was it to play in? At school, would that child have been standing in a corner of the playground or joining in a game? A striving to understand the culture and the social environment cannot be separated from the attempt to empathise with the individual.

Background history and drinking history are intimately related. In the *background* section many matters are touched on that will inevitably elicit information on drinking and drinking problems, and such information should be jotted down, rather than discarded or ignored because it does not come tidily at the right moment. The *drinking* section as well as eliciting further new information then gives opportunity to bring together relevant material that the patient has given earlier.

Family history

(1) *For both parents.* Age, health (and mental health), and occupation; date and cause of death if deceased. Quality of relationships offered to patient in childhood; parents' drinking and drinking attitudes and drinking problems; psychiatric illness. Present relationship with parents. Enquiry may also be needed into drinking problems and psychiatric illness in the wider family.

(2) *Siblings.* Basic information, social and personal adjustment or maladjustment (including drinking), present contact with patient.

(3) *Childhood environment.* Reconstruction of the home atmosphere during childhood, and the social and cultural milieu to which this home related. Parental discord, separations.

The purpose of this section is to obtain a preliminary understanding of the crucial early relationships and experiences that have contributed to the shaping of the individual's strengths or vulnerabilities, the possible dynamic meaning of alcohol (the meaning attached to alcohol because of parental drinking), and the cultural symbolism of alcohol.

Personal history

(1) *Birth.* Date of birth, any likely evidence of brain trauma which might result in brain injury.

(2) *Adjustment in childhood.* Evidence of neurotic symptoms in childhood, difficulty in relating to other children, and childhood illness. Questioning around this area may help understanding as to

whether the patient has exhibited lifelong traits of anxiety and difficulty in adjustment, and it is useful to go back to a period before the personality picture was overlaid by all the happenings related to drink.

(3) *Schooling.* Information on schooling, with particular reference to social adjustment at school – how the patient got on with other children and with teachers, and school refusal or truancy.

(4) *Occupational history and present occupation.* Chronological information on jobs held, the alcohol-exposed nature of any occupation, problems which drinking has caused.

(5) *Sexual orientation and adjustment,* and the impact of drinking.

(6) *Marriage.* Marriage and the general implications of drinking for the family have already been discussed in Chapter 3. Information should be gathered on the duration and quality of the marriage, on the impact of drinking on the marriage, and on attitudes of the spouse to the patient's drinking.

(7) *Children.* Age and sex, closeness of the patient to children and parenting abilities, any impact of drinking on the children and their reaction to the drinking.

(8) *Finances and housing.* Information both on income and on extra sources of income which help to support drinking, debts, type, and satisfactoriness of accommodation.

(9) *Leisure.* The way in which the person usually spends their leisure, involvement of drinking in leisure pursuits, and the degree to which leisure activities have been curtailed by drinking.

(10) *Forensic history.* Enquiry should be made regarding public drunkenness offences, drink driving, and all other convictions or pending charges. The relationship between the drinking and offending may need to be explored.

Previous illnesses

(1) Physical illness and accidents.
(2) Mental illnesses.

Information is needed under both subheadings, with emphasis on identification of alcohol-related health problems. Under the heading of *mental health*, specific enquiry should always be made for any history suggesting experience of depressive illness or pronounced mood swings, generalised or situational anxiety, obsessional disorder, pathological jealousy, suicide attempts, and drug taking.

Personality

Here what is required is a description of personality prior to drinking or in periods of sobriety – 'the real you'. Information is usefully elicited by open-ended questions such as:

(1) What is the *real* you like?
(2) Your good points?
(3) Your bad points?
(4) What do you want out of life?
(5) What do you expect of friends?
(6) What sort of things worry you or upset you?
(7) What really makes you happy?

Prompts such as 'Go on. Tell me a bit more' will often give revealing information at a point where the patient at first believes that there is nothing to add. An indication should be obtained on at least the following aspects of personality: self-esteem; ability to experience warm feelings and to relate to others; self-control, explosiveness, irritability; social conformity, rule-breaking, deviance; outgoingness, introversion; drive, ambition, passivity – habitual ways of coping with stress or adversity.

Drinking history

Evolution

It is unnecessary to obtain a detailed account of everything that has happened over a lifetime's drinking, but we are seeking here to understand the individual's drinking in longitudinal perspective (Vaillant, 1983; Edwards, 1989; and see Chapter 11). It is necessary to identify important milestones, and to understand the phases of the drinking career and the broadly related influences on it. This picture needs to be built up through exploring four different but closely related dimensions to the person's life, as follows:

The evolution of drinking
The task is to chart the major phases in drinking quantities and patterns, from first experiences of alcohol to the present. Useful questions may relate to such issues as:

(1) First drinking other than the occasional sip in childhood.
(2) First buying own drink.

(3) First drinking most weekends.
(4) First drinking spirits.
(5) Any periods completely off drinking.
(6) First drinking every day.
(7) First drinking eight pints of beer at a sitting, or half a bottle of spirits.
(8) First drinking in present pattern.

Evolution of drink-related problems

Apart from noting objective impacts on health and social functioning, there are two special questions that are often useful:

(1) When did you yourself first *realise drinking was a problem*?
(2) Looking back now with greater understanding, when in fact do you think drinking *really became a problem*?

With hindsight patients will nearly always distinguish between the first self-admission of there being a problem (precipitated perhaps by some catastrophic event) and an earlier date now recognisable as the period when drinking was undramatically beginning to, say, erode the happiness of a marriage or interfere with work.

Evolution of dependence

Here the task is to date the onset of a possible crucial shift in the individual's overall relationship with alcohol, their realisation that they could no longer control their drinking, that they were 'hooked'. Enquiry can then also be made as to the approximate date of onset for specific dependence symptoms such as morning shakes or morning relief drinking.

Evolution of pressures and circumstances

The dimension, which has to be charted under this heading, is concerned with an understanding of the pressures and circumstances which have caused, contributed to, or shaped the evolving drinking patterns, dependence, and problem experience. Questioning has to sense out influences that were already operating when the patient began to drink (parental example, peer group pressures, cultural influence, and so on), and then go forward to understand the subsequent impact of environment, life events, personal relations, mental state, and other relevant factors. A few examples of questioning are these:

* How did your drinking alter
  – when you first left home?;
  – when you were married?;

- after the children were born?;
- when the children left home?;
- when you were promoted to manager?;
- when you worked abroad?;
- after your spouse left you?;
- after you were treated for depression?

The typical recent heavy drinking day

Review of the evolution in drinking history, on the one hand, seeks to build understanding which is *longitudinal* – the present is understood in its historical perspective. Reconstruction of the typical drinking day, on the other hand, focuses exclusively on the present, and the cross-sectional rather than the longitudinal view (Dunn *et al.*, 1992). The styles of enquiry are correspondingly different. When reconstructing the evolution of the problem it is the broad sweep that is important, and the reconstruction of how drinking has interacted with a life path. Analysis of the typical day requires in contrast a minute and focused enquiry directed at present behaviour. This understanding should be so exact that in the mind's eye it is possible to play out a videotape of the patient's day. If necessary, the therapist should feed back to the patient what that person seems to be saying, until accurate understanding is achieved. Some guidelines for this technique of enquiry may be useful.

Establishing the notion of 'typical'

Firstly, the concept which is involved has to be conveyed to the patient. He or she is asked to identify: (1) *a recent period* when drinking was, in terms of their own definition, (2) *heavy*, with the drinking then of a kind which they would generally consider to be (3) *typical* of their recent drinking. The patient has to identify the exact period they have in mind – 'the way I was drinking until two weeks ago when I lost my job and had to cut down'. What has to be emphasised is the actuality, rather than any generalised abstractions that have no real time base. Most patients find it possible to identify such a period, but for others there is so much variability in their drinking pattern that what is typical is difficult to define, and this in itself is a reality which has to be described.

Waking and events around waking

Secondly, having explained the ground rules, it is necessary to establish at what time the patient usually wakes. Enquiry is then made as to the events immediately around the time of waking, for it is here that evidence will be obtained of withdrawal symptoms, withdrawal relief drinking, and other signs and symptoms which help to elucidate the patient's degree of dependence.

Subsequent hour by hour timetabling

Thirdly, the patient is then taken through a reconstruction of the day, as follows:

(1) *The background structure of daily activities.* For instance, what time they leave the house in the morning, what train they catch, what time they get to work, when they take their lunch break, and so on.
(2) *The timetabling of drinking.* With the framework now provided by the structure of the day, the next task is to fit in a full description of the day's drinking. What time does the patient take their first drink, how much do they drink and over what duration? This enquiry is then taken forward step by step, through the day. To a description of actual alcohol intake is in each instance added a note of where the drinking takes place, and with whom (if anyone) the patient is drinking. Note also has to be made of the patient's ideas as to the determinants of each drinking occasion – whether to relieve or avoid withdrawal symptoms, to relieve anxiety or other unpleasant inner feelings, whether in the setting of business or for the companionship of the pub, or for any other reason. A final aspect of drinking which has to be timetabled is the experience of intoxication, and whether at any point of the day the patient would consider that drink is interfering with ordinary functioning. For example, are they unable to work after lunch or falling about when they get home?

Influence of drinking on personality

Some patients are not aware that drinking alters their personality, while another will state that 'I'm an entirely different person when I've been drinking – Jekyll and Hyde'. The issue has to be examined, both in terms of positive and negative effects. Positively, someone may for instance see themselves as more outgoing, confident, and assertive when drinking. On the negative side, the effect may be irritability and loss of control over temper (including violence), suspiciousness, moroseness, self-pity, or lack of feeling for others.

Probing and checking

The following dialogue shows how an important aspect of the drinking history can be elucidated by careful probing:

THERAPIST: All right, you say you have three pints of lager at lunch-time. How long do you spend in the pub at lunch-time?

PATIENT: Twelve noon till 2 p.m., sometimes 3 p.m.

THERAPIST: More often 2 p.m. or 3 p.m?

PATIENT: Say, 2.30 p.m.

THERAPIST: Three pints in two-and-a-half hours seems quite slow drinking.

PATIENT: If I'm there 12 to 2.30 I suppose it would be four or five pints. I was thinking of when I have a short lunch hour. It's more often a long lunch these days.

THERAPIST: You say four or five pints – could it be more?

PATIENT: No, I'd get too bloated. I don't think I'd ever go above five pints.

THERAPIST: Anything else besides lager at lunch-time?

PATIENT: Probably have a couple of whiskies.

THERAPIST: Why 'a couple' – could it be more?

PATIENT: No, I'll have just a couple of whiskies to round things off when I've finished with the lager. Not more than a couple.

THERAPIST: Double or single measures?

PATIENT: Doubles.

THERAPIST: Ever leave out the whisky?

PATIENT: No, it's pretty regular.

Putting quantity consumed against time spent drinking, sometimes checking stated consumption against money usually spent, testing the stated upper limit by offering a higher or lower one, going through other alcoholic beverages than the one first named, relating the stated drinking to the company and other circumstances, all these provide useful methods for checking which can help to build up a valid picture.

Totalling the daily intake

Information on quantity drunk throughout the day can be summed to total daily intake. Because of uncertainties in size of drink poured, broad variations in alcohol content for drinks within any beverage type (beer, wine, or spirits), and international differences as to the size of a standard drink, the summated figure is best seen as an approximation rather than an exact index (Turner, 1990; Miller *et al.*, 1991). For research purposes the most satisfactory approach is to express the total in terms

211

of grams absolute alcohol, but in the clinical setting the idea of *units* provides a useful basis. A unit of intake can be defined approximately thus:

- One glass (half pint) of medium strength beer   1 unit
- Large can of strong lager   3–4 units
- One glass of wine   1 unit
- One measure of fortified wine (port or sherry)   1 unit
- One measure of spirits   1 unit

A standard bottle of wine is likely to contain about 6 units and a bottle of spirits 30 units. A British unit thus defined corresponds to about 8–10 g of absolute alcohol, but it should be stressed that this approach is intended to provide a rough and ready method of totting up the individual's alcohol consumption rather than an absolute measure. American units or 'standard drinks' contain more alcohol (11–12 g) than a British unit; and in the United States the concept has not gained such popularity as in the UK. A Canadian unit is probably about 13–14 g and an Australian unit 10 g. Various questionnaires exist specifically for recording alcohol consumption (Witte & Haile, 1996).

Bringing together the evidence for dependence

Much information relevant to establishing the degree to which the patient is alcohol dependent will have been obtained from questioning in the areas of *evolution* and *drinking day*. It is, however, necessary to have in the history a place where evidence on dependence is reviewed and brought together.

The picture of the dependence syndrome, and its degrees of variations has been fully discussed in Chapter 3 and the headings used in that chapter to describe the core elements of the syndrome provide the framework for this section of the history-taking. Brief notes are added below on the practical approach to questioning in each instance.

Narrowing of the drinking repertoire

Useful questions relate to the sameness or otherwise of drinking during weekdays as opposed to weekends, or during the working year as opposed to holidays. In determining the meaning to be given to the concept of the *typical* day (p. 209), relevant information will in passing have been collected on the degree of variability in recent drinking patterns.

Salience of drinking

Reconstructing the evolution of the patient's drinking will have implicitly provided an account of the progressive importance of alcohol in their life, and their progressive ability to discount other considerations. Attempt should also be made to sense out with the patient how salient drinking has become in the here and now. Useful questions are, for instance:

(1) Just now important has drinking become for you?
(2) Is drinking more, or less, important for you than eating?
(3) Is drinking more important than people?

A particular phrase in the patient's answers may suddenly and empathetically convey the reality of their drink-centredness, 'When my wife said she would leave me if I went on drinking, I had the sly thought, well, if she leaves me, there will be more money for drinking'.

Here it is often useful to ask a question like, 'What are the good things that drinking does for you?' In this way one gains a sense of the functional significance of alcohol for that patient – whether, for example, they see themselves as drinking for company and the pleasures of the bar-room environment, or for the 'high' state and directly pleasurable effects of intoxication, or for relief of unpleasant feelings, or for a combination of these reasons. The dependent drinker may insist that they have ceased to get any pleasure out of drinking, or even say that they hate every drink – they are caught on a treadmill.

Increased tolerance (or evidence of decreased tolerance)

Most patients will say that they can 'drink a lot without getting drunk', and the quantity which is habitually taken is itself evidence of tolerance. If at a later stage in the drinking career a severe *decline in tolerance* is being experienced, this is often reported as a worrying happening.

Withdrawal symptoms

Questioning has to deal with the frequency and intensity of the commoner withdrawal symptoms – tremor, nausea, sweating, mood disturbance. These symptoms may be experienced not only on waking, but also with partial alcohol withdrawal during the waking day. Any history of subacute hallucinatory experiences, delirium tremens, or withdrawal fits should also be noted.

Relief or avoidance of withdrawal symptoms by further drinking

Questioning must cover the frequency with which the patient drinks to relieve or avoid withdrawal and the perceived urgency for such a drink.

Subjective awareness of compulsion to drink

Matters that may bear on assessment of subjective experience have been discussed in Chapter 3. A useful technique is to focus on a specific event or situation and explore the feelings about drink experienced in this setting.

Reinstatement after abstinence

Questioning should focus on the actualities of what happened on recent occasions when the patient was off drink, and went back to drinking again – when they came out of prison perhaps, or when they came out of hospital, or when after a period of involvement with AA they 'had a slip'. How quickly were they again experiencing withdrawal symptoms or needing to take a morning drink?

Standard diagnostic systems for alcohol dependence

DSM-IV (American Psychiatric Association, 1994) and ICD-10 (World Health Organisation, 1992) criteria for diagnosis of alcohol dependence are reproduced in Box 13.1 and 13.2 respectively. These approaches are of great value in standardising diagnostic practice, nationally and inter-nationally, and they carry authority. Their drawback from the clinician's point of view is that they each picture dependence as an all-or-none rather than dimensional state – categorical formulae are proposed at the cost of clinical subtlety. The DSM-IV and ICD-10 approaches are in many ways similar. In the accompanying text ICD mentions 'narrowing of repertoire' and 'subjective awareness of compulsion to use', but does not include these elements in its diagnostic rubric. If a history has been taken in the detail outlined above, more than enough information will have been gathered to enable formal diagnostic decisions to be made within either official system.

Questionnaires for measuring dependence

A number of standardised instruments have been designed which can be used to rate the individual's degree of alcohol dependence (Skinner, 1981; Skinner & Allen, 1982; Hesselbrock et al., 1983; Davidson & Raistrick, 1986; Davidson et al., 1989). The practitioner will do well to gain a working familiarity with just one such approach so that scores can be readily related to their clinical meaning. The Severity of Alcohol Dependence Questionnaire or SADQ (Stockwell et al., 1979), has been widely employed both for clinical and research purposes. On the

SADQ's 60-point scale, scores of around 20–30 suggest that the patient is entering a range of severe dependence. A questionnaire has been developed for rating severity of dependence as represented in patient records (Månsson *et al.*, 1993).

Box 13.1. DSM-IV Criteria for substance dependence (American Psychiatric Association 1994, reproduced by kind permission)

A maladaptive pattern of substance use, leading to clinically significant impairment or distress, as manifested by three (or more) of the following, occurring at any time in the same 12-month period:

(1) tolerance, as defined by either of the following:

    (a) a need for markedly increased amounts of the substance to achieve intoxication or desired effect

    (b) markedly diminished effect with continued use of the same amount of the substance

(2) withdrawal, as manifested by either of the following:

    (a) the characteristic withdrawal syndrome for the substance . . .

    (b) the same (or a closely related) substance is taken to relieve or avoid withdrawal symptoms

(3) the substance is often taken in larger amounts or over a longer period than was intended

(4) there is persistent desire or unsuccessful efforts to cut down or control substance use

(5) a great deal of time is spent in activities necessary to obtain the substance . . .

(6) important social, occupational, or recreational activities are given up or reduced because of substance use

(7) the substance use is continued despite knowledge of having a persistent or recurrent physical or psychological problem that is likely to have been caused or exacerbated by the substance (e.g., current cocaine use despite recognition of cocaine-induced depression, or continued drinking despite recognition that an ulcer was made worse by alcohol consumption)

Box 13.2. ICD Criteria for substance dependence (World Health Organisation 1992, reproduced by kind permission)

Diagnostic guidelines

A definite diagnosis of dependence should usually be made only if three or more of the following have been experienced or exhibited at some time during the previous year:

(a) a strong desire or sense of compulsion to take the substance;

(b) difficulties in controlling substance-taking behaviour in terms of its onset, termination or levels of use

(c) a physiological withdrawal state . . . when substance use has ceased or been reduced, as evidenced by: the characteristic withdrawal syndrome for the substance; or use of the same (or a closely related) substance with the intention of relieving or avoiding withdrawal symptoms

(d) evidence of tolerance, such as that increased doses of the psychoactive substance are required in order to achieve effects originally produced by lower doses . . .

(e) progressive neglect of alternative pleasures or interests because of psychoactive substance use, increased amount of time necessary to obtain or take the substance or to recover from its effects

(f) persisting with substance use despite clear evidence of overtly harmful consequences, such as harm to the liver through excessive drinking, depressive mood states consequent to periods of heavy substance use, or drug-related impairment or cognitive functioning; efforts should be made to determine that the user was actually, or could be expected to be, aware of the nature and extent of the harm

---

Bringing together the evidence for alcohol-related disabilities

Questioning in this section should be aimed at involving the patient themselves in an audit. They should now be able to build a comprehensive picture of the way in which alcohol has adversely influenced their life. Each relevant fact is adduced with the patient's exploration of the significance of the fact and the degree to which alcohol was involved. The final listing of damages is therefore one in which each item has been included only with the patient's testing and agreement. It ends up as their list, their audit, rather than it being the therapist's private clinical note.

Testing each item: the 'agreed' audit

The introduction to this section of history-taking could be as follows:

> Let's try to bring together the ways in which alcohol may have been having any sort of bad effect on your life – on your physical health or your nerves or your job or your marriage, or anything else. You've already told me a lot about separate problems, but now let's try to make out the whole list.

If, for example, the impact of drinking on the patient's marriage were to arise in a particular case, the discussion might be as follows:

THERAPIST: You told me that your wife walked out on you because of your drinking.

PATIENT: If it hadn't been for the drinking we might have made a go of it. I'm not saying we *would* have made a go of it. We *might* have made a go of the marriage.

There is a question here which could be explored with this patient later at greater length, but for purposes of this initial history it is sufficient to establish that the patient accepts as a fair assessment that without the drinking he 'might have made a go of the marriage'. A clumsy inter-rogation that faced him with no more than a sort of yes/no alternative would not have given him an opportunity to convey and define in a per-sonally meaningful way the impact of drinking on marriage.

Playing back the audit

What has been worked through is, at this stage, brought together and the patient is played back a summary of what seems to have been estab-lished – either fully established or accepted only with reservations. The summing-up has to be made with opportunity for interruptions and discussion.

A standardised questionnaire for measuring intensity of problem experience

The Alcohol Problems Questionnaire or APQ (Drummond, 1990) is a standardised inventory which exists in a fuller version and includes

217

sections on marriage, children, and employment, and in a shorter version which excludes those areas. The APQ can make a useful contribution to the overall assessment with the meaning of any scored items discussed with the patient.

History of help-seeking for drinking problems and assessment of motivation

Enquiry should be made both about help sought by the patient in the past, and help being given at present. It is then essential to understand the patient's reasons for coming to this present consultation – the pressures they see themselves as experiencing (for instance, a court order, or threats from a spouse), what crisis may suddenly have precipitated the immediate help-seeking, or what inner sense of need is driving the motivation. Once more, the process of history-taking is an experience for the patient as well as its giving information to the therapist. The patient is exploring the question of why he or she is in this room, and themselves trying to understand the ambiguous, confused or contradictory motivations that have brought them here. Such knowledge is an important basis for later work. The history has to be taken with awareness that motivation is always ambivalent – the patient wants both to go on drinking and to stop drinking. It is these conflicting forces that have to be identified, rather than the reality of conflict being evaded.

Prochaska and DiClemente's concept of 'stages of change' (Prochaska & DiClemente, 1984) has been appreciated by many clinicians as providing a useful framework when assessing the individual's motivation, while Rollnick *et al.* (1992) have developed a 'readiness to change' questionnaire. Read simply, this approach suggests that it is possible to place patients in one of the change categories of pre-contemplation, contemplation, action, and maintenance. We will return to these issues when discussing how psychological interventions may be used to enhance motivation for change (p. 285).

Physical examination and investigations

Physical examination and laboratory investigations will be part of the assessment routine in a medical setting. In a social work or probation office this aspect of assessment is clearly not within expected practice, but there will be advantage in such agencies ensuring that the patient receives a physical examination from a doctor, with the results fed back.

218

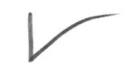

This insistence on the importance of making a medical connection may go against the usual working methods of some non-medical agencies and be seen as burdensome. However, the likelihood of physical disorder in the patient with a drinking problem puts that person in a different category from most social work clients.

History-taking with the patient: the essential framework

In Table 13.1 the essential structure for history-taking is laid out. In the first column, major areas of enquiry are tabulated, using the same headings employed previously. The second column seeks to help the practical business of history-taking by providing a few important reminders as to what has specially to be kept in mind during the process of interview – a series of working notes on technique. The third column provides reminders as to the purpose of the whole exercise and of individual sections. If the sense of purpose is lost, there is danger both of the history becoming inordinately long, and at the same time of its failing in its essential goals.

Initial assessment with the spouse

We now come to discussion of why it is important to interview the spouse, or significant other, as part of the initial assessment procedures, how this interview is to be handled, and its content. It is often helpful if the patient or client can be interviewed by one member of the team, while the spouse is being seen by another, with the information and perspectives then later brought together for joint appraisal and formulation. If that kind of support is not available the therapist may decide to see both husband and wife at this early stage in assessment. There can be advantages in seeing them separately rather than somewhat uncertainly fusing two accounts. Later, however, added insights may be gained through a joint interview.

An outline of the scheme is given at the end of the chapter, and again the detail should not be allowed to intimidate the therapist who is working under extreme constraints of time. With practice, things are simpler than they first seem. Given that many of the issues to be discussed in this part of the chapter parallel matters considered earlier with the patient, the emphasis will so far as possible be on brevity.

Although this chapter deals with the spouse, the value of, at times, also obtaining a story from other informants should be remembered – from another family member, from a friend, or from an employer.

Table 13.1. *Summary scheme for history-taking with the patient*

Area of enquiry	Matters to be kept in mind	Essential purposes
The whole exercise	History-taking is conducted within a patient-therapist *interaction*. The quality of this interaction must purposively be developed so as to *invite the surrender of defences*. A history must *serve the needs of both therapist and patient*.	**For the patient:** *the initiation of therapy*, in terms of (1) the accomplishment of a self-review which *factually arrays and inter-relates a wide variety of experiences* (with drinking and its impact placed in context), and (2) an *undefended exploration of the meaning of those facts*, together with (3) laying the *foundations of a therapeutic relationship*. **For the therapist:** (1) the provision of initial understanding which will be the basis for *developing with this patient the treatment goals and treatment programme*, (2) building the relationship, and (3) a basis for *therapeutic training* and the continued growth of awareness and skills. **Overall:** to provide (1) essential understanding of *the person in their own right, of their present as* continuous with *their past*, and (2) the *context for* understanding the drinking history.

Family history
Both parents, childhood environment

To search after what the home felt like and who was there: 'the street in which it stood'.

Preliminary understanding of crucial early relationships and experiences which may have contributed to the individual's strengths and vulnerabilities, the way they will relate to people, and the dynamic and cultural meaning they will give to alcohol. Understanding of possible genetic influences.

Personal history
Birth, adjustment in childhood, schooling, occupational history, sexual adjustment, marriage, children, finances and housing, leisure, forensic history.

. . . what it feels like to have lived this life . . .

Serving the overall purpose of this dialogue while in passing some information will be obtained on drinking and its consequences, which has later to be ordered.

Previous illness
Physical and mental

Serves the overall purpose as above.

Personality

. . . and to be this person

Crucial explorations to serve the overall purpose.

Drinking history

Throughout – put drinking against background history

Evolution

Four strands of enquiry:
(1) drinking pattern
(2) dependence
(3) drink-related problems
(4) pressures and circumstances

To sense the broad dynamic of an evolving story: *the longitudinal perspective*

Typical recent heavy drinking day.
Waking and events around waking: the timetable of drinking, influence on personality, totalling the daily intake.

(1) Establish the *notion* of the typical day.

(2) The need to focus down on small actualities.

(3) The need to check and probe.

To understand the present in fine detail: *the cross-sectional view.*

Table 13.1. (cont.)

Area of enquiry	Matters to be kept in mind	Essential purposes
Bringing together the evidence for dependence.	To look for *coherence*	An understanding as to whether dependence is *present*, and if so its *degree*.
(1) Narrowing of repertoire		
(2) Salience of drinking		
(3) Tolerance		
(4) Withdrawal symptoms		
(5) Relief or avoidance of withdrawal by drinking		
(6) Subjective awareness of compulsion		
(7) Reinstatement after abstinence		
Bringing together the evidence for alcohol-related disabilities	Testing each item for the patient's agreement	Building a broad and comprehensive picture of the way in which alcohol has adversely affected the patient's life – a *shared audit*
Physical health, mental health, social functioning, and functioning within the family		
History of help-seeking for drinking problems: motivation		
Past and present	Motivation is a matter of ambivalence	To understand why the patient is in this room and the work on motivation that will have to be done.

Permission has always to be obtained from the patient. The occupational physician will want to define the limits of confidentiality which may pertain in that special consultation setting (see p. 339).

Making contact

The spouse who is asked to come for interview may be glad to attend or may come along only with reluctance. A wife may herself have formed the view that her husband's drinking is in some sense a 'family problem', while another woman may see the problem as being solely in her husband's behaviour and be resistant to seeing herself as other than passive victim. Before the therapist starts to guide the discussion into a loosely formal structure, the spouse should be given time to talk freely and to feel assured that their personal needs are going to be listened to attentively.

It is useful to be alert to some of the commoner ways in which the spouse's account may deviate from anything which could fairly be considered the independent and objective truth. Spouses will, for instance, be found who will exaggerate their partner's drinking, and this either because of a conscious wish to blackguard a reputation, or because of a profound anxiety about drinking and drunkenness which at times may lead to something approaching delusional misinterpretation. At the other extreme, a wife or husband may in the face of their partner's appalling and long-continued drinking insist that all is well, either because they are frightened of the drinker's anger if they divulge the truth, or because of subconscious reasons. The more bizarre distortions are not common, but they can give rise to a great deal of puzzlement when they occur. It may be months before the treatment team tumbles to the fact that the client's plaintive insistence on their sobriety is valid, and the partner's account based on a desire to obtain a divorce. But the importance of the issue that is being raised here is to be seen not in terms of the extreme case, but in the reminder that with every case (and each partner), one is presented not with abstract chronicles but with accounts coloured by the active involvement in the story of both people who are talking.

Personal history of the spouse

Family and personal history

The worth of routinely making such enquiry (and the handicap that results from not asking such questions), is illustrated by the following dialogue:

THERAPIST: How much did your parents drink?

WIFE: I went through in childhood everything I'm going through now. How my mother put up with it none of us ever understood. I'd say for years my father never came home sober, and my mother put up with it. He'd come home blinding and swearing and just looking for a fight, and my mother took it year in and year out.

The extent to which this woman is acting out her mother's role is a question vital to any understanding of her (and her husband's) present position, and yet if no one bothers to ask about her parents, she may feel that it is not relevant to tell anyone about her childhood.

Spouse's account of the partner's drinking history

Evolution

The spouse's picture of the evolution of the patient's drinking problem may be the same as the patient's account, or they may be able to offer additional insights.

> He won't tell you this, but I've always felt that he's never liked the attention I've given to the children. I think it was soon after our first son was born that I noticed my husband's drinking. He didn't know how to fit back into the family. Sounds funny, but I've always thought *he* wanted to be the baby in the family.

Present pattern of drinking

To suppose that the spouse can be the independent informant who can give a printout on the quantity and frequency of the patient's drinking is usually unrealistic. It is unlikely that the spouse will be able to give a picture of the present drinking pattern in anything approaching the detail of the patient's account of their 'typical drinking day'. What the spouse can in fact usefully describe is the frequency with which the patient behaves in a way that can be summarised as 'unacceptable' (Orford & Edwards, 1977). A spouse may be able to identify withdrawal symptoms and know that the patient is shaky and retching in the morning, or these symptoms may go unobserved.

224

Problems and hardships

The spouse may or may not be in a position to know what alcohol-related problems the patient has experienced, but it is worthwhile to ask in outline about such matters as illnesses, accidents, lost jobs, debts, forensic involvement, and so on. There are, however, a range of other matters relating to the patient's drinking which the spouse may be uniquely well-equipped to speak about, and these concern the direct impact of the drinking on the family and the spouse themselves – the *hardships* which are being experienced (Orford & Edwards, 1977).

Here are some indications as to the areas of questioning that may be useful.

(1) *Has drinking made the patient unreliable?* The word 'unreliable' may, for the spouse, exactly catch the frustration of what has been experienced, and a question phrased in this manner then leads directly into matters they want to talk about.

> Yes. That's it exactly. It's everything from you have the dinner ready and she's not there to eat it, to that dreadful time last year when we were all lined up for the summer holiday and she disappeared. You can never believe what she's telling you, never trust her to do what she says she is going to do.

(2) *'Rowing on and on'* Here the typical story is of the husband coming home after pub closing time, waking his wife up, and then embroiling her in a smouldering row which goes on for hours. She learns to expect these recurrent scenes in which he recapitulates all her faults and shortcomings, and with the wife knowing of no way to cut into or terminate these dreary replays. Jealous accusations are often part of the content.

(3) *'Turning nasty'* The spouse may come to recognise that at a predictable stage of intoxication *bonhomie* suddenly passes over to a mood of anger or violence. They may know that in such moods the patient will start breaking up the furniture, or assaulting the spouse or the children.

(4) *Money* Commonly the financial hardships and uncertainties experienced by the spouse are part of the chronic strain of living with someone with a drinking problem. It may be a matter of taking money from a purse, the housekeeping money not being provided, of the bills not being paid. Possessions may have been sold or pawned.

(5) *'Useless in the evening'* The story here is of the drinker who gets home in the evening and who does not engage in rowing or violence, but who pushes aside the supper and then night after night slumps

drunkenly asleep in an armchair. They may be found there in the morning.

(6) *Wetting the bed* Bed-wetting is a not uncommon feature of a drinking problem, and in an advanced stage the patient may soil themselves. And in a state of drunken confusion they may get up and urinate in a corner of the bedroom.

Coping

The *coping mechanisms* that the spouse may employ have been discussed in Chapter 4. Enquiry should be made into the ways in which the spouse is dealing with the patient's drinking and the types of mechanism that they are deploying. It is useful to think in terms of different styles, such as circumvention, attack, manipulation, spoiling, constructive management, and constructive help-seeking, although it is likely that in many instances some mixtures of styles will be perceived (Orford & Edwards, 1977). This type of understanding can provide a useful basis for later therapeutic work. The spouse begins to see patterns in their own behaviour, and to realise the degree to which they may be persevering in unproductive or counter-productive responses, and the possibilities of more constructive reaction.

Rounding off the interview

It must be stressed again that any assessment interview is properly a therapeutic encounter, whether that interview is with the person with the drinking problem or with the spouse. For the spouse, the interview should be an opportunity to bring order and understanding to muddled and painful happenings, the chance to discover or express feelings and often a conflict of feelings, a confirmation of worth as an individual, and a sensing of ways in which they may have compounded the problem. When this interview is being rounded off, it is necessary to show some response to the feelings that have been awakened.

Assessment with the spouse: the essential framework

Table 13.2 displays the essential framework for history-taking with the spouse, in a format parallel to that used for assessing the patient given earlier.

Area of enquiry	Matters to be kept in mind	Essential purposes
The whole exercise	Establishing the objective facts is important	*For the spouse:* (1) the review of happenings and feelings in a way that begins to make sense and to have shape (2) awareness of self as more than passive participant or victim (3) laying the foundations for future therapeutic work
	Feelings and interactions also matter	*For the therapist:* (1) further understanding of the needs of the spouse (2) further understanding of the marital interactions (3) collateral information
Personal history of the spouse	A history has to be taken of this person in their own right; to know who this person is; where they are coming from, what is brought to the marriage	Understanding how these heritages interact with current problems and determine present needs.
The drinking problem	The objective facts are only to be sensed through the colouring which this witness must bring to a situation in which he or she is personally involved	To sense the outlines and dynamics of the drinking story, the picture of the present drinking, and the extent of hardship
	The account given by the spouse of hardships experienced needs different headings than the patient's account of alcohol-related problems	To enable the spouse to express grief and anger and ambivalences of feeling, and to know that it is safe to share these experiences
Coping	The range and mixture of mechanisms that are being deployed	Understanding the stage of development in the marital interaction and possibilities for more constructive response

Patient and spouse: assessment as asset

The assessment procedures both with the patient and their spouse constitutes a considerable investment of their time and that of the people conducting these procedures. Significant work has been accomplished in terms of building relationships and self-understanding, and the material gathered constitutes an essential base for planning and action. It should at this point again be emphasised that these initial assessments are designed to provide insights and information to be used, and to be employed in guiding the practical next steps forward. A well-conducted assessment is an immensely valuable therapeutic asset on which further to build.

The case formulation

The diagnostic interview or interviews with the patient, interviews where possible with the spouse or additional informants, reports from other agencies, the results of laboratory tests, and any other enquiries are between them going to provide a mass of information. That information has to be synthesised into an initial case formulation. Lots of separate pieces may give many separate and partial insights, but it is crucial that the attempt should then be made to stand back and perceive the whole predicament. Formulation is the attempt to *understand*, and a well-constructed formulation is a creative act of empathy rather than just an ordering of information under headings.

There are in fact several reasons for believing that this additional investment of time is worth the demand. The therapist is directionless until the formulation is made. Furthermore, even if after data-gathering has been completed and the therapist has a sense of understanding the patient, when the notes are put aside for a few weeks and the patient re-attends, the freshness of understanding has often faded unless the formulation has been written. The original formulation will also be of great use if a case is reopened after a gap of a year or two, or if the patient is eventually taken over by someone else. Construction of a detailed formulation is invaluable as a training exercise.

Besides these various ways in which the formulation is of use to the therapist or therapeutic team, it is equally to be conceived as a basis for discussion with the patient and spouse – a basis for sharing and feedback on the assessment work which has been accomplished together.

A formulation should not be of inordinate length or it defeats its purpose. The format proposed here is to be taken only as a starting point, to be amended or scaled down according to individual professional needs and feasibilities.

Headings for a formulation

Diagnosis

It is preferable that this heading should be taken as an invitation to a *full listing* of diagnosis rather than just a statement of 'the' diagnosis. The necessary subheadings are as follows:

(1) Alcohol dependence – its presence or absence, and if present its degree of development, with an outline of the supporting evidence.
(2) All alcohol-related disabilities (medical, psychological, social).
(3) Ancillary diagnoses, including underlying or accompanying psychiatric conditions and physical disorders.

Description of personality

It is preferable to attempt a brief description of personality, rather than to use such phrases as 'personality disorder' within the diagnostic listing above. The aim is to summarise provisional insights regarding both personal strengths and vulnerabilities.

Present social situation

(1) Marital status, marital interactions and rewardingness of the marriage, wife's coping, and role of children in the present situation.
(2) Employment.
(3) Accommodation.
(4) Leisure.
(5) Religious involvement.
(6) Forensic status.

Drinking

(1) *History of the drinking problem.* Synopsis.
(2) *Aetiology of the drinking,* in terms both of more distant determinants and more recent influences.
(3) *The typical drinking day.* Summary description and estimate of usual daily intake.
(4) *The balance of present motivations.* Appraisal of patient's current losses and gains from drinking, and degree of motivation.
(5) *History of help-seeking.*

The family's health and well-being

Problems currently affecting spouse or children

Further information needed

A list, for instance, of what further information has to be sought from the patient or other informants, other agencies to be contacted, specialist opinion to be obtained, or specialised diagnostic procedures to be arranged.

Goals

On the basis of what has already been laid out in the preceding sections of the formulation it should be possible to set up a series of specific treatment goals. As with diagnosis, what is required is a list rather than a single monolithic statement.

Action steps

Under this heading are set out in objective terms the steps that have to be taken to achieve the stated goals. The actualities should be listed, rather than any vague generalisations such as 'treat the alcoholism'. This is an aspect of the formulation that must be designed in co-operation with patient and family.

Prognosis

Prognosis should be written in terms of an informed, balanced and well argued weighing of probabilities.

The formulation as shared exercise

Reference has already been made to the necessity of the formulation serving the needs of the patient as well as the therapist. Before making final notes on the formulation there should have been an interchange in which the therapist says, 'What we have talked through is valuable . . . I see it this way . . . What we ought to do is perhaps this . . . How do you see it? . . . Can we agree then . . .'. Such discussion ensures that not only is the therapist standing back from the data and gaining a whole view, but the patient is doing the same, and they are doing so together.

References

American Psychiatric Association (1994) *Diagnostic and Statistical Manual of Mental Disorders*, 4th edn. Washington: American Psychiatric Association.

Compton, W. M., Cottler, L. B., Dorsey, K. B., Spitznagel, E. L. & Mager, D.E. (1996). Comparing assessment of DSM substance dependence disorder using CIDI-SAM and SCAN. *Drug and Alcohol Dependence* **41**, 179–88.

Cottler, L. B., Robins, L. N. & Helzer, J.E. (1989). The reliability of the CIDI-SAM: a comprehensive substance abuse interview. *British Journal of Addiction* **159**, 653–8.

Cottler, L. B. & Compton, W. M. (1993). Advantages of the CIDI family of instruments in epidemiological research on substance use disorders. *International Journal of Methods in Psychiatric Research* **3**, 109–19.

Davidson, R. & Raistrick, D. (1986). The validity of the Short Alcohol Dependence Data (SADD) questionnaire: a short self-report questionnaire for the assessment of alcohol dependence. *British Journal of Addiction* **81**, 217–22.

Davidson, R., Bunting, B. & Raistrick, D. (1989). The homogeneity of the alcohol dependence syndrome: a factor analysis of the SADD questionnaire. *British Journal of Addiction* **84**, 907–15.

Departments of Psychiatry and Child Psychiatry, The Institute of Psychiatry and the Maudsley Hospital London (1987). *Psychiatric Examination: Notes on Eliciting and Recording Clinical Information in Psychiatric Patients.* Oxford: Oxford University Press.

Drummond, D. C. (1990). The relationship between alcohol dependence and alcohol-related problems in a clinical population. *British Journal of Addiction* **85**, 357–66.

Dunn, J. N., Seilhamer, R. A., Jacob, T. & Whalen, M. (1992). Comparisons of retrospective and current reports of alcoholics and their spouses on drinking behaviour. *Addictive Behaviours* **17**, 543–55.

Edwards, G. (1989). As the years go rolling by. Drinking problems in the time dimension. *British Journal of Addiction* **154**, 18–26.

Griffin, M. L., Weiss, R. D., Mirin, S. M., Wilson, H. & Bouchard-Voelk, B. (1987). The use of the Diagnostic Interview Schedule in drug dependent patients. *American Journal of Drug and Alcohol Abuse* **13**, 281–91.

Hasin, D. S. (1991). Diagnostic interviews for assessment: background, reliability, validity. *Alcohol Health and Research World* **15**, 293–302.

Hesselbrock, M., Babor, T. F., Hesselbrock, V., Meyer, R. E. & Workman, K. (1983). 'Never believe an alcoholic?' On the validity of self report measures of alcohol dependence and related constructs. *International Journal of Addiction* **18**, 593–609.

Kranzler, H. R., Kadden, R. M., Babor, T. F., Tenner, H. & Rounsaville, B. J. (1996). Validity of the SCID in substance abuse patients. *Addiction* **91**, 859–64.

Månsson, M., Hansson, M., Hoberg, A.-L. & Berglund, M. (1993). Severity of alcohol dependence, rating by patient records. *Alcohol and Alcoholism* **28**, 347–51.

MacGrady, R. G., Rogler, L. H. & Tryon, W. W. (1992.) Issues of validity in the Diagnostic Interview Schedule. *Journal of Psychiatric Research* **26**, 59–67.

Miller, W .R., Heather, N. & Hall, W. (1991). Calculating standard drink units: international comparisons. *British Journal of Addiction* **86**, 43–7.

Novey, S. (1968). *The Second Look*. Baltimore: Johns Hopkins Press.

Orford, J. & Edwards, G. (1977). *Alcoholism: A Comparison of Treatment and Advice, with a Study of the Influence of Marriage*. Maudsley Monograph Number 26. Oxford: Oxford University Press.

Prochaska, J. O. & DiClimente, C. C. (1984). *The Transtheoretical Approach: Crossing Traditional Boundaries of Therapy*. New York: Daw-Jones Ireven.

Rollnick, S., Heather, N., Gold, R. & Hall, W. (1992). Development of a short 'readiness to change questionnaire' for use in brief, opportunistic interventions among excessive drinkers. *Addiction* **87**, 743–54.

Segal, D. C., Hersen, M. & Van Hasselt, V. B. (1994). Reliability of the Structured Clinical Interview for DSM-III-R; an evaluative review. *Comprehensive Psychiatry* **35**, 316–27.

Skinner, H. A. (1981). Primary syndromes of alcohol abuse: their measurement and correlates. *British Journal of Addiction* **76**, 63–76.

Skinner, H. A. & Allen, B. A. (1982). Alcohol dependence syndrome: measurement and validation. *Journal of Abnormal Psychology* **91**, 199–209.

Stockwell, T., Hodgson, R., Edwards, G., Taylor, C. & Rankin, H. (1979). The development of a questionnaire to measure severity of alcohol dependence. *British Journal of Addiction* **74**, 79–87.

Thom, B., Brown, D., Drummond, C., Edwards, G., Mullan, M. & Taylor, C. (1992). Engaging patients with alcohol problems in treatment: the first consultation. *British Journal of Addiction* **87**, 601–11.

Turner, C. (1990). How much alcohol in a 'standard drink'? An analysis of 125 studies. *British Journal of Addiction* **85**, 1171–5.

Vaillant, G. E. (1983). *The Natural History of Alcoholism*. Cambridge: Harvard University Press.

Witte, J. S. & Haile, R. W. (1996). Agreement in alcohol consumption levels as measured by two different questionnaires. *Journal of Studies on Alcohol* **56**, 406–9.

World Health Organisation (1992). *The ICD-10 Classification of Mental and Behavioural Disorders: Clinical Descriptions and Diagnostic Guidelines*. Geneva: World Health Organisation.

14

Withdrawal states and treatment of withdrawal

Withdrawal in perspective

Different needs of differing patients

On the one hand, there are many patients who, although they have sustained serious problems as a result of their drinking, have not contracted the dependence syndrome and will experience no significant physiological disturbance on withdrawal. A further important sector of patients will show dependence to a slight or moderate degree, but will not suffer from withdrawal symptoms that are to any major extent incommoding. On the other hand, there are patients who are going to feel wretched on withdrawal, and a small group for whom withdrawal will precipitate life-threatening disturbance.

Given diversity in possible withdrawal experience, it makes no sense to approach the treatment of withdrawal in terms of a fixed regime for all-comers. A spectrum of likely withdrawal experiences suggests the need for a spectrum of treatment approaches as corollary. Many patients will need no medication at all to help them come off alcohol while for many others withdrawal can be safely managed on an out-patient basis with minimum drug cover. In only the minority will withdrawal require admission to hospital, but for some of those patients the effective use of medication will be vital. The clinical significance of withdrawal is firstly, therefore, the demand it makes on the clinician to see the different needs of different patients and to manage minor withdrawal states without unnecessary fuss, while at the same time learning to recognise the necessity for very great care in treating the potentially dangerous situation. This chapter will discuss treatment in terms of different regimes for different intensities of need.

Significance of withdrawal as barrier to 'coming off'

Some patients will present themselves as unable to come off alcohol because of their incapacity to cope with the withdrawal symptoms. This plea may be entirely genuine. A patient who has previously experienced an attack of delirium tremens may know full well that when they are in a state of severe relapse there is a grave risk of precipitating a further attack of delirium if they attempt abruptly to stop drinking. Their pleas for admission should be heeded. However, there are patients with less severe degrees of dependence whose belief that they cannot stop drinking without coming into hospital should be kindly resisted. It is important for such patients to learn that they can cope with withdrawal at home, with minimal ado, and without repeated admissions which reinforce the idea of incapacity to deal with relapse themselves. Unnecessary admissions that mean invalidism and time-off work must be avoided.

Withdrawal and teamwork

Given that drugs may have to be prescribed for out-patient withdrawal, and given also the potential seriousness of the major withdrawal experience which demands in-patient admission, it is evident that the medical practitioner has an important role to play in treatment of these conditions. If the case is primarily being handled by non-medical staff, this implies the need for good medical liaison. The social worker in a voluntary agency must, for instance, know when to make the quick out-patient referral, or call on the advice of the GP with whom there is a working relationship.

Detoxification in context

Mere drying out is not by itself an effective way of helping a patient and, whatever is done about withdrawal, only has its meaning within the context of other strategies for aiding the patient. When plans for withdrawal are being made at the same time as initial assessment and goal-setting, the withdrawal phase is easily placed within the wider frame. When, however, withdrawal is being dealt with in response to relapse and in an atmosphere of crisis, it is easy to react precipitously and forget the context within which decisions about withdrawal treatment ought to be made. Questions that should be asked in such circumstances centre on what *use* the patient is to make of this help (either as out-patient or in-patient), and what the patient's expectations are of this particular aspect of the contract to help. What plans has the patient got for the far side of withdrawal? Treatment of relapse is discussed further in Chapter 15.

A checklist for detoxification in the community

It should be possible safely and effectively to detoxify the majority of patients in the community (Hayashida *et al.*, 1989; Collins *et al.*, 1990; Stockwell *et al.*, 1991). This section will consider the ways in which community or out-patient detoxification of the not too severely dependent patient can be managed.

Does the patient want to come off alcohol?

To put this item first in the checklist may seem an over-emphasis of the obvious, but it is not uncommon to see medical prescribing that suggests a confusion of logic. The doctor has given the patient drugs to treat withdrawal because the doctor believes that the patient ought to come off alcohol, rather than because the patient seriously intends to come off alcohol. The patient leaves the interview with a prescription for a bottle of tranquillisers which they will use to supplement their continued alcohol intake.

Is it safe to conduct withdrawal in an out-patient setting?

This decision is made without difficulty when, as commonly happens, it is obvious that the patient has not got a severe dependence syndrome. They are, for instance, suffering from morning shakes of only moderate intensity which have been present for not much longer than six months, and one month ago they came off alcohol for two weeks on their own initiative without any untoward happenings. A brief review with the patient of such points as these will usually settle the question of whether out-patient withdrawal is appropriate. A similarly quick answer can be reached in the other direction if there is a previous history of major withdrawal experience and the patient has now reinstated dependence of serious degree. It is decisions in the middle ground that set difficulty and which call for the most experienced skill. Handling this problem will, as ever, depend on a relationship with the patient that allows open discussion of the issues involved. Such a patient may come into hospital for an admission of only two or three days 'to see how things go', or alternatively they may opt initially to try detoxification at home provided they have good support.

In addition to severity of dependence, a number of other specific pointers may offer further guidance regarding the safety of a community 'detox'. Has out-patient detoxification failed previously and, if so, why? Is there any specific medical reason why community detoxification may be hazardous – for example, a history of delirium tremens or withdrawal seizures? Is the home environment sufficiently supportive, both in terms of family or friends who may summon help if needed, and in terms of support for treatment of the drinking problem? (This is discussed further, below.)

A summary of the indicators that might suggest that detoxification is more safely and effectively conducted on an in-patient basis is given in Box 14.1.

Box 14.1. Contra-indications to a community detoxification

- Severe dependence

- History of delirium tremens or withdrawal seizures

- Previous failed community detoxification

- Unsupportive home environment

Is there likely to be a withdrawal experience which requires treatment?

If it is necessary to make sure that the patient is not so dependent as to preclude the out-patient approach, it is also necessary to ensure that they are indeed suffering at all from a dependence syndrome, or from dependence of more than minimal degree. Otherwise, one may fairly talk about treatment of their drinking problem and the strategies they may apply for abstinence or ameliorated drinking, but there is no sense in setting up a withdrawal regime when there is no significant withdrawal disturbance to be treated. This might again seem a too obvious point if it were not common to find patients routinely medicated with minor tranquillisers without any enquiry being made into their true needs.

What is the best time?

It may be asking too much for a man or woman with a busy job to try to achieve successful withdrawal in the midst of engagements and in the full setting of usual drinking pressures. Discussion may suggest that the patient set aside a long weekend or take a holiday specially for this purpose. To suggest this degree of forward planning may usefully help to focus commitment.

Is there adequate support?

Although there are plenty of people who at some time in their lives have been so determined to deal with their drinking that they have come off alcohol in such adverse surroundings as a drink-laden doss house, it is always useful to think through with the patient how environmental supports may be deployed to maximise the chances of success. If there is a husband or wife to give support, that person should be brought into the discussion and the active engagement of the spouse may have benefit for both partners. This may also be the moment when a patient will be particularly able to accept the usefulness of AA – getting out, for instance, to an AA meeting and hearing how others dealt with this problem, or a phone call from an AA member giving a feeling of contact and fellowship, with a follow-through to more continuing involvement. The hospital doctor must also ensure that the GP is kept in the picture. Support from the hospital may imply the offer of daily appointments over the period of a few days, and staff should be prepared to make a home visit if necessary. If there is no other social support available, day-patient facilities for a short period may be helpful.

Use of drugs

Some practical aspects of the use of drugs in out-patient withdrawal will be briefly discussed in this section, both so as to provide background information for the person other than the doctor who wants to understand this aspect of the patient's treatment, and so as to emphasise points of immediate medical concern.

Given that assessment suggests that a major withdrawal state is not a risk, but that there is reason to believe that some degree of withdrawal symptoms is going to be experienced, then most patients within this band of the dependence spectrum are going to need a minor tranquilliser prescribed. The same drug may be used for daytime and night-time sedation. Within this spectrum there will, however, be a range of severities, so therapy may involve a range of drug doses with the emphasis always on avoiding needless over-medication.

There are a number of different drugs that are effective for this purpose. A drug of the benzodiazepine group should be considered as the first choice. It is best for the individual doctor to become familiar with one drug, so as to develop a sense of the likely needed dosages in particular circumstances, rather than their switching from drug to drug. Among the benzodiazepines, chlordiazepoxide (trade name Librium) may be prescribed in a dose of say 5 to 10 mg three or four times per day.

Although chlormethiazole (trade name Heminevrin) has been popular in the past, and may still have a role in in-patient detoxification, it is contraindicated in the out-patient context. This is because of the potentially fatal interaction with alcohol in the case of the patient who continues drinking (McInnes, 1987). Chlormethiazole is not licensed for prescription in the United States.

The dose and frequency of medication should be discussed with patient and spouse, and explicit instructions written down. A prescription should not be given for more than three to seven days, and prescribing should not be allowed to trail on unnecessarily once the patient has withdrawn. A community detoxification regime does not need to be longer than one week. The patient should be cautioned against the risks of driving when under the influence of drugs.

Prescription of vitamins is not a routine part of withdrawal treatment within this severity range, but may sometimes be indicated on other grounds.

A checklist for in-patient treatment of withdrawal (other than delirium tremens or withdrawal seizures)

In this section the treatment of the greater part of the spectrum of withdrawal states seen in the in-patient setting will be discussed, but treatment of delirium tremens and of alcohol withdrawal seizures will be held over for discussion in the next section. The checklist here bears on medical and nursing practice.

Remember that in the in-patient setting (as with out-patient), a wide range of withdrawal states will be encountered

It is inappropriate for a ward to operate in terms of any fixed drug regime. At the time of admission a patient-specific withdrawal regime has to be set up for each case, and this regime must be flexible in response to unfolding events.

Monitoring is very important

Competent routine ward monitoring provides the basis for treatment which is alert, flexible, and able rapidly to be escalated in case of need.

There is much to be said for the use of standardised scales to facilitate this process, and a number of suitable instruments are available. For example, the Selective Severity Assessment Scale (SSA; Gross *et al.*, 1973) provides precise instructions for rating 11 variables: eating disturbance, sleep disturbance, agitation, hallucinations, tremor, sweats, clouding of consciousness, quality of contact, temperature, pulse, and convulsions. The revised Clinical Institute Withdrawal Assessment for Alcohol scale (CIWA-Ar; Sullivan *et al.*, 1989) is a more recent, 10 item, derivation of the SSA, which has been refined and modified in various ways. Careful monitoring, combined with supportive care, can reduce the need for medication (Shaw *et al.*, 1981).

A sensible ward procedure may be for the nurses to make at least eight-hourly observations on all withdrawing patients for the first three days, but this may need to be more frequent during the first 24 hours. Observations may be discontinued with the senior nurse's approval if all areas are normal. Every now and then a patient who has given an incomplete history and who is expected to show only mild withdrawal will unexpectedly develop more severe symptoms. Routine observations over the first few days are therefore essential.

In addition to rating withdrawal symptoms, breath alcohol should be measured when the patient arrives on the ward, and again an hour or so later. This allows an estimation of the actual BAC, and also confirms the rate of fall of blood alcohol. This is important for several reasons. Firstly, if estimated blood or breath alcohol is high, there may be a danger of interaction with prescribed medication during the first few hours of admission, and particular care must be taken with prescribing during this period. Secondly, if the patient has consumed a significant amount of alcohol immediately before admission, their blood alcohol levels may still be rising. This should generate even greater caution in the prescribing and administration of medication immediately after admission.

Environment

That the environment should be properly supportive is as important here as when the patient is detoxifying at home. General and psychiatric nursing skills have to be employed to help the patient through what may be a few unpleasant days, and the ability of the patient to tolerate this experience will depend in part on the sort of friendliness which they are being offered. To mobilise support from other patients and from visiting relatives can also be valuable.

Drug treatments

The possible use to be made here of a number of different drugs will be considered separately.

Minor tranquillisers

The same types of drugs can be prescribed here as for ambulatory treatment, but in a setting which allows close monitoring and where the severer grades of withdrawal are sometimes being dealt with, considerably larger doses may on occasion be employed. There is an old saying that the proper dose of any drug is *enough*, and that certainly applies in these circumstances. The skilled use of a drug with the intention of ameliorating severe withdrawal distress or aborting risk of delirium is a matter of titrating the drug dose against the symptoms. The withdrawal symptoms occur because the level of alcohol in the brain is falling, and these symptoms will be ameliorated when the level of prescribed drug is high enough to compensate for the fall in alcohol. What one is in fact doing is substituting a monitored drug intoxication for an alcohol intoxication, and it is in those terms necessary and rational, in the severe case, to press the drug dose boldly.

With a benzodiazepine, in severe withdrawal, one may have to give quite large doses. For example, a dose of 40 to 60 mg chlordiazepoxide, three or four times a day, or even more than this, may be required. If there is immediate need to bring severe symptoms under control, then lorazepam may be given by intramuscular injection, with an initial dose of, say 25–30 µg/kg. Alternatively, diazepam may be given by slow intra-venous injection or per rectum (as a suppository or enema).

If chlormethiazole is given, the dose may be pressed up to say 600 mg of chlormethiazole base, four times daily by mouth. (Note that chlormethiazole syrup contains chlormethiazole edisylate, and that 250 mg chlormethiazole edisylate in syrup is therapeutically equivalent to approximately 192 mg chlormethiazole base as a capsule. If in doubt about dosage, current information should be obtained from the manufacturer or the relevent national formulary.) In the in-patient setting, this drug can be safely and effectively employed in the treatment of alcohol withdrawal. However, there is no particular advantage over the benzodiazepines and in-patient practices are often seen as a model to copy in primary care. It may, therefore, be best avoided.

It should again be stressed that what is 'enough' is determined by clinical observation of response rather than by any rule book. If the patient becomes excessively drowsy or if there is a large fall in blood pressure, drugs should be cut back or temporarily withheld. Such an approach is far more in the patient's interests than a blind reliance on heavy mixed drug schedules, which will be unnecessarily extreme in many instances, and yet insufficient in other cases.

If it has been necessary in the acute phase to load the patient with a drug, one is then in effect subsequently carrying out a drug withdrawal rather than an alcohol withdrawal procedure. And this implies gradually tailing off the drug dose at a rate that will not produce significant drug withdrawal symptoms. The rate of reduction must once more be patient-specific and in accord with monitored symptoms. Problems may in particular arise if withdrawal from a large dose of chlormethiazole is carried out too quickly, with confusion or delirious symptoms arising. However, there is evidence that few, if any, patients actually require medication with a benzodiazepine for more than two days (Saitz et al., 1994), and regimes of longer than 7–10 days are rarely if ever necessary for uncomplicated alcohol withdrawal.

Vitamins

With patients who have had a heavy alcohol intake there is the risk of an acute Wernicke's encephalopathy developing with disastrous suddenness (see Chapter 8), and it is therefore a wise prophylactic measure to give thiamine (vitamin B1) supplements. These may be given orally, for example in a dose of 100 mg daily, but there is evidence that absorption is particularly poor in this group of patients (Thomson et al., 1970). Parenteral administration (either intramuscular or slow intravenous) is therefore to be preferred, particularly where there is specific cause for concern (Cook & Thomson, 1997). For example, in cases of malnutrition, peripheral neuropathy, or signs and symptoms of a Wernicke-Korsakoff syndrome, it would seem to be particularly important to employ this approach. The correct dose is a subject of debate, but one pair of ampoules of high potency parenteral B vitamins, once or twice daily, for three to five days, is probably effective in preventing the onset of Wernicke-Korsakoff syndrome (Majumdar, 1980; Bligh & Madden, 1983). A higher dose may be required in established cases (Nakada & Knight, 1984; Lindberg & Oyler, 1990).

Administration of parenteral vitamins has become much less popular following reports of very rare, but sometimes severe, adverse reactions (O'Brien, 1995). However, it must not be forgotten that Wernicke's encephalopathy is potentially fatal, and that the sequelae can be severely disabling. In a properly supervised in-patient setting, where some patients may be at particular risk of Wernicke-Korsakoff syndrome, the balance of risks and benefits will usually be in favour of parenteral vitamin supplementation.

Major tranquillisers
Phenothiazines and other major tranquillisers have no part to play in the treatment of this spectrum of withdrawal, and only add to the risks.

Specific treatment to avert withdrawal seizures
The effective use of minor tranquillisers should be sufficient to minimise the development of serious withdrawal seizures, and it is usually neither necessary nor useful to give additional medication for this purpose. (See below for further discussion of this matter.)

The treatment of delirium tremens

This section deals with technical issues that are mainly the concern of medical and nursing staff, but it may again be of interest to other professionals to acquaint themselves with at least the outlines of how such problems are handled.

The best hope here is in fact that the condition will not arise and not have to be treated. If severe withdrawal is adequately managed with appropriate drug doses the risk of delirium tremens will in many instances be aborted. However, despite the best efforts, ward admission and alcohol withdrawal will sometimes precipitate delirium tremens, and cases of already established delirium will also sometimes present directly for admission. Once a fully developed attack of delirium tremens is underway, it is uncertain whether any treatment will actually shorten the course of the disorder, but there is persuasive evidence that the difference between competent and less competent treatment may be the survival as opposed to the death of the patient. The dangers of death from delirium tremens should not be exaggerated, but they exist.

The following are matters to be kept in mind when treating this condition (and see also Box 14.2).

What setting for treatment?

Given the risks to life, patients suffering from this condition should have the benefit of being treated in a setting where the medical and nursing staff are as experienced as possible. When a case occurs on a psychiatric ward there may be uncertainty as to whether the patient should remain on that ward or be transferred to a general medical unit. The decision can only be made in the light of an appraisal of the skills and resources available in either setting.

242

Box 14.2 Important requirements in the treatment of delirium tremens

- In-patient environment, preferably with experienced staff
- Careful assessment and monitoring for comorbid physical and psychiatric disorders – especially head injury, intercurrent infection, liver disease and hepatic coma, gastrointestinal bleeding, and acute Wernicke-Korsakoff syndrome
- Chlordiazepoxide is the preferred drug treatment
- Careful monitoring of body temperature, fluids, electrolytes, and blood sugar
- Parenteral vitamin supplementation
- Availability of emergency medical facilities

But whatever the ward on which the patient is to be treated, the basic elements which the setting must provide are much the same. First-rate nursing is required, both for observation and for care. The situation must be one where a potentially disturbed patient can be cared for without staff becoming flustered, and there must be precaution against a patient sustaining accidental injury whilst in a state of confusion. A safe nursing environment must be established with no possibility of the patient falling out of the window or wandering off the ward. A patient who is only uncertainly in contact with reality is going to be helped by friendliness, reassurance and by good room lighting rather than a side-room with shadowy corners.

Depending upon the mental health legislation of the country concerned, it may be necessary to consider formal admission if the patient refuses to stay in hospital. The risks to such a patient, should they be allowed to take their own discharge, would be considerable and there should be no hesitation to arrange an assessment for compulsory detention. In the UK, this would be under a section of the Mental Health Act (1983). Note that it is the delirium tremens, not alcohol dependence, which would justify detention against the patient's will.

What underlying or complicating conditions may be missed?

Those patients who die in delirium tremens perhaps most often do so as a result of a medical complication that has been overlooked. Such oversight, unless actively guarded against, can easily come about when all energies are being concentrated on dealing with the immediate and acutely worrying presentation. The patient is probably in no condition to give an accurate history or an account of other symptoms.

The conditions, which may have to be recognised, are many (and have already been outlined in Chapter 6), and no checklist can substitute for full initial examination and subsequent continued watchfulness. But conditions specially to be borne in mind include the possibility of head injury, intercurrent infection (particularly chest infection), liver disease and hepatic coma, gastrointestinal bleeding, and the acute onset of the Wernicke-Korsakoff syndrome. The picture may also be complicated if the patient has been taking barbiturates or another depressant.

What drug to use for specific treatment?

Much the same considerations apply here as with choice of drugs for treatment of less severe withdrawal symptoms. A great deal of research has been aimed at determining which drug is likely to be most useful in treating delirium tremens, and the evidence is still conflicting. On the whole it seems best to employ a drug with cross-tolerance to alcohol, and hence one that effectively *substitutes* for alcohol. Chlordiazepoxide may be given in a dose up to 400 mg daily by mouth in divided doses. Where a rapid response is required, it may be necessary to supplement this with intramuscular, intravenous or rectal medication, as described above. As ever, an intravenous drug should not be used if avoidable. The dose of chlormethiazole will usually be in the region of 600 mg by mouth, four times daily (but see the note above regarding the dosage of chlormethiazole syrup, which is slightly different) with higher doses employed with care if indicated. Phenothiazines and other major tranquillisers may increase the risk to life, although some clinicians do prescribe them in delirium tremens, to control acutely disturbed behaviour (see for example, Chick, 1989) or hallucinations (Fish, 1991).

The use of an intravenous chlormethiazole infusion is worthy of especial mention, because of the particular dangers associated with its use. It is rarely, and in our experience virtually never, necessary to resort to such treatment if oral chlordiazepoxide has been employed boldly in conjunction with good nursing care. Where it is employed, we would urge that it should only be when high doses of oral chlordiazepoxide have failed to control the delirium, and where the uncontrolled withdrawal state itself poses a serious risk to the safety of the patient. The correct protocol is for 24–60 mg/minute (as a 0.8% solution of chlormethiazole edisylate) until shallow sleep is induced. This should then be reduced to the lowest possible rate to maintain shallow sleep with spontaneous respiration. Such treatment should never be employed unless adequate resuscitation facilities are available, and then only with constant monitoring of cardio-respiratory function and consciousness level. Sudden changes in cardio-respiratory function or consciousness are a notorious and unpredictable complication of such treatment and may have fatal consequences in the absence of unceasing vigilance. Prolonged treatment should be avoided as it may be associated with accumulation of the drug, electrolyte imbalance, and delayed recovery. At intervals, the flow of the infusion should therefore be reduced, in order to check that consciousness lightens rapidly. Especial care must be taken where drug clearance is reduced because of hepatic impairment or where cerebral, pulmonary, or cardiac function are compromised, and in the elderly. Drug interactions (especially with other depressants, such as chlordiazepoxide) are also a potentially fatal concern. If these warnings have not discouraged the reader from ever using this treatment, then the manufacturer's data sheet, and an appropriate formulary (for instance the British National Formulary) should be consulted for further advice before prescribing or administration of intravenous chlormethiazole.

Fluids and electrolytes

Patients who are over-active, sweating, and feverish (and perhaps also suffering from gastro-intestinal disturbance), are candidates for serious disturbances in fluid and electrolyte balance which must therefore be monitored. A dangerous fall in potassium level must be averted, and there have been suggestions that decreased magnesium levels are a particular likelihood in delirium tremens (Turner *et al.*, 1989). Blood sugar levels should also be watched. Although a drip may have to be set up, so far as possible fluid and electrolyte correction should be managed by oral administration – keeping a drip in position with a delirious patient can set problems.

Vitamins

Given the dangers of a Wernicke-Korsakoff syndrome, there can be no doubt that the patient with delirium tremens should receive heavy intravenous or intramuscular doses of thiamine for several days.

Life support

Emergency facilities must be available in the event of acute circulatory failure. A rare complication is hyperthermia with the temperature suddenly rising to 40.5 °C or more. Hepatic coma is sometimes precipitated when the previously malnourished patient begins to take protein.

Alcohol withdrawal seizures

Seizures usually occur within the first 24 hours of admission (Turner *et al.*, 1989) but they may also happen during the course of delirium (see Chapter 6). They are less likely to develop if the patient has been adequately sedated, and the same basic drug treatment as for withdrawal symptoms is in general the correct prophylaxis for withdrawal seizures, rather than additional anti-convulsant medication being given. However, opinions differ on this matter and there may be an argument for prescribing anti-convulsant medication for patients whose past history suggests a particular risk of withdrawal seizures (Turner *et al.*, 1989). If a sequence of seizures occurs or status epilepticus develops (a run of seizures in continuous succession), intravenous medication will have to be given to bring the situation rapidly under control, and the usual measures deployed as for any patient suffering from seizures.

Illustrative case history

A 33-year-old man, living alone, asked his social worker for help with 'coming off' alcohol. A previous episode of withdrawal, a year earlier, had failed because he recommenced drinking whilst still taking medication prescribed for his withdrawal symptoms. He therefore reluctantly agreed that on this occasion he would go into hospital for detoxification. On arrival on the ward he was intoxicated, with a BAC of 350 mg/100 ml. An hour later a repeat measurement indicated a decrease to 335 mg/100 ml, at which point the patient was starting to sweat and suffering from a coarse tremor. Regular observations of withdrawal symptoms were commenced using the CIWA-Ar and chlordiazepoxide was prescribed, commencing with a cautious dose of 25 mg in view of the high breath alcohol.

In view of the evidence of poor nutritional status, a high dose B complex vitamin preparation was prescribed, for intramuscular administration once daily for five days.

Over the first 24 hours, a total of 250 mg chlordiazepoxide was administered to the patient orally and this was effective in keeping him reasonably comfortable, albeit he was rather sleepless for the first night on the ward. Gradually lower doses of chlordiazepoxide were prescribed over succeeding days and the drug was discontinued completely after five days on the ward.

The patient was discharged after 10 days. By this time, after encouragement and advice from the ward staff, he had made his own arrangements to be admitted to a residential rehabilitation facility in another part of the country. Arrangements had also been made by the medical staff for him to receive investigation and treatment for a suspected peptic ulcer. The ward occupational therapist had taught him some basic anxiety management techniques, as he had indicated that he often drank in response to symptoms of anxiety, due to various life stresses.

Withdrawal symptoms in summary

From what has been said in this chapter it must be evident that the clinical skills required effectively to respond to the range of alcohol withdrawal pictures that will be encountered involve the ability to deploy a range of techniques apposite to varied presentations. The proper use of drugs can sometimes be very important, but this should not lead to any neglect of the importance of support and encouragement. The trust and the relationships established during the treatment of the crisis can be valuably carried through to the next phase of treatment.

References

Bligh, J. G. & Madden, J. S. (1983). Managing alcohol dependence. *Practitioner* **227**, 82–85.

Chick, J. (1989). Delirium tremens. *British Medical Journal* **298**, 3–4.

Collins, M. N., Burns, T., Van den Berk, P. A. H. & Tubman, G. F. (1990). A structured programme for out-patient alcohol detoxification. *British Journal of Psychiatry* **156**, 871–4.

Cook, C. C. H. & Thomson, A. D. (1997). B-complex vitamins in the prevention and treatment of Wernicke-Korsakoff syndrome. *British Journal of Hospital Medicine.* (In press.)

Fish, D. N. (1991). Treatment of delirium in the critically ill patient. *Clinical Pharmacology and Therapeutics* **10**, 456–66.

Gross, M. M., Lewis, E. & Nagarajan, M. (1973). An improved quantitative system for assessing the acute alcoholic psychoses and related states (TSA and SSA). In *Alcohol Intoxication and Withdrawal: Experimental Studies*, ed. Gross, M. M., vol. 35, pp. 365–76. New York: Plenum.

Hayashida, M., Alterman, A. I., McLellan, A. T., O'Brien, C. P., Purtill, J. J., Volpicelli, J. R., Raphaelson, A. H. & Hall, C. P. (1989). Comparative effectiveness and costs of inpatient and outpatient detoxification of patients with mild-to-moderate alcohol withdrawal syndrome. *New England Journal of Medicine* **320**, 358–65.

Lindberg, M. C. & Oyler, R. A. (1990). Wernicke's encephalopathy. *American Family Physician* **41**, 1205–9.

Majumdar, S. K. (1980). Chlormethiazole and utilisation of vitamin B1 in chronic alcoholics. *European Journal of Clinical Pharmacology* **18**, 361–2.

McInnes, G. (1987). Chlormethiazole and alcohol: a lethal cocktail. *British Medical Journal* **294**, 592.

Nakada, T. & Knight, R. T. (1984). Alcohol and the central nervous system. *Medical Clinics of North America* **68**, 121–31.

O'Brien, P. (1995). Parenteral vitamin therapy in alcoholism. *Psychiatric Bulletin* **19**, 789–96.

Saitz, R., Mayo-Smith, M. F., Roberts, M. S., Redmond, H. A., Bernard, D. R. & Calkins, D. R. (1994). Individualized treatment for alcohol withdrawal. A randomized double-blind controlled trial. *Journal of the American Medical Association* **272**, 519–23.

Shaw, J. M., Kolesar, G. S., Sellers, E. M., Kaplan, H. L. & Sandor, P. (1981). Development of optimal treatment tactics for alcohol withdrawal. I. Assessment and effectiveness of supportive care. *Journal of Clinical Psychopharmacology* **1**, 382–8.

Stockwell, T., Bolt, L., Milner, I., Russell, G., Bolderston, H. & Pugh, P. (1991). Home detoxification from alcohol: its safety and efficacy in comparison with inpatient care. *Alcohol and Alcoholism* **26**, 645–50.

Sullivan, J. T., Sykora, K., Schneiderman, J., Naranjo, C. A. & Sellers, E. M. (1989). Assessment of alcohol withdrawal: the revised clinical institute withdrawal assessment for alcohol scale (CIWA-Ar). *British Journal of Addiction* **84**, 1353–7.

Thomson, A. D., Baker, H. & Leevy, C. H. (1970). Patterns of 35 S-thiamine hydrochloride absorption in the malnourished alcoholic patient. *Journal of Laboratory and Clinical Medicine* **76**, 34–45.

Turner, R. C., Lichstein, P. R., Peden, J. G., Busher, J. T. & Waivers, L. E. (1989). Alcohol withdrawal syndromes: a review of pathophysiology, clinical presentation, and treatment. *Journal of General Internal Medicine* **4**, 432–44.

15

The basic work of treatment

The structure of this chapter will be as follows. The meaning given here to the term 'basic work' will first be defined. The significance of the therapeutic relationship will be discussed. Some guiding principles to provide a frame within which the therapy will be conducted are outlined and the likely content of the basic therapeutic work is considered with emphasis on a person-specific approach. Attention is then given to such issues as how the effort to achieve sobriety is for the patient to be made worthwhile, how to deal positively with relapse, basic work with the family, and matters relating to the duration and termination of treatment. A note is given on basic approaches in the generalist setting. The chapter is rounded with a summary, which brings together ideas on these various fundamentals of the treatment process.

What is meant by 'basic work'?

Special techniques, such as various psychotherapies, cognitive and behavioural therapy, or the use of drugs, can all make contributions to an individual's treatment programme (Miller & Heather, 1986; Chick & Cantwell, 1994; Babor, 1995; Heather, 1995a; Edwards & Dare, 1996; see Chapter 17). It is these approaches that offer the conventional headings for discussion, while the undramatic basics of the helping process tend to be passed by, or dismissed as the background to the application of specialised techniques. It is, however, vital that attention should be given to the subtle and important range of happenings that occur whenever patient and therapist interact – the what, when, and how of what is felt and said and done between them. Otherwise we are at risk of throwing out as packaging the essential content of the parcel. Here is how a patient saw what happened between himself and a doctor:

I remember when I first met that doctor. She seemed friendly but when I tried to con her, she laughed and told me to get my priorities right. Typical alcoholic thinking – just told myself that she didn't understand, and I didn't bother to turn up for the next appointment. What happened next? I get a letter, not one of those form-letters that hospitals send out, but a personal letter from this doctor saying something like, 'I know it's difficult. I don't want to push you into anything, but I'll be in the clinic on Friday afternoon if you want to talk about things further'. So I went back to tell her she didn't understand!

Concern for the impression made at the first encounter (Thom *et al.*, 1992), the ability to combine being 'friendly' with confrontation, finding a phrase like 'priorities' to sort out complexity, the way a letter is written (Batel *et al.*, 1995), these are examples which point to what is meant by 'basic work'.

Interventions are only likely to produce movement when in alignment with the real possibilities for change within the individual, the family, and social setting (Vaillant, 1983, 1993). The basic work of therapy is largely concerned with nudging and supporting movement along these 'natural' pathways of recovery. We need a more developed sense of people's innate capacity for recovery and the possible dimensions of recovery, rather than a belief that we can impose therapies on people who are to be marched along at our dictate. The clumsy therapist is like someone who tries to carve a piece of wood without respect for the grain. The basic work of treatment requires immense respect for that grain, and therapy must always be matched to individual needs.

This chapter will be written largely in terms of the patient or client who is aiming at abstinence rather than at modification of drinking. That latter question is dealt with in Chapter 19. Much of what is said in this chapter is generally applicable, whatever the chosen goal.

The relationship

The relationship between patient and therapist is fundamental both to what can be achieved in any one therapeutic session and to what changes can be won over time (Luborsky *et al.*, 1985; Carroll & Rounsaville, 1993). It begins to be built at the first moment of contact, is developed during the assessment interview (or interviews), is vital to the effectiveness of the initial counselling and goal-setting, and continues thereafter as an important component of therapy (Edwards, 1996). 'What is said' matters, but it cannot be abstracted from the feelings between the two people who are doing the saying and the listening.

Take, for instance, the following remarks by a therapist, which might be necessary at a certain point in an individual's treatment:

> You know that I believe you can stop drinking and make sense of your life, but things can't just drag on. You've been coming up here regularly to talk about your problems for the last six months, and we are both aware that you're now becoming badly caught up in this business of "I'll start tomorrow . . . the day after". Here's a challenge. I'm nòt giving you an appointment for next week but instead am going to propose that you come back in six weeks and show me that by then you have stopped these binges and started instead to do some of those things with your family that you have been talking about. I want you to show yourself that you can succeed, and that will be a great feeling. It's time to make a start. You *can* make a start.

That same form of words may have three different types of impact. The impact may be negative, with the patient reinforced in their sense of hopelessness. The second alternative is for the patient in effect not to hear what is said, because no words spoken within a meaningless relationship can matter – if they bother to come back in six weeks' time, it will be with nothing having changed, and with what was said in that previous session blandly neutralised. Lastly, there is the possibility that the challenge is taken and used as a turning point, but this outcome can only be expected when the relationship positively matters. At worst, the word 'relationship' is devalued into a catch-phrase of professional jargon, and yet every now and then one senses again the intensely important reality of what is being talked about.

Work with drinking problems requires awareness of how relationships are made and used, but there is little that is unique to alcohol problems in this regard. The same basic skills are needed in any area of therapy and the general nature of a therapeutic relationship will not be discussed here in detail. It may, however, be useful to list a number of considerations that derive from psychotherapeutic principles (Luborsky & Crits-Christoph, 1990; Malan & Osimo, 1992), but which have to be thought through when working with drinking problems (Levin & Weiss, 1994). These issues are summarised in Box 15.1

Showing warmth and empathy

Warmth cannot be invented, and a show of pretended warmth will be transparent. The ability to express genuinely warm feelings towards the patient may be easy, or may be frustrated by what the patient or the therapist themselves brings to the encounter, for instance, the patient's expectation of rejection or the therapist's unease with deviant behaviour. Warmth has to be felt and worked towards, and it is possible positively to make the effort to reach this experience. When warmth is genuinely experienced, it still has to be conveyed, and there are skills in the use of voice and gesture, as well as in learning how to convey warmth in words which are not cloying.

Box 15.1. The therapeutic relationship

The quality of the relationship between therapist and client is funda-mental to what can be achieved.

- The ability to show empathy
- Avoiding possessiveness and the lure of directiveness
- Conferring worth and giving hope

Possessiveness and directiveness

The seeming helplessness of the patient who is caught up in drinking and their pleas for rescue, if not guarded against, may set up a relation-ship in which the patient is invited to slip into the regressed role of a child. The therapist takes the position of the perplexed and guilt-ridden parent, loaded with responsibility to save the child from its wilful destructiveness. The patient's successes belong to the therapist and, at the same time, the patient's failures are felt as personal failures by the therapist. Such a relationship is the antithesis of one that encourages growth towards autonomy. Directiveness may work in the short-term as the patient is carried along by the therapist's will and demand, but progress of that kind is unlikely to be sustained. The patient will sooner or later rebel and drinking is the likely act of rebellion. There is a dis-tinction between the directiveness of telling the patient what to do and reinforcement of the expectation that the patient can meet the goals which they have themselves set up.

Conferring worth and giving hope

The way in which the patient's bad feelings about themselves are to be handled within the relationship is another important question. Feelings of worthlessness, helplessness, pessimism, and unresolved guilt are common in the person who has experienced years of excessive drinking, and can handicap the attempt at recovery. Bad feelings have to be brought into the open and the covert as well as the overt statements which indicate these attitudes identified. The therapist's job is not then to give cheery and false comfort that will carry no conviction, but to attempt by many small strategies to help towards better feelings. Much of what can be achieved depends on the central, unspoken, and yet tangible qualities of the relationship itself, 'What really helped me to turn the corner was that this particular nurse seemed to have faith in me. She believed that I could do it and I couldn't let her down. She always had time to listen'.

Work with the patient: some guiding principles

What actually happens when, after the initial assessment, formulation, and goal-setting, the client and therapist, on a series of later occasions, sit down together and talk? Here are some principles which can guide the work and they are summarised in Box 15.2.

Box 15.2. Working with the patient: guiding principles

- Seek to maintain continuity of purpose. Use the initial formulation and goal-setting, check on what has been achieved, set further goals in concrete terms
- Be flexible, listen to what the patient brings to the session, but identify leading issues for the session
- Be aware of what is happening in the therapeutic relationship
- Hold onto the family perspective
- Monitor progress and engage the patient in self-monitoring
- Keep a balance between dynamics and realities
- Maintain a balance of emphasis between drinking and other areas for work

---

Maintain continuity of purpose

Both patient and therapist have to maintain a sense of progress and purpose, and avoid confusion and drift. Recovery needs a maintained sense of direction. This is achieved in a number of ways:

(1) *Make use of the initial formulation and goal setting.* The initial exercise in clarification of understanding and purpose should be referred back to as the continued basis for action (see p. 228).

(2) *Emphasise what has been achieved.* At each session, it is useful for the therapist to help the patient identify what has been achieved since the last meeting and thus reinforce the patient's own sense of achievement – for instance, so many days or weeks of abstinence, a difficult situation dealt with successfully, a new job started, an outing with the family, or new aspects of self-understanding.

(3) *Set the next task for the short-term.* The meeting also has to identify what are to be the next steps, with the patient making a commitment to attempt these steps. The work plan is of no value if it is only in terms of generalities, such as 'getting some other interests going' or 'trying to be more understanding of the wife's point of view'. Generalities cannot provide a programme for action. What is needed is a series of explicit, practical, and attainable goals that can be checked at the next meeting.

(4) *An eye on the slightly longer* term. Although it is useful to concentrate on the short-term (AA's 'day at a time'), patients will also, to varying extent, want to see further ahead, and be helped forward by thoughts of what things may look like in six months or a year hence. The person who thinks concretely will be happier to plan their steps in such visible terms as new possessions, while someone else may chart their progress in terms of personal changes and changes in relationships.

Be aware of the relationship

The importance of the therapeutic relationship has already been noted, and continuing thought has to be given to what is occurring in this regard. Is the therapist, for instance, being edged into a too authoritarian role, or being moved towards argument or sterile intellectual debate?

Hold onto the family perspective

Despite intentions, it is easy to become too focused on the individual and to discover after some months that the needs of the family and the relevance of the home situation have been allowed to slip from sight, with adverse consequences. If the patient has a family, what is happening within the family and within other close relationships has to be discussed and plans made for continuing work with the people involved.

Monitor progress

Implicit in the idea of commitment is the expectation that commitment will be met, but the process only works if the therapist checks on what is agreed. It is helpful for the patient to feel that their progress is being monitored, and periodic reporting to the therapist can be supported by an element of self-monitoring. The patient may, for instance, be asked to keep a daily diary, with headings to deal with such issues as drinking (Miller *et al.*, 1981), craving, 'tricky situations', and the use of leisure time.

Maintain a balance between dynamics and realities

The treatment approach, which is outlined in this chapter, embraces a concern with psychodynamics, cognitive-behavioural aspects, and external realities. There is danger in putting too heavy an emphasis on one area while others are neglected (see p. 318).

Keep a balance between drinking and other issues

Each interview is likely to reinforce the agreed drinking goal and monitor progress along the drinking dimension. Work towards recovery also has to be planned, pursued and monitored along other dimensions, often bearing on enhancement of the quality of sobriety. It is when therapist or patient focuses too much on one sector to the cost of any other that things go wrong (see Chapter 19).

The therapeutic work

So much for a discussion of the general framework. With those headings in mind we can now go on to look at some likely detailed content of the therapeutic work.

Working on the drinking problem.

According to the phase of recovery to which the patient has progressed, this heading will have different meanings. It should again be emphasised that this discussion is worded in terms of the patient who is aiming at abstinence, although with due modification the same principles apply to work toward a controlled drinking goal. For instance, at the earliest stage the immediate question is how the patient who is aiming at abstinence is to come off drink and be helped where necessary with detoxification (see Chapter 14), while for the patient who has chosen the goal of controlled drinking, the immediate task is to get the drinking under control (Chapter 18). Whichever the chosen goal, the patient has to be presented with the unambiguous message that dealing with the drinking problem is a high priority. In terms of Prochaska and DiClimente's 'stages of change' model (Prochaska & DiClimente, 1984), much of the initial work under this heading may be concerned with helping patients to move from 'precontemplation' to 'contemplation', 'preparation' and then on to 'action' and 'maintenance'. Many therapists find that this model provides them with a useful map for charting individual progress, although at the theoretical level there is debate as to the validity of this segmentation (Davidson, 1992; Sutton, 1996). A further psychological approach relevant to this phase of work, and which will be discussed later in more detail (p. 286), is that of *motivational interviewing* (Miller & Rollnick, 1991; Rollnick *et al.*, 1992; Davidson, 1996). Motivation will be built and nurtured by encouraging the patient to review in detail the rewards that are likely to come with sobriety and the negative consequences that will result from continued drinking. Some patients may find a self-help manual useful (Heather *et al.*, 1990).

When the patient is off alcohol – focusing again primarily in the present discussion on the abstinence goal – there is important work to be done directly on the drinking problem, and this is the time for consolidation rather than for sitting back. The patient's basic understanding of the nature of their drinking problem (and the nature of dependence) has to be rehearsed and reinforced. This is not accomplished by the therapist giving a lecture, but by their pointing up a discussion, 'Just how do you *understand* this drinking problem? How would you explain to another person what's different between your relationship with alcohol and their drinking?' Work on ambivalence is also a continuing task rather than something ever settled once and for all, 'What would you lose now if you went back to drinking? What, so far, looks like the best thing that's coming out of sobriety?'

Discussion will usefully focus on questions such as the degree to which the patient is thinking about or craving for alcohol, the cues and circumstances that trigger these subjective experiences, and the ways in which the patient copes with such feelings (Marlatt & Gordon, 1985; Gossop, 1996). Personal coping mechanisms must be identified and it is important to teach patients to think in these terms and rehearse the strategies that are going to be employed in difficult situations. He or she has to learn to sense the reality of these mechanisms as an important personal armoury to be kept in good repair and used whenever there is any threat to sobriety. Much of the psychological underpinning of this phase of the work will come from a relapse prevention approach (see

p. 290). There may also be work to be done in terms of dealing with relapse (p. 126).

Mental health

A patient or client will often bring up problems related to their 'nerves' – anxiety, phobic symptoms, irritability, jealousy, depression, or difficulty in sleeping. During the initial weeks (or even months) of sobriety, these symptoms may still be related to withdrawal, and can therefore be expected gradually to clear. What at first appear to be handicapping phobic symptoms may, for instance, fade out with two to three months of sobriety. In practice the contribution made to the patient's 'nerves' by the biological processes of withdrawal will, over the initial period of sobriety, be inseparable from symptoms that may stem from the patient's rediscovery of what it is like to be their real self, unshielded by alcohol. Their real self may be anxious and irritable, but for years alcohol has blotted out, exacerbated, or confused these underlying propensities.

No matter which of the above factors may explain the patient or client's psychological discomfort, the best immediate response is not heedlessly to offer drugs, but to employ a commonsense and supportive approach. The message that has to be carried to the patient is firstly the optimistic one that such symptoms can generally be expected to ameliorate as the weeks go by, and secondly the realistic one that it may be necessary and possible for them to learn to live with their 'nerves' without resort to a chemical answer. A reflex assumption that has been reinforced over many years' drinking has to be overcome – psychic distress is part of the human condition and not something that has to be immediately and chemically ablated. The patient is, as it were, too anxious about being anxious.

The patient is then likely to be helped if together with these basic messages, some ideas are offered as to how distress is to be ameliorated more constructively than by resort to tranquillisers. This may entail further effort by the patient to deal with circumstances that are generating stress, for instance, anxiety about debts, housing or employment, which can only be relieved by the problems being positively met. The patient may be helped by learning a relaxation technique, or by developing a variety of simple coping strategies such as listening to music, going for a walk, or telephoning a friend.

While the basic approach to many psychological problems is best made in this low-key fashion, the therapist must also keep an eye open for the presence of more serious disturbances (see Chapter 6) that may require very active attention.

Social and family adjustment

A wide range of problems may need to be discussed and monitored under this heading, as the patient works towards agreed goals. If such topics are not spontaneously brought up by the patient during the session, it may be wise for the therapist on each occasion to make at least a general enquiry as to what is happening within the family, how things are going at work (or as regards looking for a job), and how leisure is being spent. Financial problems, housing or any court proceedings may also need to be checked on. Work along these lines is essential to the process of recovery, and the therapist needs to be as much interested in monitoring what is being achieved in these directions as in talking about the drinking itself or any psychological problems. Basic work with the family is discussed later in this chapter (p. 264).

Physical health

Particularly in the early stages of sobriety, there may be problems in the patient's physical health that require attention or referral, and which must not be lost from sight because of all else that is on the agenda. A feeling of rediscovered physical well-being may be one of the prime rewards of sobriety, and work under this heading should therefore entail not only dealing with ill health, but efforts positively to enhance good health.

Slotting in more specific treatments

The use of the more specific treatment approaches, which are discussed in Chapter 17, requires discretion and timing. Only on the basis of an understanding of the individual and their progress, is it possible to judge whether any added help is needed or likely to be effective. Questions of this type should therefore be in the therapist's mind from the first session onwards – is it appropriate to set up a behaviour therapy programme? Should disulfiram be prescribed? Is it now, after six months, timely to think of psychotherapeutic help? Every session, besides its immediate contact, is also potentially a routing point.

Making the effort worthwhile

No one is likely to achieve long-term success in dealing with a drinking problem unless sobriety (or ameliorated drinking) proves to be a personally rewarding experience (Vaillant, 1983; Edwards *et al.*, 1992).

258

Alcohol can only be given up grudgingly if its surrender is a loss with no gain. If all that is won by the effort to stop drinking is a grey and empty existence, it will not be long before there is a relapse. When sobriety is unrewarding there is also the danger that alcohol will be substituted by uncontrolled gambling or by excessive use of tranquillisers or sedatives. Many patients move spontaneously towards discovery of rewards, and two general patterns of development can often then be seen – either a wide new engagement in life or, alternatively, a much narrower substitute activity. The first of these two pathways – the wide new engagement – is in fact often a re-engagement in life rather than an entirely new series of moves, and is characteristic of the person who had a positive involvement in life before the emergence of the drinking problem overwhelmed these enjoyments. The second pathway – that of narrower substitute activity – more often characterises the recovery of the person who never, at any previous period, achieved any great base of enjoyment. In this instance, it is not that a happy pattern of living was overwhelmed by drinking, but, on the contrary, that the drinking problem initially developed in the setting of unrewarding relationships and activities. Recovery may be marked by an almost frenetic commitment to one particular interest.

When no rewarding pattern of new involvement develops in the wake of sobriety and as the months go by there is instead a continued complaint that 'it was better when I was drinking', thought has to be given to what can be done to obtain constructive movement. The therapist's role is firstly that of identifying the problem and encouraging the patient to identify small real steps towards a solution and to take those steps. This is often a stage where the family again needs to be involved. Beyond commonsense advice, there are various other lines of approach. For instance, the passivity and pessimism that stands in the way of a determined attempt to find rewards seems often to have the characteristics of a learnt expectation of failure – 'I just can't get on with people, I'm no good at anything'. Even one small limited success may begin to offer a new sense of possibilities – success generalises (see p. 320). Efforts may usefully be concentrated on finding reward in one relationship, or a sense of achievement can come from learning how to be a good cook or from taking the children fishing, and so on. One strand of activity suggests, enables, and interacts with another. As ever with goal-setting, detailed and factual planning of steps is likely to be required, rather than general declarations of intent.

On other occasions, the rewards of sobriety take a turn for the better after a major life change that is more or less accidental or very purposely brought about, such as a shift to a new locality, a new job, the break-up of a marriage, or a new relationship. These are the kind of solutions that tend traditionally to be looked on with suspicion as 'geographical escape', with the problems in no way resolved but taken along to be acted out again in the new personal setting. Such strategies are, admittedly, in some instances no more than unprofitable escapism, but it is wrong automatically to take a negative view of what is likely to be achieved by these large shifts. At times the patient is precisely right in taking the bold and simple view that 'what is wrong is living in this street', and the move to the new house, with the decorating, furniture buying and pride in ownership, the shared family involvement, the escape from the old social environment, and all the drinking friends who used to knock on the door, marks the start of a new epoch.

The therapeutic use of the concept of alcoholism as a disease

A proportion of patients may find the concept of alcoholism as a disease (Jellinek, 1960) helpful to recovery. Such a formulation can serve as an idea around which that patient organises understanding of his or her condition and a personal programme of recovery. This concept is central to the philosophy of AA (see Chapter 16).

The advantages inherent in such a simple definition of the problem can for many patients be considerable. There is comfort in the view that they are suffering from a condition that can be understood within much the same model as diabetes – guilt is relieved and acceptance of the inexorable fact that the only remedy for this disease is to stop drinking offers a clear personal goal. Seen in these terms the disease is 'incurable', and recovery is a lifetime programme centred around vigilant avoidance of the first drink.

The disease concept is sometimes seized on as a revelation by a patient who has previously been thrashing around chaotically for a way of understanding their seemingly totally irrational drinking, with self-defeating attempts to 'control' that drinking. Embracing the disease concept can in such instances provide a dramatic turning point. There are, however, therapists who are unhappy with this formulation or unwilling to work within its constraints. They see the disease concept as inviting the patient to avoid self-responsibility – 'It's a disease, I can't help it'. They may also see it as a formulation that detracts attention from a wide spectrum of drinking behaviours and alcohol-related problems and psychological processes, and over-emphasises the dependence element.

While this debate continues, the question remains how best to help the individual patient. From the therapeutic angle the reasonable position to take must be that there are different ways of formulating problems that will be more or less helpful to different patients and with which different therapists will be more or less comfortable. The patient can be rendered a disservice if the therapist insists on a dogmatic view of either kind. In reality the risk of damage is usually obviated by the patient shopping around until a model of understanding is found that suits that person best.

How to deal positively with relapse

Relapse is a common event (Hunt *et al.*, 1971). This statement will be interpreted pessimistically if one has misread the treatment of drinking problems as being only about rapid and maintained 'success'. More often real success involves trial and error along the way. Dealing with and learning from relapse is commonly part of the process of recovery, but such a view is not to be read as favouring a *laissez-faire* attitude. Relapse has to be taken seriously by patient and therapist alike, but in another sense it has also to be demystified. It is a piece of behaviour to be objectively understood rather than a fall from grace. The relationship needs therefore to be trusting enough for relapse to be talked about rather than hidden and denied, and trust should be such that the patient and family can turn for help if relapse occurs rather than their avoiding all contact because of shame and feelings of failure.

Relapse can take many different forms. It may be precipitate and explosive, or it may be a matter of a slow slide; the pace of relapse is often directly related to the degree of dependence. The patient may then stay relapsed for months or years, and the AA member of 20 years' standing may seem tragically to have lost all their gains. However, the relapse may be short-lived, with the patient pulling back after a day or two. Beyond the surface description of these different patterns, there is then the question of the cause and meaning of the occurrence, and it is these inner significances which, in the individual case, have to be examined if there is to be profit from the experience and recovery is to move forward.

Some of the commoner circumstances of relapse are set out below, but in reality the determinants are often likely to be multiple (Marlatt & Gordon, 1985).

An initial and ambivalent sobriety overthrown

Here one is dealing with the patient who relapses in the early days of treatment because they have not as yet satisfactorily sorted out the balance of their motivations. They are in two minds as to whether or not they want to stop drinking, and the relapse indicates that there is still important initial work to be done in sorting out these ambivalences. Motivation has got to be strengthened (Tober, 1991).

Insufficiency in coping mechanisms

Here the same surface picture has a different inner meaning and different therapeutic implications. This type of patient has, to a greater extent, overcome their ambivalence, but they are unskilled in defending their sobriety. They know what they want to do, but are caught out and fail in their intentions. Effort has to be directed at better learning of coping mechanisms.

Failure to find sobriety rewarding

Sobriety has not been consolidated and no satisfactory substitutes have been found for drinking. This is the type of relapse that occurs after perhaps 6 to 12 months of uneasy sobriety. The need is to work again on the reward of sobriety.

Disturbance of mood

Relapse is, in such instances, an indication that the patient has been unable to cope with an upset in mood. The patient may have experienced a transient patch of gloom, anxiety, or irritability, that has overwhelmed their defences, or they may be prone to cyclical mood swings. Depressive illness is a not uncommon cause of relapse, and the possibility of hypomanic illness may also have to be considered.

Overcome by events

In such instances, an event or series of events proves too much for the individual's defences. Rather than drinking being a response to catastrophic happenings, the more usual story is of an event which, to the outsider, might seem trivial, or a cluster of seemingly minor troubles. For instance, the patient has had a row with her husband and, that same morning, the water tank in the roof has leaked, and the desire to bring back a bottle of gin from the supermarket is irresistible. To dismiss such a story as 'just a bundle of excuses' is unhelpful. Its analysis tells us that for this woman, ordinary marital discord gives rise to feelings of insecurity that are hard to bear, and that when subjected then to a little extra stress, she will be without any means of coping other than resort to drink.

Failure in vigilance

Sometimes it seems that the patient has been careless. They were half aware that it would be dangerous to go to that party, but such considerations were less important than the prospect of fun. They knew that it would be risky to start drinking in such a setting, but by the time the party was in full swing, they 'thought they could get away with it'. This lack of vigilance is often related to a fading of memory; the pains previously experienced with drinking are now rather distant, while the pleasure of a glass of wine is immediate.

The study of a particular incident will thus often reveal the need and possibilities for targeted further work with the patient. But it also frequently points to the need for further examinations of family interactions, rather than either the cause or prevention of relapse being issues to be analysed only in terms of the individual.

Whether relapse is insidious or abrupt, it is a happening to be *used* in treatment. The usefulness of the experience is, however, lost if the incident is met inappropriately; for instance, if it is passed by as trivial and unimportant, interpreted as reason for pessimism and surrender of therapeutic effort, or taken as occasion for abandonment of the patient's and family's active responsibility with an unnecessary retreat to hospital. Relapse is best met with no retreat from expectations of the patient's self-responsibility. That responsibility now includes getting out of the relapse, working out its meaning, and setting things up so that further relapse is less likely.

Many relapses are short-lived, with the patient regaining sobriety before harm is done. It is potentially misleading to use the same word to describe the happenings when a patient takes a few drinks one evening and then stops drinking again completely, as opposed to their sliding into a rapid reinstatement of dependence and being once more in the grip of very threatening drinking – some therapists prefer to distinguish between 'lapse' (transient or minor) and 'relapse' (major and perhaps with reinstatement of dependence). A lapse may lead on to the relapse, but this is not the inevitable march of events. And what the therapist at first views as 'lapse' may be the patient's tentative move toward re-establishment of normal drinking.

As well as therapy seeking to enable patient and family to learn from the incident, there may be immediate work in seeking to minimise the harm done by any such occurrence. They should have learnt that one drink can be dangerous, rather than their having been fed the idea that one drink spells inevitable disaster. Such a myth may harmfully perpetuate a self-fulfilling prophecy of a different kind, with the patient believing that after the one drink all is lost so that they may as well go on drinking (the 'abstinence violation effect', Marlatt & Gordon, 1985).

Damage must, however, be averted and the patient has, for instance, to avoid losing their job and should get back to work as soon as possible. Where there are particular dangers to physical health, such as may be present if the patient is suffering from pancreatitis or liver disease, then the sooner drinking is stopped the better. Relapse may sometimes pose dangers of suicide if the patient believes that 'the last chance has gone'.

Basic work with the family

The importance of the family dimension in the initial assessment and goal-setting, and the value of the initial interview with the spouse have already been discussed (p. 219).

Work with the spouse

The spouse's behaviour patterns may have become stuck in a rut, and be producing no benefit, and sometimes just trying a change of tack can help. Constructive help-seeking and constructive management seem on the whole to be more effective than continued attack or manipulation (Orford & Edwards, 1977), but it is impossible to lay down absolute rules as to how best a spouse should cope in varied situations. Much will depend on what that particular spouse believes to be within their resources. It may generally be beneficial if the spouse can reach a decision as to what they definitely will not do, and what are their limits. For instance, they may decide as an act of definite policy that they will abandon arguing and nagging, or that they will not give their partner money nor go out and buy them drink. It is the open identification of a set of intentions, the sense of something to do, the drawing up of a personal programme, that is useful in such a situation.

It is often helpful to hold a few joint sessions to try to ensure that mutual goals are understood and that there is shared commitment to constructive change. This can be used to give the sense of a new start, with an emphasis on the positive, on identifying what is good in the marriage, what each in practical terms wants from the other and what each will give to the other partner.

There is no evidence that a routine, major therapeutic intervention with the spouse is of benefit. It is better to develop the discrimination that allows deployment of resources where they are needed. The basic approach that is being proposed with the spouse is therefore relatively low-key, but judgement is necessary to identify a range of circumstances where more must be done. For instance, if a wife is in acute danger of violence, there must be an immediate response, and a crisis may have to be dealt with by providing shelter for her and children forthwith.

Help for the children

The best help for the child is restoration of the happiness of the home. The fact of a previously alcohol-dependent parent ceasing to drink, of rowing and violence no longer being the continuing experience, can be dramatically beneficial to the child's happiness and well-being (Lynskey *et al.*, 1994). The extent to which a child can grasp and utilise the possibility of happiness depends on the degree of previous hurt, and on whether there have been continuing elements of warm feeling and good contact despite all the distress. Sometimes the changes are evident within a week. The teacher notices that the child is concentrating at school, the mother knows that a child has stopped bed-wetting or will say, 'It's lovely, they're talking to their dad again'. More often the changes are going to be seen over a longer period, and the restoration of confidence will take many months, with the previously drinking parent hurt and discouraged because their children have not sooner come towards them.

Given that help for the problem drinking parent (and the partner) may be of indirect benefit to the children, other ways of aiding the children have also to be considered, especially where there is no immediate treatment response from the adult (Zeitlin, 1994). There can be instances where urgent thought has to be given to removal of the child from the home as an immediate measure of physical protection, or where high priority has to be given to social work supervision of an intensity which can monitor the child's safety (on p. 162 we give a case example of such a situation). The procedures of the 'at risk' register may have to be invoked. The decisions that have to be made call, as ever, for balanced judgement. Taking a child out of its home unnecessarily is to no one's benefit, while a careless decision in the other direction can be disastrous. What must be borne in mind is the unpredictability of a parent's drunken behaviour – the dangers of a sudden aggression directed against a child causing appalling damage. Such a problem is often best dealt with by a case conference which can bring together everyone with knowledge of the family. At a certain stage the decision may be made that temporary removal of the child from the home is desirable to allow escape from the continuing stresses, even if actual violence is not threatened. As far as possible the alcoholic parent as well as the spouse should be involved in the discussion, so that the move is not seen as punitive (see also Chapter 4).

As regards individual help for the child remaining in the disturbed home, much the same range of approaches is applicable as with a child or young person facing any other disturbing home influence. The offer of a good and confident relationship is itself valuable, but with a child who is of an age to verbalise problems it is helpful to discuss directly the parent's drinking – to listen to and offer understanding of the child's distress, to find some more satisfactory way of looking at the parents and of coping with the anger and hurt, to offer straightforward information, to discuss the child's role within the family, what the child 'can do to help' and the limits of those possibilities, and to aid towards good friendships outside the home. Children too have their coping mechanisms, which can be adaptive or maladaptive.

There may be occasions when older children should be involved in family therapy in a formal sense, but the skills necessary to handle the interactions of children and parents in such a forum should not be underestimated. More often what is useful is the home visit or series of home visits where children can experience a family discussion in a natural setting, and where family members drop in and out as they feel like it. The role of Al-Ateen (a self-help group deriving from AA and Al-Anon) is discussed in Chapter 16.

The use of therapeutic groups

The place of group therapy as a special technique to be deployed at the stage when the patient is consolidating their recovery is discussed in Chapter 17. AA and Al-Anon also provide group experience. But groups can also have their place in the basic work of treatment, and many therapists would see involvement in groups at an early stage of the treatment process as being useful for information giving, shared solution of problems, and support. There is no evidence that more intensive group work at these earlier stages brings special benefit.

Spacing of appointments

There is no one rule for the spacing of appointments, and some patients will need to be seen more frequently than others. In general, the emphasis on autonomy and self-determination is best supported by giving more spaced rather than more frequent appointments, with escalation into a routine of intensive intervention thus resisted. It may be useful to ask the patient when they next want to be seen, without accidentally implying that the therapist 'doesn't care'. Much must depend on the thoroughness and purposiveness of the initial assessment and exercise in goal-setting. It is better to put investment in that direction, with similarly purposeful but spaced follow-up, than to start from an incomplete assessment with a follow-through that lacks direction despite frequency of contact. If more specialised treatment such as a cognitive-behavioural programme is under way, then the frequency of contact will be increased.

As for how long a session should last, this again must be individually determined. On many occasions, a 20–minute interview can give sufficient time for a focused monitoring of progress, while in other instances, it may be necessary to find 45–60 minutes for listening and detailed discussion.

The treatment organisation should also have the capacity to respond to emergency and be able to see the patient who experiences a crisis between their fixed appointments. It may, however, be unhelpful to agree to see a patient on a sort of free-demand basis if it is judged that their demands are witness to their over-dependence on other people; it would be better to encourage them to meet their own crises and keep to the schedule of appointments.

When a patient fails to keep an appointment there should be an administrative mechanism that ensures that they are not then lost from sight. A personal letter offering a further appointment should be written or a phone call made, and if contact is not re-established a home visit should perhaps be arranged. When all else fails the patient should still be left with the indication that the door remains readily open.

Duration and termination of treatment

The duration of treatment may be proposed by the therapist but it is effectively determined by the patient. There are patients who appear to have benefited from one or two sessions and who decide this is all they need, while at the other extreme there are those who want to maintain at least intermittent contact over years.

A man aged 63 had first been seen for help many years previously when he was in severe difficulties with his alcohol dependence. He was at that time admitted briefly for detoxification, and was then in contact with a community-based counselling centre for two years. He continued thereafter to drop in for an occasional chat, and 12 years after initial contact he came along to discuss his son's drinking. A few years later he made contact again because his wife had died and he was finding it difficult to face life alone – he did not think there was any danger of his drinking, but he wanted to 'find someone who would listen'. Feelings of guilt and remorse relating to his drinking days had been stirred up.

In many cases it may be good policy never formally to 'discharge' a patient but to stress the continued availability of help as and when it should be needed, and to couple this with the offer of yearly follow-up appointments. Such an approach is more appropriate for the patient who has had serious and multiple problems than the person whose initial problems were slighter and more quickly resolved.

A fixed course of so many sessions over so many months cannot in reality meet the needs of an enormously varied patient population. Judgement needs to be made in terms of the patient's progress along a number of dimensions of recovery, the likelihood of further useful work, the timeliness of a move that further emphasises the patient's ability to handle their own responsibilities, and negotiation on timing between therapist and patient. Rather than there then being a 'this is the end of your treatment' type of announcement, what is said might often be something like this:

> We've been meeting each month for the last eight months, and you've achieved a great deal. If you agree, what I would now suggest is that we meet again just before Christmas – that's five months hence. But if for any reason you wanted to see me earlier, 'phone and let me know.

The question arises in a different form when making this decision in a case where after six months of work the drinking has continued unabated, than when substantial progress has been made. Does one 'terminate treatment' on the grounds that the patient is failing to benefit or show commitment to change? In general rather than such a situation being an indication for termination of treatment, it more often suggests the need for reassessment of what is being done. There is no profit in stumbling on aimlessly and without therapeutic movement, but the response to continued drinking should be constructive and considered, rather than an angry discarding of an unsatisfactory patient.

Basic work in the generalist setting

This chapter and the book as a whole for the most part focuses on how to respond to drinking problems of significant severity and dealt with by professionals with more than a few minutes of time to deploy. Help given in the primary care, general hospital ward, or other generalist frontlines is, however, of such importance as to make it mandatory to enter a note on this matter within a chapter that discusses 'basic work' (Bien *et al.*, 1993; Anderson, 1995; Heather, 1995b). These issues are taken up again within the service planning context in Chapter 20.

Here what needs to be underlined is that within the generalist setting the basic skills that are required relate firstly to case identification (Chapter 12). The professional working in a specialist clinic is likely to have the task of case recognition already accomplished for them – in that the referral letter will tell them that this is a patient with a drinking problem. Not so the GP or other generalist working in settings where the patients come unsorted and unlabelled and the challenge is to recognise heterogeneous drinking problems that can exist in all shades of degree.

The majority of cases dealt with in these types of generalist setting will be of lesser severity than those encountered by the specialist. In most instances the appropriate treatment will be brief intervention directed at milder or earlier alcohol-related pathologies, or at excessive alcohol intake where there is as yet no evidence of adverse consequences. With the case identified, the necessary skills include the ability to give succinct and intelligible advice to encourage explicit and targeted change (for instance, bringing down weekly intake to 21 units or, say 170 g absolute alcohol per week for men and 14 units or 110 g for women, with concomitant lowering of liver enzymes). Along with the advice should go monitoring and feedback to the patient. The generalist will also on occasion be identifying and dealing with more severe drinking problems or alcohol dependence, and decisions will have to be made as to when and from what direction specialist support should be sought.

Basic work: bringing the ideas together

It would be misleading to present a carefully ordered flow chart or series of ordered steps to describe the basic work of treatment, for this would contradict the message that what is most required is the flexibility to meet the needs of the individual patient as their recovery evolves. But with that caution in mind, it may be useful to summarise a checklist of ideas.

(1) Assessment with patient and spouse is the initiation of therapy, and a shared experience.

(2) The case formulation orders the material obtained in the assessment and is again shared with patient and spouse.

(3) Goal-setting must be negotiated in similar terms. Goals must be specific and cover non-drinking as well as drinking issues. There must be an invitation to a tangible commitment to working towards those goals.

(4) The therapeutic relationship is enormously important and must

be skilfully fostered. The therapist must learn how to show warmth and give hope, but they should not be be lured into over-directiveness either with patient or spouse. Self-responsibility should be fostered.

(5) Some basic therapeutic principles should be borne in mind – continuity of purpose and sense of movement must be maintained; salient questions must be identified at each interview, with the patient allowed to define what is of importance; and the family perspective must be maintained. Therapy requires continuous monitoring and the patient may usefully engage in self-monitoring. Balances have to be struck both between focus on reality and dynamics, and between drinking and other topics. Commitment may at various points need to be re-examined. An eye has constantly to be kept on the development of the relationship.

(6) The actual content of the interview includes work on the drinking problem and attention to problems in the areas of mental and physical health and social adjustment.

(7) Each interview, as well as being concerned with the continuing basics of treatment, is also an occasion for deciding whether it is timely to signpost the patient towards any more specialised type of help.

(8) The effort towards recovery by patient and spouse has to be worthwhile. They must be helped to sense out the gains, and a sobriety that is only negative will not be maintained. The *quality* of sobriety is important. Strengthening of the patient's motivation is basic to therapy.

(9) Relapse is not to be considered a taboo subject. If relapse does occur it should be possible to learn from the event. The many different patterns, causes, and meanings of relapse must be understood.

(10) Basic work with the family may also be needed. This includes meeting the immediate needs of spouse and children, as well as work that facilitates conjoint efforts towards the patient's recovery.

(11) The pacing and intensity of help must be kept under review and ultimately tailed off, perhaps with the offer of an 'open door' rather than formal closure of the case. What must be guarded against is an automatic escalation into heavy intervention. Once there has been full assessment and careful and agreed goal-setting, much may then often be left to patient and family with monitoring and encouragement and a little talking through.

(12) Basic treatment is an alliance with the natural processes of recovery. It is a matter of discovering rather than imposing possibilities

for change, a matter of teaching map-reading skills rather than pushing people along a path which we dictate.

References

Anderson, P. (1995). *Alcohol and Primary Health Care. European Series No.64.* Copenhagen: WHO Regional Office for Europe.

Babor, T. F. (1995). The social and public health significance of individually directed interventions. In *Alcohol and Public Policy: Evidence and Issues*, ed. Holder, H. D. & Edwards, G., pp.164–89. Oxford: Oxford University Press.

Batel, P., Pessione, F., Bouvier, A.-M. & Rueff, B. (1995). Prompting alcoholics to be referred to an alcohol clinic: the effectiveness of a simple letter. *Addiction* 90, 811–14.

Bien, T. H., Miller, W. R. & Tonigan, J. S. (1993). Brief interventions for alcohol problem: a review. *Addiction* **88**, 315–36.

Carroll, K. M. & Rounsaville, B. J. (1993). Implications of recent research on psychotherapy for drug abuse. In *Drugs, Alcohol and Tobacco: Making the Science and Policy Connections*, ed. Edwards, G., Strang, J. & Jaffe, J. pp. 210–21. Oxford: Oxford University Press.

Chick, J.& Cantwell, R. (eds) (1994). *Seminars in Drug Misuse.* London: Gaskell.

Davidson, R. (1992). Prochaska and DiClimente's model of change: a case study. *British Journal of Addiction* 87, 821–2.

Davidson, R. (1996). Motivational issues in the treatment of addictive behaviour. *Psychotherapy, Psychological Treatments and the Addictions*, ed. Edwards, G. & Dare, C., pp. 173–88.Cambridge: Cambridge University Press.

Edwards, G. (1996). Addictive behaviours: the next clinic appointment. *Psychotherapy, Psychological Treatments and the Addictions*, ed. Edwards, G.& Dare, C., pp. 94–109. Cambridge: Cambridge University Press.

Edwards, G., Oppenheimer, E. & Taylor, C. (1992). Hearing the noise in the system. Exploration of textual analysis as a method for studying change in drinking behaviour. *British Journal of Addiction* 87, 73–81.

Edwards, G. & Dare, C. (1996). *Psychotherapy, Psychological Treatments and the Addictions.* Cambridge: Cambridge University Press.

Gossop, M. (1996). Cognitive and behavioural treatments for substance abuse. *Psychotherapy, Psychological Treatments and the Addictions*, ed. Edwards, G. & Dare, C., pp. 158–72. Cambridge: Cambridge University Press.

Heather, N. (1995a). *Treatment Approaches to Alcohol Problems. European Series No.65.* Copenhagen: WHO Regional Office for Europe.

Heather, N. (1995b). Interpreting the evidence on brief interventions for excessive drinkers: the need for caution. *Alcohol and Alcoholism* 30, 287–96.

Heather, N., Kisson-Singh, J. & Fenton, W. (1990). Assisted natural recovery from alcohol problems: effects of a self-help manual with and without telephone contacts. *British Journal of Addiction* **85**, 1177–85.

Hunt, W. A., Barnett, L. W. & Branck, L. G. (1971). Relapse rates in addiction programs. *Journal of Clinical Psychology* **27**, 455–6.

Jellinek, E. M. (1960). *The Disease Concept of Alcoholism.* New Brunswick: Hillhouse Press.

Levin, J. D. & Weiss, R. H. (Eds.) (1994). *The Dynamics and Treatment of Alcoholism: Essential Papers.* Northvale: Jason Aronson.

Luborsky, L. & Crits-Christoph, P. (1990). *Understanding the Transference.* New York: Basic Books.

Luborsky, L., McLellan, A. J., Woody, G. E., O'Brien, C. P. & Anerback, A. (1985). Therapist success and its determinants. *Archives of General Psychiatry* **42**, 602–11.

Lynskey, T .M., Fergusson, D. M. & Horwood, J. (1994). The effect of parental alcohol problems on rates of adolescent psychiatric disorder. *Addiction* **89**, 1277–86.

Malan, D. H. & Osimu, F. (1992). *Psychodynamics Training and Outcome.* New York, Basic Books

Marlatt, G. A. & Gordon, J. R. (1985). *Relapse Prevention: Maintenance Strategies in the Treatment of Addictive Behaviour.* New York: Guilford.

Miller, W. R., Gribskov, C. J. & Mortell, R. L. (1981). Effectiveness of a self-control manual for problem drinkers with and without therapist contact. *International Journal of the Addictions* **18**, 1241–54.

Miller, W. R. & Heather, N. (Eds.) (1986). *Treating Addictive Behaviours: Processes of Change.* New York: Plenum.

Miller, W. & Rollnick, S. (1991). *Motivational Interviewing: Preparing People to Change Addictive Behavior.* New York: Guilford.

Orford, J. & Edwards, G. (1977). *Alcoholism. A Comparison of Treatment and Advice, with a Study of the Influence of Marriage.* Maudsley Hospital Monograph No.26. Oxford: Oxford University Press.

Prochaska, J. O. & DiClimente, C. C. (1984). *The Transtheoretical Approach: Crossing Traditional Boundaries of Therapy.* Homewood: Dow Jones/Ireven.

Rollnick, S., Heather, N., Gold, R. & Hall, W. (1992). Development of a short 'readiness to change questionnaire' for use in brief, opportunistic interventions among excessive drinkers. *Addiction* **87**, 743–54.

Sutton, S. (1996). Can 'stages of change' provide guidance in the treatment of addictions? A critical examination of Prochaska and DiClimente's model. *Psychotherapy, Psychological Treatments and the Addictions*, ed. Edwards, G. & Dare, C., pp. 184–205. Cambridge: Cambridge University Press.

Thom, B., Brown, D., Drummond, C., Edwards, G., Mullan, M. & Taylor, C. (1992). Engaging patients with alcohol problems in treatment: the first consultation. *British Journal of Addiction* **87**, 601–11.

Tober, G. (1991). Helping the pre-contemplator. In *Counselling Drug Problems*, ed. Davidson, R., Rollnick, S. & MacEwan, I., pp. 21–38. London: Routledge.

Vaillant, G. E. (1983). *The Natural History of Alcoholism.* Cambridge, MA, Harvard University Press.

Vaillant, G. E. (1993). *Wisdom of the Ego.* Cambridge MA: Harvard University Press.

Zeitlin, H. (1994). Children with alcohol misusing parents. In *Alcohol and Alcohol Problems*, ed. Edwards, G. & Peters, T. J., pp. 139–51. *British Medical Bulletin No. 50.* Edinburgh: Churchill Livingstone.

16

Alcoholics Anonymous

AA was founded in the USA in 1935 by two alcoholics (Wilson, 1994) and first began to establish itself in the UK in the late 1940s. There are more than 3000 groups in Great Britain and over 88,000 groups in 134 countries worldwide. The estimated world membership is upwards of two million. It has helped countless individuals (often when professional intervention has failed), is a repository of astonishing experience and subtle and often humorous wisdom, and has had a profound influence in humanising social attitudes towards people with drinking problems. AA is thus an enormous potential resource, and it is a dereliction of duty if patients go through treatment without AA ever being mentioned, or worse still if they are deflected from AA involvement by some negative statement born of ignorance and misunderstanding – 'I think you would find it all too religiose'.

The therapist must be willing to find out how AA operates and what its beliefs are, and the best way of doing so is to pay a personal visit to an open meeting of AA – a meeting open to all-comers, as opposed to closed meetings which are restricted to AA membership.

AA meetings

The AA meeting is of central importance to AA's functioning. It has a unique atmosphere, marked by a seeming informality but with an underlying and purposeful method of working. The number of people at a meeting will vary from group to group, but is typically around 10 to 20. Some of those present will have been attending AA for years, while the man or woman sitting in the back row may have just walked hesitantly through the door for the first time. A chairman will have been elected for that evening and they will probably be sitting at a table with one or two members who have been asked 'to give their stories'. The newcomer will notice a lot of friendly greeting and talking.

The meeting will start with the chairman saying 'My name is . . .' (only first names are used), 'I am an alcoholic'. These words carry immense implications – the speaker is not ashamed of his/her alcoholism, but without reservation, acknowledges their condition as an inalienable fact. The starting point of the evening is thus one individual's reaffirmation, for all present, of what in AA terms must be the starting point of recovery for every individual, namely the admission that he or she is suffering from 'alcoholism'.

The chairman will then read the AA preamble.

Alcoholics Anonymous is a fellowship of men and women who share their experience, strength, and hope with each other that they may solve their common problem and help others to recover from alcoholism. The only requirement for membership is a desire to stop drinking. There are no dues or fees for AA membership; we are self-supporting through our own contributions. AA is not allied with any sect, denomination, politics, organization or institution; does not wish to engage in any controversy, neither endorses nor opposes any causes. Our primary purpose is to stay sober and help other alcoholics to achieve sobriety. (Leach & Norris, 1977)

With these preliminaries out of the way, the first speaker of the evening will then be called. Their introduction will again be in terms of 'My name's . . ., and I'm an alcoholic'. He or she will speak for 20 to 30 minutes, giving an account of their personal background and then going on to describe the development of their drinking problem, the sufferings they endured or inflicted on others, the deceptions and pre-varications of their drinking days, and then often some final turning-point or 'rock bottom' experience. They will go on to describe their introduction to AA and their recovery within the programme of that fellowship, and their evolving understanding of the meaning of AA as a way of life. Within this biographical format different speakers each develop their own approach, and the ability of the person who has never given a public speech in any other setting to make a personal statement, which is both moving and convincing, is no doubt related to the unwritten guidelines which propose that a personal *story* should be given, rather than an abstract lecture. The story, which is told in unadorned manner by the person with fairly recent experience of recovery, seems often to be better received than the highly polished performance by the person who has told their story many times, but who is by now rather distanced from the acuteness of their experience. And stories that deal with recovery, and which offer practical hints on how to work at recovery, are likely to be better received than long drawn-out accounts of drinking days.

These life stories are followed by comments and personal statements from the floor. Themes are caught up and explored by the listeners, who often stress their identification with the speaker's story – 'That happened to me too . . .'. No one is forced to speak and it is realised that for weeks the new member may want to do no more than sit and listen.

Reference is often made during the meeting to 'the twelve steps', which enshrine the basic ideology of AA (Alcoholics Anonymous, 1977). These steps are:

(1) We admitted we were powerless over alcohol – that our lives had become unmanageable.

(2) Came to believe that a Power greater than ourselves could restore us to sanity.

(3) Made a decision to turn our will and our lives over to the care of God *as we understood Him.*

(4) Made a searching and fearless moral inventory of ourselves.

(5) Admitted to God, to ourselves, and to another human being the exact nature of our wrongs.

(6) Were entirely ready to have God remove all these defects of character.

(7) Humbly asked Him to remove our shortcomings.

(8) Made a list of all persons we had harmed, and became willing to make amends to them all.

(9) Made direct amends to such people wherever possible, except when to do so would injure them or others.

(10) Continued to take personal inventory, and when we were wrong, promptly admitted it.

(11) Sought through prayer and meditation to improve our conscious contact with God *as we understood Him* praying only for knowledge of His will for us and the power to carry that out.

(12) Having had a spiritual awakening as the result of these steps we tried to carry this message to alcoholics and to practice these principles in all our affairs.

A speaker may comment on the meaning that any one of these steps has had for them personally and describe their efforts to achieve this step. For instance, the meaning to be given to step (2) with its idea of 'a Power greater than ourselves' often attracts discussion, with an interpretation in terms of an open and individually determined concept of God – the 'God *as we understood Him*', of steps (3) and (11). This seemingly theistic formulation does not in practice debar an atheist from finding help in AA.

The formal proceedings end with the meeting saying together what is known as the Serenity Prayer:

God grant me the serenity
To accept the things I cannot change
The courage to change the things I can
And the wisdom to know the difference.

The members then chat and exchange news over tea or coffee, and subtle but positive effort is likely to be made to put the new attender at their ease and draw them into contact. Frequently the new member will after some weeks find a 'sponsor' who will offer personal advice and a special degree of availability – a phone number to contact, an arrangement to meet in the evening to attend an AA meeting, and so on. The sponsor is also a role model.

Besides the meetings themselves, much else is potentially on offer. Members may start to visit each other at home, go out to meals together or share other social activities. Old drinking friends are dropped, and new friends found who think and talk AA. In some localities routine meetings will be supplemented by study groups, and AA literature shared and passed around. Regional and national AA conventions may be attended, and the more experienced member may give time to 'twelfth-stepping' (acting as sponsor and working with new members); they may help with prison or hospital groups, or offer availability as a speaker at meetings of community organisations.

The 'Minnesota Model'

AA itself is a worldwide network of self-help groups, with no allegiance to any other institution. However, it has been extremely influential upon the working of many individuals and organisations, particularly in North America where its principles have been applied to institutional forms of treatment now known commonly as the 'Minnesota Model' (Cook, 1988a; see Chapter 20).

In some countries, entry into this form of treatment may begin with an 'intervention' in the client's home. This strategy, directed mainly at the drinker who denies having any problem with alcohol, requires the gathering of family, friends, colleagues, and significant others under the direction of a trained therapist. The unsuspecting 'alcoholic' then arrives home to be confronted by the assembled gathering. The aim of the confrontation, in which each person presents examples of the drink related harm that they have witnessed, is to challenge the drinker's denial that they have a problem, and to encourage them to enter a suitable programme of treatment. Such interventions may be very effective

276

when expertly managed, but could easily be destructive and counter-therapeutic if ill-considered or attempted by the inexperienced. However, they illustrate the principle that, in the first instance, treatment may have to be taken to the problem drinker, rather than expecting the drinker to seek help themselves in the clinic or treatment centre.

Whether or not an 'intervention' has been employed as the starting point, the typical Minnesota Model treatment package commences with a residential phase, typically lasting one to two months, with a packed programme of group therapy, lectures, work assignments, daily reading groups, and other activities, notably attendance at AA meetings. The staff are mainly, or even entirely, comprised of recovering 'alcoholics' and drug 'addicts' who have themselves worked through the 12 steps and demonstrated a commitment to abstinence for a period of some years. Such individuals, even in recovery, would consider themselves to be suffering from 'alcoholism' or 'chemical dependency' and the terms 'problem drinker' or 'drug misuser' would be quite alien in these settings.

In addition to 'alcoholics', residents in such centres will usually also include addicts to other drugs, who will work through the programme of Narcotics Anonymous (NA). A range of 'behavioural' addictions are also treated in many such centres, including eating disorders, relationship or sexual addictions, and a diverse group of other problems.

Following the residential phase of treatment, the 'alcoholic' may be encouraged to participate in a programme of aftercare offered by the same institution. One of the great strengths of this approach, however, is its ability to link people in to their local AA groups for long-term or lifelong support. No other approach to the treatment of drinking problems can boast an international network of support groups on such a scale as this.

The Minnesota Model has been criticised in some quarters as being expensive and ineffective. In fact, it need not be any more expensive than other residential approaches to treatment, and is potentially cheaper than in-patient units which provide expensive medical and nursing care. Such evidence as has been published suggests also that it is no less effective than many other treatment programmes (Cook, 1988b).

Essential processes

What are the essential processes through which AA operates? There have been many attempts to answer this question, and in summary the following dimensions can probably be identified.

Coherent, flexible ideas

A coherent but flexible set of ideas is offered (an ideology), which can relieve the individual's sense of hopelessness and explain the nature of their problem. They are suffering from 'the disease of alcoholism', which is pictured as metaphorically akin to an 'allergy to alcohol'. Their constitution is such that they will react to this drug differently from other people. They can never be 'cured' but the disease will be 'arrested' if they do not drink again. Lifetime abstinence must be their only goal. It is the first drink that they cannot risk.

Action programme

AA offers an action programme, and 'the twelve steps' outline the actions that have to be taken. The 'alcoholic' must join AA and stay close to AA. They will be advised to take things 'one day at a time' and to work for short-term goals. The stories and discussions they listen to at AA meetings and the guidance from their sponsor will provide them with many hints on coping and problem solving. Their first priority is to deal with their drinking, but the programme will also require them to examine psychological problems – their guilt, their 'resentment', their tendency to blame others, their 'stinking thinking'. AA is 'a selfish programme' and each individual is working for sobriety for their own sake and not to please anyone else, and they thus give no hostages to fortune. If they relapse they are not rejected but may return any number of times to try again. The programme will finally include 'twelfth-stepping', but by then members should have learnt that in the process of helping other people they will help themselves and confirm their own strength; it is not, however, their job to proselytise, 'pull people down lamp-posts', or put their own sobriety at risk.

Rewards of sobriety

AA carries the message that sobriety is rewarding, and helps the individual to discover these rewards. It gives them new friends, introduces them to a new social network, relieves their loneliness, helps them to structure and employ their time, removes a stigma, and confers on them a sense of personal worth. If they have been sober for one day, they have been a success. Through AA they may ultimately achieve serenity, with sobriety a way of life.

Possibility of recovery

AA's ideology is persuasive and an approach to recovery is made to appear possible. This last heading bears on each of the previous headings. AA does not 'work' through an abstract set of ideas, but through those ideas being found persuasive by the individual. The most apt theoretical definition of the disorder and the pathways to recovery would remain useless if AA did not have the ability to persuade the new member that AA is about him or her as an individual, can meet their problems, and show them personally the way ahead. AA can carry this conviction because its members so evidently know what they are talking about; they too have been through it all and know every stratagem of deceit and denial, while at the same time bearing tangible witness to the possibility of success.

Who will affiliate with AA?

Like other approaches to treatment, AA is not a panacea. Its membership is almost exclusively composed of people who have suffered from moderate or severe alcohol dependence, and group cohesion is therefore built around total acceptance of the abstinence goal. The person who is not dependent and who does not wish to aim for abstinence is unlikely to find AA compatible.

The drinker who goes to a meeting where everyone is of another social background is also unlikely to feel at home, although this problem can be met by the individual shopping around until they find a group of people with whom they can identify. Different AA meetings vary in composition; some operate with a wide mix of social backgrounds, while others seem tacitly to have recruited their membership with a bias toward a particular socio-economic stratum. Also, some groups will emphasise the spiritual aspect of AA ideology much more than others. It may therefore take some time and perseverance for the new member to find the group that most suits their needs. Some groups may have a particular reputation for being helpful to the newcomer, who may be guided in their direction.

It is always difficult to predict who will and who will not find AA helpful and patients should be advised to go along to meetings and see for themselves whether AA offers an answer.

The therapist and co-operation with AA

As was stated earlier, the therapist should, whenever appropriate, sign-post the way to AA. This not only implies being able to provide the appropriate phone number (which is available in the local telephone directory), and perhaps being able to effect a direct introduction to an AA sponsor with whom the patient is likely to identify, but also means having the knowledge and sympathy which will enable them to convey to the patient that attending some AA meetings is likely to be eminently worthwhile. The therapist will know that only a minority of their patients (perhaps no more than 5 to 10%) will enter into a full and pro-longed relationship with AA, but even a lesser exposure can be beneficial. The therapist who, on occasion, is able to attend AA open meetings will enhance their credibility as informant and build up valuable contacts with local groups.

Co-operation is, of course, a two-way business, and AA needs to understand the workings of the local services and be able to make a direct referral for professional advice if assistance is thought necessary. Many centres have established a fruitful two-way relationship of this sort, and at the national level AA has set up mechanisms for liaison with hospitals and prisons. A centre which is offering a normal drinking goal for some of its patients will, however, need to talk through this aspect of its work with AA, if misunderstanding is to be avoided. Another difficulty can stem from the anti-drug attitude of some AA members, which may result in advice to a new member that they should stop taking anti-depressant drugs, or disulfiram, against their own best interests. At the extreme, some AA members may be so convinced that AA offers the only true pathway to recovery as to make co-operation with other agencies difficult. But such difficulties are rare, and with open communication and mutual respect, problems can usually be sorted out.

The relationship of AA to the in-patient unit is discussed in Chapter 20.

Research on AA

Although there is a considerable research literature on AA, definitive studies proving (or disproving) its efficacy are lacking. This is a result of the methodological problems that are inherent in the study of a voluntary programme of self-help with which people may affiliate, or from which they may disaffiliate, at will (Bebbington, 1976; Glaser & Ogborne, 1982). The evidence of efficacy is therefore largely suggestive, being based upon popularity, personal testimony, and perceived benefit rather than scientific proof (Edwards, 1995). Surprisingly, there is somewhat more evidence (although still far from being definitive) to support the contention that there is an aggregate level effect of AA, in reducing alcohol related problems in the population as a whole (Babor, 1995).

A detailed analysis of research on AA is beyond the scope of this book, but the interested reader should consult the review by McCrady and Miller (1993).

Learning from AA

Claims for the success and universality of AA can easily be exaggerated, and its emphasis on the disease concept may be out of tune with the model employed by some therapists. But there can be no doubt that as well as the direct benefit which AA offers to individual drinkers, it also has much to teach the therapist about the processes that aid and influence recovery. There is wisdom to be borrowed from AA.

Al-Anon

Al-Anon is an organisation that is independent of, but allied with, AA (Al-Anon Family Groups UK and Eire, 1980). It is a self-help group that caters for the families of 'alcoholics' – for 'anyone who loves an alcoholic'. It has its own 'twelve steps' that mirror AA thinking. Quite often, an AA meeting will be going on in one room and an Al-Anon meeting in the next room, with everyone getting together afterwards over the tea and biscuits.

The functioning of Al-Anon will not be discussed here in detail, because its principles and methods of working have much in common with AA. That Al-Anon can fulfil an extremely important function does, however, need to be emphasised, and the therapist should again be able knowledgeably to point the way. Al-Anon may give immediate relief, for example, to the wife who has been struggling by every stratagem to stop her husband from drinking, and who has in the process been experiencing stress and frustration. Al-Anon will teach her to 'let go' and to give up the hope of trying to control her husband's behaviour or solve his problem for him. He must find his own answers to *his* own problem, and similarly, she must examine *her* own behaviour – the only behaviour that she is directly able to control or alter is, indeed, her own.

Al-Ateen

Al-Ateen is a self-help group operating along AA lines that aims to help the teenage children of families where there is an alcoholic parent. To date, this organisation has become more widely established in North America than in the UK or other parts of Europe. That children living in such families are often experiencing distress and conflict cannot be doubted (see Chapter 4), and Al-Ateen potentially meets the needs of a group that the professional services involved with the parents may all too easily pass by.

Other self-help groups

Although AA is the largest and best known self-help group for people with drinking problems, on a local basis other self-help groups may be available. In the UK, for example, there is a special group for doctors and dentists (the 'British Doctors and Dentists Group'; Anonymous, 1995). This profession-specific self-help group is often more approachable for a practitioner who may have fears of traditional AA groups, not least that they may meet their patients at the meetings. However, the group does have a close affinity to AA.

Other groups have deliberately set out to take a different approach to AA. For example, Secular Organizations for Sobriety (SOS) and Rational Recovery (RR), in the United States, have taken a non-religious stance (Connors & Dermen, 1996).

References

Al-Anon Family Groups UK and Eire (1980). Help for families of problem drinkers. *Health Trends* **12**, 8.

Alcoholics Anonymous (1977). *Twelve steps and Twelve Traditions*. New York: Alcoholics Anonymous World Services.

Anonymous (1995). The British doctors' and dentists' groups: over two decades of successful work. *Addiction Counselling World* **6**, 26–7.

Babor, T. (1995). The social and public health significance of individually directed interventions. In *Alcohol and Public Policy: Evidence and Issues*, ed. Holder, H. D. & Edwards, G., pp. 164–89. New York: Oxford University Press.

Bebbington, P. (1976). The efficacy of Alcoholics Anonymous: the elusiveness of hard data. *British Journal of Psychiatry* **128**, 572–80.

Connors, G. J. & Dermen, K. H. (1996). Characteristics of participants in Secular Organizations for Sobriety (SOS). *American Journal of Drug and Alcohol Abuse* **22**, 281–95.

Cook, C. C. H. (1988a). The Minnesota model in the management of drug and alcohol dependency: miracle method or myth? Part I. The philosophy and the programme. *British Journal of Addiction* **83**, 625–34.

Cook, C. C. H. (1988b). The Minnesota model in the management of drug and alcohol dependency: miracle method or myth? Part II. Evidence and conclusions. *British Journal of Addiction* **83**, 735–48.

Edwards, G. (1995). Alcoholics Anonymous as mirror held up to nature. In *Psychotherapy, Psychological Treatments, and the Addictions*, eds. Edwards, G. & Dare, C., pp. 220–39. Cambridge: Cambridge University Press.

Glaser, F. B.; Ogborne, A. C. (1982). Does AA really work? *British Journal of Addiction* **77**, 123–9.

Leach, B. & Norris, J. L. (1977). Factors in the development of Alcoholics Anonymous (AA). In *Treatment and rehabilitation of the chronic alcoholic*, ed. Kissin, B. & Begleiter, H., pp. 441–543. *The Biology of Alcoholism*, vol. 5. New York: Plenum.

McCrady, B. S. & Miller, W. R. (Eds.) (1993). *Research on Alcoholics Anonymous. Opportunities and Alternatives*. Brunswick: Rutgers Centre of Alcohol Studies.

Wilson, W. (1994). The society of Alcoholics Anonymous. *American Journal of Psychiatry* **151**, 259–62.

17

Special techniques

Introduction

No single treatment approach is effective for all individuals with drinking problems (Institute of Medicine, 1990). It is now accepted that some treatments are more effective than others for certain patients, but which treatments work? In an influential review, Miller and Hester (1986) highlighted the fact that the effectiveness of treatment methods being widely used in alcohol treatment programmes, particularly in the USA, were not supported by controlled research. However, treatment methods with proven efficacy were at that time not commonly being used in treatment settings. We take the Miller and Hester (1986) review as usefully indicative, but in the light of evolving evidence, judgement on which treatment works must be subject to continuing scrutiny. There is a difference between 'no evidence' for efficacy (e.g. AA) and controlled evidence that a particular treatment is no better than no treatment. Our basic plea is that treatment choices should wherever possible be research based while at the same time a spurious scientism should not be allowed to inhibit the efforts of the individual therapist who is trying to help the individual patient in difficult and unique circumstances. Box 17.1 summarises our judgement as to the extent of current research-underpinning for different treatments.

In this chapter, five broad approaches to the treatment of drinking problems are discussed – motivational interviewing; cognitive-behavioural therapy; relapse prevention; psychotherapy; and pharmacotherapy. This will be prefaced by an account of the stages of change model that are relevant. The aim is to outline different techniques and discuss their value and limitation; no attempt will be made to go into details about their application. Anyone wanting to acquire the necessary specialist clinical skills will do best to train under the guidance of someone familiar with such methods.

Box 17.1. Special treatments for drinking problems: an appraisal of their research underpinning

- *Psychological treatments* including motivational interviewing, broad-spectrum cognitive-behaviour approaches, relapse prevention and community reinforcement. Well supported by research.

- *Individual psychotherapies* other than cognitive-behavioural. Little or no research support – deploy with discrimination.

- *Group therapy.* Probably useful for basic support, but efficacy as a treatment of choice not supported.

- *Marital therapy.* Not supported as a routine treatment of choice.

- *Alcoholics Anonymous.* The impact of Alcoholics Anonymous has not as yet been conclusively researched.

- *Disulfiram.* Not without side-effects, but useful in some circumstances.

- *Anti-craving drugs* including naltrexone and acamprosate. Research suggests promise.

What are described as 'special techniques' may be considered routine by some practitioners, while others would place a lesser emphasis on these approaches from that given here. The adjective 'special' is still useful to differentiate these methods from the basic approaches discussed in Chapter 15, and most experienced therapists would agree that whatever the special approach thus favoured, it is only valuable within the context of the general therapeutic work discussed in that chapter.

Stages of change

The 'stages of change' model, which acknowledges the pivotal role of the patient in the process of behavioural change, describes five discrete stages of change that can be applied both to an understanding of drinking behaviour and to the practical work of treatment (Prochaska & Di Clemente, 1986; Prochaska *et al.*, 1992). These stages are: *precontemplation, contemplation, determination, action and maintenance* (see p. 218). In the *precontemplation* stage individuals are not considering a change in their drinking habits in the next six months. They may present to treatment services because they are under pressure from a partner, family, employer, or GP. Individuals in the *contemplation* stage recognise that they have a problem and begin to consider the implications for change. They have not yet made a commitment to take action and may remain at this stage for long periods if they do not resolve their ambivalence to change. Individuals in the *determination* stage are intending to take action and may already have tried to cut down on their alcohol consumption. Having made a decision to change, individuals move forward into the *action* stage. They make a commitment to change and try to modify their drinking behaviour, often needing considerable support and encouragement. In the *maintenance* stage individuals seek to maintain the changes in order to prevent relapse.

The stages of change model was first put forward as a linear schema and then as a circular or revolving-door model. Because individuals usually relapse, and re-enter the cycle, often moving through the stages several times before achieving long-term maintenance, Prochasksa and DiClemente (1992) have more recently presented a spiral model.

Prochaska and DiClemente's model provides a useful and practical framework in the treatment setting. It is helpful for the therapist to consider the degree to which the patient is prepared to change. Thus patients in the precontemplative stage are not impossible to treat and patients in the action stage will not always succeed. The view that relapse is part of the process helps to avoid a sense of failure, and allows it to be seen as part of the natural process rather than as a catastrophe. This model has intuitive appeal and has been influential in guiding clinical practice (Davidson, 1992). However, the discrete categorisation of the various stages is perhaps over-simplified and artificial, and the model is possibly best viewed as a model of ideal change that may be helpful in the design of interventions (Sutton, 1996).

Motivational interviewing

Since its original description as a therapeutic technique for use with problem drinkers, motivational interviewing has emerged as a practical and acceptable treatment approach for individuals who are reluctant to change and who are ambivalent about changing. It draws on strategies from client-centred counselling, cognitive therapy, systems theory and the social psychology of persuasion (Miller & Rollnick, 1991). The therapist does not assume an authoritarian or confrontational role, but seeks to create a positive atmosphere conducive to change. The overall goal is to increase the intrinsic motivation of the patient, leaving them with the responsibility to effect their own change. It is helpful to view motivational interviewing in the context of the stages of change model. In the early stages, patients are helped to explore their ambivalence to address reasons for change, using strategies derived from client-centred counselling, such as open-ended questions, reflective listening, affirmation, and summarising. Self-motivational statements are elicited from patients in order to help them to develop a perceived discrepancy or dissonance between their present behaviour and their stated goals. Motivational interviewing develops and amplifies this discrepancy, ultimately allowing the patient to present the reasons for change without feeling coerced. Motivational interviewing has been found to be effective in reducing alcohol consumption in problem drinkers in a variety of health settings including primary care and general hospitals (Bien *et al.*, 1993). The six elements commonly used in brief interventions have been summarized by the acronym FRAMES: feedback, responsibility, advice, menu, empathy and self-efficacy (Miller & Sanchez, 1993).

Cognitive-behavioural therapy

The cognitive-behavioural approach to treatment is based on the assumption that it is the problem drinking that is to be treated, as opposed to the psychoanalytic view that the drinking is a symptom or symbol of an underlying psychodynamic conflict or neurosis. Implicit in this approach is the belief that problem drinking is mainly a learned behaviour and that treatment involves replacing the maladaptive pattern of drinking behaviour with more appropriate drinking or abstinence. Cognitive-behavioural psychology also highlights the role of expectations about alcohol in the development of drinking and its consequences.

Broad spectrum approaches

A further development of the cognitive-behavioural approach has been the inclusion of training in skills thought to be lacking in patients with drinking problems. Drinkers may for instance use alcohol to cope with anxiety or anger or as a result of negative cognitions associated with low self-esteem and depression. Such individuals may benefit from specific techniques including relaxation training, anger management, and cognitive restructuring. These approaches are not specific to alcohol problems, but find their application as treatments aimed at dealing with postulated psychological causes of excessive drinking. Within this spectrum at least the following kinds of intervention can be listed.

(1) *Social skills training and assertiveness training.* Some patients with drinking problems are handicapped by an underlying inability to function confidently in social situations, and treatment by role playing, desensitisation or other behavioural methods may ameliorate this situation. Assertiveness training comes under this heading – the patient who is unassertive may find it difficult to say 'no' to an offered drink, and one element in therapy may involve teaching them to rehearse saying 'no'. Social skills training that includes assertiveness training is an extremely effective method of treatment for alcohol problems (Holder *et al.*, 1991). However, it requires a certain level of cognitive functioning and patients with alcohol-related brain damage will not benefit from this approach.

(2) *Problem-solving skills.* Individuals with drinking difficulties frequently have handicaps in solving problems and will then cope by denial or by further drinking. Training in problem-solving skills is similar to social skills training and aims to help the patient to develop alternative coping strategies for use in high risk situations (Monti *et al.*, 1989).

(3) *Relaxation training.* Many patients report that they initially began to drink in order to relieve feelings of anxiety. Anxiety disorders are not uncommon among such individuals (see Chapter 6). Teaching of relaxation by simple psychological techniques may be useful for a tense patient who drinks to relax, and can offer an alternative method of coping with cravings.

(4) *Anger management.* Without alcohol, many patients experience difficulties coping with and expressing their anger. Training in anger management can be of benefit, particularly if carried out in conjunction with assertiveness training (Heather, 1995).

(5) *Cognitive restructuring.* Often patients will attribute their alcohol use to extrinsic factors such as stress and are not aware that their own negative thoughts are implicated (Beck *et al.*, 1993). Cognitive restructuring helps the individual to interrupt the series of thoughts that would usually lead to drinking and to replace them with positive thoughts. This is an effective treatment which should be used routinely as part of a cognitive-behavioural programme. It is particularly successful when used in combination with social skills training (Oei & Jackson, 1982).

Behavioural self-control

Behavioural self-control is particularly effective in helping individuals at the less severe end of the dependence spectrum to reduce their alcohol consumption. Initially the therapist and client negotiate sensible limits of alcohol consumption and the client keeps a drinking diary or fills out a self-monitoring card to record all drinks taken. A craving diary or daily activity diary can also be helpful. Clients are then taught techniques for reducing the rate of drinking and are helped to identify triggers to drinking, in particular negative moods (boredom, anxiety, depression), positive moods (excitement, happiness), and external cues (meeting with friends, particular time of day, a particular place). Behavioural self-control training can be used in the individual or group setting, and self-help manuals are available (Heather, 1995).

Cue exposure

This approach is based on the principles of classical conditioning and borrows from a treatment strategy that was developed for phobias, obsessive-compulsive disorder, and other anxiety disorders. The patient is exposed to conditioned stimuli or cues which have previously precipitated craving or excessive drinking, and encouraged either not to drink or not to drink excessively. For instance, they may be asked to carry around with them a bottle of whisky and sniff at it without drinking, or the therapist may accompany them on outings to a bar, or they may be asked to take sufficient alcohol to activate craving and then desist from further drinking. Cue exposure reduces the likelihood that the stimulus will trigger a response in the future and improves the individual's self-efficacy. It can be combined with coping skills (Monti *et al.*, 1989) or incorporated into a relapse prevention programme (Drummond & Glautier, 1994).

Aversion therapies

Aversion therapies, based on the principles of classical conditioning, came to the fore in the 1930s and are of historical importance because they fostered an optimistic interest in 'alcoholism' treatment at a time when little else appeared to be promising. The act of drinking alcohol is paired with a variety of unpleasant experiences, and the individual should show an automatic negative response when later exposed to alcohol. Such counter-conditioning techniques have included chemically-induced nausea (using emetine and apomorphine), apnoea (using intravenous succinylcholine), electric shock, and covert sensitisation (Miller & Hester, 1986).

There is little evidence that chemical aversion does establish a classical conditioned response, and the favourable results reported in the literature are more likely to be due to the artefact of patient selection, rather than any special effect – a patient would need to be highly motivated to volunteer for such an unpleasant experience in the name of treatment. As the dangers and unpleasantness of chemical aversion outweigh any supposed advantages, this treatment should now be abandoned. Succinylcholine induced apnoea (cessation of breathing) as a treatment should be discarded completely. It is also questionable whether electric shock treatment, which is associated with considerable pain, is an ethical mode of treatment.

In covert sensitisation, the patient is taught to associate the sight or taste of alcohol with unpleasant images, which they learn actively to conjure up. This method is suited to an abstinence goal and is recommended for use on an individual basis as the best results are thought to be achieved when the images are specific to the individual. Covert sensitization is an effective treatment (Holder *et al.*, 1991) and its success can be predicted from the degree of conditioning established during treatment (Elkins, 1980).

The community reinforcement approach

This approach is based on the principles of instrumental learning and the emphasis is on manipulation of real-life rewards in the patient's environment. The family's positive reactions, aid with job-finding, membership of a social club, and other social rewards are presented to the patient as contingent on treatment success, and the therapeutic team accepts responsibility to ensure that such rewards are in fact on offer (Hunt & Azrin, 1973; Azrin, 1976). This technique was initially used with in-patients, but has been employed with out-patients and with supervised disulfiram (see p. 298). It is effective, particularly for drinkers with serious problems. However, the full treatment package is expensive and time-consuming.

Relapse prevention

Some aspects of relapse have already been discussed in Chapter 15 (p. 261) in relation to the basic work of treatment. The term, relapse prevention, refers to a wide range of techniques many or all of which are cognitive or behavioural in their thrust, but it is convenient to give relapse prevention its own heading. This approach has its origins within a theoretical model of relapse proposed by Marlett and Gordon (1985). Within this, perspective relapse is not viewed as an inexplicable catastrophe, but as an event that takes place through a series of cognitive, behavioural, and affective processes. One of the main objectives of the relapse prevention programme is preventing a lapse from becoming a relapse (see p. 263). Relapse is viewed as an untoward event, which is to be avoided by careful forward planning and by the design of an individual relapse prevention programme. Patients themselves are active partners in identifying high risk situations that are associated with a potential for relapse. Intra-personal factors such as negative and positive emotional states, inter-personal conflict and social pressure can all be determinants of relapse. The patient then has to learn more effective coping mechanisms including cognitive strategies, or personally planned substitute activities and rewarding use of leisure. Strategies will thus involve both learning how to avoid unnecessary risks and how to deal positively and confidently with inevitable risks. Relapse prevention essentially addresses itself not just to changing a self-destructive habit, but beyond that to the maintenance of change. The approach is applicable both to abstinence and the normal drinking goal.

Marlatt and Gordon also discussed life-style imbalance. The individual experiencing feelings of self-deprivation may be particularly likely to relapse in high risk situations. Cognitive factors such as rationalisation or denial come into play when individuals are craving and are used to legitimise the drinking behaviour and to reduce feelings of guilt and anxiety. Covert planning of relapse through a series of seemingly irrelevant decisions is also described in this model. Beyond Marlatt and Gordon's pioneering formulation several other authors have now contributed to elaboration of the relapse prevention model. (Annis, 1986; Litman, 1986; Wanigaratne *et al.*, 1990; Daley, 1991).

Cognitive-behavioural 'packages'

Anyone working with drinking problems will recognise that they are a very heterogenous population and that different approaches are needed for different patients. It is best to carry out an individual assessment and on the basis of this assessment to identify the type of treatment best suited to that person. Thus a treatment 'package' may usefully incorporate several cognitive-behavioural techniques tailored to the individual's need.

Psychotherapy

Drinking and its psychodynamic meanings

In the past, some psychoanalytic writing has suggested that the dynamic meaning of drinking can be pronounced upon in universal terms – for instance, excessive drinking as always being a suicidal equivalent. Such a dogmatic view of the psychodynamics of drinking is

291

as unhelpful to work in this field as are any fixed formulae for dynamic interpretations in the general field of psychotherapy.

Drinking and excessive drinking will in fact have different meanings for different patients, and often multiple meanings for any one patient. Without seeking to pre-empt the need to explore the individual there are some recurrent themes with which it is useful to become familiar. Some of these themes are set out briefly below, but this list is by not exhaustive:

(1) Drinking may be an indicator of identification with a heavy-drinking parent or other key figure in the patient's childhood. The patient is, as it were, destined to act out someone else's life rather than their own. Other people in the patient's present surroundings are also being set up as actors in the old play, for instance, the wife is being forced into the same role as the patient once saw his mother play in relation to his own alcoholic father. The acutely traumatic early experience of the child in an 'alcoholic' family, with the many unresolved conflicts of love, hate, rage, and pity, are particularly likely to result in a patient continuing to define relationships in terms of the play that they still desperately hope to resolve.

(2) Related to the general framework proposed above, one may identify a variety of common sub-plots. A man with a drinking problem may, for instance, seek defeat, punishment, or even destruction through drink, because they see themselves (their father) as deserving such fate. They may be seeking to inflict punishment on others, believing that at some level their mother destroyed their father and that she (and now the patient's own wife) are in a sense dreaded enemies. He may see drinking as giving power, because his father was only powerful when drunk. However, drinking may also point directly to interpersonal dependency conflicts – the patient wants to be powerful and independent but also wants to be a dependent child who is sick, erring, and repeatedly forgiven.

(3) Patients sometimes seem to use alcohol as a way of entering a blissful state of reverie where they can engage in fantasy and wish fulfilment. The real world is too difficult. Alcohol is valued for its subjective effect, and it becomes symbolised as all-warm, mother-like or milk-like. The drink is then an indicator of the patient's general difficulty in consistently maintaining an engagement with the real adult world.

The meanings given to alcohol are not only individually determined and shaped by early personal experience, but are also often coloured by culture. The need to be sensitive to the special meanings that a woman may give to her drinking also needs to be noted, for symbolic meanings may differ between the sexes.

Psychotherapy is not a panacea and its deployment may pose particular difficulties for those with alcohol and other addiction problems (Davison, 1996). Insight-oriented psychotherapy has not been shown to be an effective treatment for drinking problems in controlled trials. Yet, it has something to offer the carefully selected patient, and may on occasion be essential to that improvement in the quality of sobriety, which is such an important adjunct to recovery. The therapist who with modesty, open-mindedness, and guidance, engages in such work is also personally going to benefit and will round out their understanding of the extraordinarily complex human processes, which often lie behind a drinking story.

Indications for psychotherapy

The position that is taken in this section on the place of psychotherapy is in tune with the overall emphasis which is being given to the importance of approaching each patient in terms of their unique needs. This is the way in which an experienced nurse therapist described her use of psychotherapeutic insights:

> Most of the time I am not 'doing psychotherapy', at least overtly. I doubt whether most of my patients would regard themselves as 'being in psychotherapy'. I am in fact making use of psychotherapeutic principles in every interview – I am working through and with a relationship, and dealing with defence mechanisms. But all this work goes on in a setting which emphasises the need to keep one's feet on the ground, deal with drinking, pay the bills, get the children to school.

Such deployment of dynamic skills in the every day clinical setting merges with more formal and intensive psychotherapeutic strategies. We do not favour the routine and intensive deployment of formal psychotherapy as a treatment for drinking problems. The psychotherapeutic intervention that is always put into top gear for every patient and family from the earliest stages, not only represents an uneconomic and undiscriminating deployment of resources, but may damage the individual and family's capacity to generate their natural and spontaneous ways of working for, and consolidating, recovery. Such a perspective must not be misinterpreted as antipathetic to psychotherapy. On the contrary the position which is being taken is both that an understanding of dynamic principles must underpin basic work in this area, and that formal psychotherapy can on occasion have an important part to play. The argument is, however, that formal psychotherapy is not universally applicable and that its deployment requires timing and discrimination.

Different therapists will have their own views as to whether suitability for psychotherapy is determined restrictively or more freely. What should particularly be cautioned against is the danger of forgetting that suitability for psychotherapy does indeed have to be determined by careful assessment. The enthusiasm of those not specially trained in general psychotherapeutic work may lead to the prescription of psychotherapy for a patient whom no experienced psychotherapist would regard as a suitable patient for such engagement. Many psychotherapists will make the offer of psychotherapy actually conditional on the patient achieving a stable period of sobriety or other life changes.

Here is an example of a referral to psychotherapy which was timely and proved useful:

> A woman aged 45 years had presented three years previously with heavy non-dependent drinking in the setting of a painful marital breakdown. After a year's total abstinence from alcohol she had for two years been drinking in a moderate and controlled fashion. She was now contemplating remarriage, but was worried that she might in this new relationship re-enact what she sensed as being life-long problems in close relationships with men. Her father had been a strong but distant figure whom she had been taught greatly to admire, but towards whom her feelings had been very ambivalent. After two assessment interviews by a psychotherapist, she was offered a contract in terms of relatively short-term psychotherapy (six months with weekly sessions) which was to focus on her problems with key relationships, and her conflicting needs to be dominated together with her resentful and destructive responses to the people whom she manoeuvred into this role.

The alcohol team may have appropriate psychotherapeutic skills within its own resources, or it may be necessary to make referrals to psychotherapy specialists. This type of problem may, however, also be ideal for training staff in techniques for brief psychotherapy, with the time of the experienced psychotherapist then devoted to case supervision rather than to the treatment of referred cases.

Group therapy

Group therapy has been widely employed in the treatment of drinking problems even to the extent of sometimes being viewed as the treatment of choice (Falkowski, 1996). Despite this there is little evidence that classical group psychotherapy has a lasting impact on drinking behaviour.

In the alcohol field a diversity of activities is likely to be operating under the broad label of 'group work' and relapse prevention and cognitive-behavioural treatment are commonly delivered in this way.

At their simplest such groups would be of the kind described in Chapter 20, as often having a place within the therapeutic structure of a treatment centre. Such groups tend to have an open rather than a closed membership as patients are admitted and discharged. At the other extreme one may find practitioners who will work with closed groups of, say, 8–10 patients selected for their homogeneity (all women, for instance, or all of the same social background), and who will run these groups in terms of orthodox group therapy principles.

One can identify variations on some general themes as to the type of the work which is likely to be accomplished in group sessions. There may first be value simply in group *education* – patients for instance learn about the nature of dependence. A second important and general theme is *problem solving* – this may relate to such reality issues as how to find a job or deal with debts, or may focus on inter-personal and dynamic issues. Rehearsal of *relapse prevention strategies* is often a useful part of group work as patients share ideas with each other on how sobriety is to be consolidated and relapse avoided. Cohesion of group sentiment can assist in *definition of goals*, in overcoming *resistance* and in *strengthening of motivation*. Lastly the fellowship of the group and the opportunity to share problems may very generally contribute to support and help to overcome feelings of isolation.

The therapist should be willing to take responsibility for excluding any patient who comes to a group when intoxicated. Having anyone who has been drinking participate in a group usually causes such anxiety and anger as to rule out the possibility of constructive work.

Marital and family therapy

Alcohol problems have a far-reaching influence on family life, and are in turn affected by family dynamics. Many different types and intensities of family approach have been employed in the treatment of drinking problems, varying from informal chats with husband and wife, to sophisticated therapeutic interventions based on a specific theory. Other family members besides the husband and wife may be involved in therapeutic sessions. Over recent years there have been many advances in family therapy techniques and in the application of those techniques to this specialised sector of practice and there is evidence that marital or family therapy improve short-term outcomes. It is therefore important that anyone working with drinking problems should have some familiarity with family therapies. Two types of treatment, behavioural marital therapy and spouse therapy, have been shown to be effective.

Behavioural marital therapy

This method uses techniques such as behaviour contracting, teaching of communication, conflict resolution skills, and behaviour rehearsal to maintain abstinence (or reduced drinking) (O'Farrell, 1993). Some programmes incorporate a disulfiram contract where the problem drinker takes disulfiram every day observed by the spouse. Behavioural marital therapy has been shown to improve drinking outcomes at 18 months, and to maintain marital stability and satisfaction (O'Farrell *et al.*, 1993). Interactive couples' group therapy is another technique which shows promise (Bowers & Al-Rehda, 1990).

Spouse therapy

Here the spouse is helped to encourage the problem drinker to seek help and is taught behavioural reinforcement strategies to support abstinence or reduced drinking. Spouse therapy is effective in improving treatment retention (Heather, 1995).

Psychodrama

The use of psychodrama in the treatment of drinking problems has its advocates. Although special training is required for the skilled application of this approach, less complex role-playing techniques are more easily learnt. Patients may benefit greatly from group exploration of how they would, for instance, say 'no' to a drink, deal with anger or provocation, or manage a job interview.

Therapies for sexual problems

The sexual problems that may underly or result from excessive drinking are too often overlooked, and insufficient help is therefore given with these problems. Specialised techniques exist for assisting with such difficulties. Although it is unlikely that the therapist who was working on drinking problems will be able to come fully trained in the application of sex therapies, he or she should be conversant with what such approaches have to offer and should be able to make appropriate referrals.

Pharmacotherapy

Over recent years there have been major advances in understanding the neuropharmacological basis of alcohol dependence (see Chapter 2), and this has been paralleled by the introduction of newer pharmacotherapeutic agents, in particular drugs with anti-craving properties.

Pharmacotherapy should not be used in isolation but in conjunction with psychosocial treatments. This chapter will summarise current knowledge on the older (disulfiram) and newer drugs in the field. Alcohol withdrawal has been discussed in Chapter 14. This section of the present chapter will in turn discuss: disufiram (an alcohol-sensitising agent); drugs that attenuate drinking behaviour (anti-craving drugs); drugs used to treat psychiatric disorders associated with alcohol dependence; and finally amethystic agents.

Disulfiram

Since its introduction in the late 1940s, disulfiram (trade name Antabuse) has been used extensively in the treatment of alcohol problems. Disulfiram blocks the breakdown of alcohol at the acetaldehyde stage by inhibiting the hepatic enzyme aldehyde dehydrogenase or ALDH (see p. 23). This leads to an accumulation of acetaldehyde in the body and to the disulfiram-ethanol reaction, characterised by flushing of the face and upper trunk, throbbing headache, palpitations, tachycardia, nausea, vomiting, and general distress. With large doses of alcohol arrythmias, hypotension and collapse may occur. The reaction usually starts within 10 to 30 minutes of drinking and can last several hours. The severity varies greatly – it may be so slight that the patient 'drinks through it', or so severe as to be life-threatening. Patients with cardiac failure, coronary artery disease, hypertension, hepatic or renal impairment, respiratory disease, diabetes or epilepsy, should not be given disulfiram. In the event of a severe reaction and cardiovascular collapse the patient should lie down and the foot of the bed should be elevated. A vasopressor (blood-pressure raising drug) may be needed. Intravenous vitamin C or an antihistamine have also been recommended as antidotes. Patients prescribed disulfiram should carry a medical card with emergency instructions. The practice of exposing patients to a challenge dose of alcohol as a therapeutic test is not routinely justified.

The rationale of this treatment is that a patient cannot drink while under protective cover of the drug and they will thus only have to make a daily decision to take the medication rather than have to resist the sudden temptation at any moment to drink. Disulfiram is thus not primarily a conditioning treatment, though a variety of secondary learning processes may be involved.

Although disulfiram is used for its deterrent action, it also has effects on the central nervous system, inhibiting dopamine ß-hydroxylase and increasing concentrations of dopamine in the mesolimbic system. Patients taking disulfiram have reported a reduction in desire for alcohol.

297

Disulfiram is usually given in a daily dose of 100–200 mg. It is absorbed slowly, and therefore must be taken for a few days so as to build up a satisfactory blood level. Side-effects include initial lethargy and fatigue, vomiting, an unpleasant taste in the mouth and halitosis, impotence, and unexplained breathlessness. Other less usual side-effects include psychosis (usually accompanied by delirium), allergic dermatitis, peripheral neuritis, and hepatic cell damage. Disulfiram also interacts with other drugs enhancing the effect of warfarin, and inhibiting the metabolism of tricyclic antidepressants, phenytoin, and benzodiazepines such as diazepam and chlordiazepoxide. It is therefore a drug which should only be used with discretion and its dangers should not be discounted.

Despite the many years during which disulfiram has been in use, it is still difficult to form a view as to its place in treatment. Most studies of disulfiram have been of short duration, used small numbers of 'severe alcoholics', were not methodologically sound, and were associated with some form of coercion – from the courts, clinics, or from doctors (Hughes & Cook, 1997). Results have been equivocal but the multi-centre trial of Fuller and co-workers (1986) suggested that unsupervised oral disulfiram may help to reduce the frequency of drinking in men who are not abstinent, but who are reasonably motivated. It has been argued that this 'harm reduction' effect is a clinically important one (Heather, 1993). Supervised oral disulfiram appears to be effective when incorporated into a comprehensive treatment programme, when used in association with a contingency management plan, a community reinforcement approach (Azrin et al., 1982), or counselling (Chick et al., 1992).

The disadvantages of disulfiram include the potential dangers of the drug-ethanol reaction, side-effects of the drug, and a covert message that more basic therapeutic work is not needed. However, some patients find disulfiram helpful, especially in the early stages of abstinence. Others may prefer to take a low maintenance dose over many years and yet others will use it intermittently to cover high risk periods, for instance the executive going to a conference where they know they will be exposed to much entertaining.

In the light of present evidence the best results with disulfiram are probably likely to be seen when one or both of the following conditions are fulfilled. Firstly, the use of the drug should be explained to, and negotiated with, the patient so that the taking of these tablets becomes not only acceptable but wanted; the patient is not being muzzled, or surrendering autonomy, but making a free decision to engage in this type of treatment. Secondly, an acceptable degree of supervision should be set up (the tablet taken in the doctor's office, for instance, or in the medical room at work, or under the eyes of the wife), or a contingency management plan or therapeutic contract established. Disulfiram has been used quite widely in this way within industrial treatment programmes, and in the United States within court treatment programmes.

Disulfiram is also available in a long-acting implant form but research evidence in favour of this route of administration is negative. The technique involves implantation of disulfiram pellets beneath the skin by means of a surgical operation conducted under local anaesthetic. The preparation is not officially approved in all countries. The pellets sometimes work their way to the surface and are scratched out, and unpleasant septic complications can occur. Pharmacologically effective blood levels of the drug are not obtained, and any success which results must depend more on expectancy than chemistry. The occasional patient may, however, be found who has great faith in this treatment and who will regularly attend for a three-monthly implant – a patient who, for example, has experienced frequent imprisonment for drink-related crime, and who believes that only with this seeming extreme of external control can further trouble be avoided

Drugs that attenuate drinking behaviour

Below are notes on two drugs, naltrexone and acamprosate. Their emergence as substances targeted at the treatment of drinking problems has occurred only over the last few years. Controlled research results to date are promising, but we would warn against incautious enthusiasm at this comparatively early stage.

Naltrexone

The opioid receptor antagonist, naltrexone, in a dose of 50 mg daily, has been shown to be an effective adjunct to out-patient psychosocial treatment of individuals with alcohol dependence (O'Malley et al., 1992; Volpicelli et al., 1992). In these North American studies, naltrexone improved abstinence, decreased relapse, and diminished alcohol consumption over a 12-week treatment period. The optimal dose and duration of treatment with naltrexone need further exploration, as do the effects of long-term treatment. It is possible that compliant patients are more suited to naltrexone and that some individuals will benefit from continued treatment (O'Malley et al., 1996).

Naltrexone is a reasonably safe drug. Side-effects include nausea, vomiting and abdominal pain, headache, reduced energy, joint and muscle pain, and sleeping difficulty. Loss of appetite, diarrhoea, constipation, increased thirst, chest pain, increased sweating, increased energy, irritability, chills, delayed ejaculation and decreased potency are less frequent side-effects. Liver function abnormalities and reversible thrombocytopaenia (reduction in platelet count) have been reported but are rare.

How does naltrexone work? Alcohol is thought to be reinforcing because it stimulates brain opioid activity. Opioid antagonists, such as naltrexone, should theoretically block or reduce the effect of alcohol on opioid receptor activity, and decrease the pleasure or 'high' experienced by drinkers. This mechanism would explain the lower rates of drinking or relapse in the naltrexone groups in the American studies. Another putative mechanism invoked to explain the effect of naltrexone on relapse is that it increases the aversive effects of alcohol (e.g. nausea), increases intoxication for a given dose, or a combination of the two.

Acamprosate

Acamprosate (calcium bis acetyl homotaurinate, trade name Campral), has been used in the treatment of alcohol dependence in France for several years. Clinical trials suggest that it may help to prevent relapse in alcohol dependent patients when used as part of a therapeutic programme (Paille *et al.*, 1995; Sass *et al.* 1996; Whitworth *et al.*, 1996). Acamprosate is a safe drug that does not interact with alcohol or diazepam and appears to have no addictive potential itself. The recommended treatment dose is 1998 mg daily for body weight over 60 kg and 1332 mg daily for body weight under 60kg. Acamprosate should not be prescribed to individuals with renal insufficiency or severe hepatic failure, nor to women who are pregnant or breast-feeding.

The mechanism of action of acamprosate is uncertain (Littleton, 1995). It has been reported to stimulate inhibitory GABA transmission and to antagonise excitatory amino acids, particularly glutamate (see Chapter 2).

Selective serotonin reuptake inhibitors (SSRIs)

SSRIs are amongst the newer antidepressants that have relatively few side-effects. A variety of SSRIs including fluoxetine and citalopram, have been shown temporarily to reduce alcohol consumption by about 20% in social drinkers and early problem drinkers. The results with alcohol dependence are less clear cut. This effect of SSRIs is independent of their action on mood and is not yet fully understood. These drugs may have a place in the treatment of problem drinkers with alcohol-related cognitive impairment (Litten & Allen, 1991). The evidence to date does not support their routine use in clinical practice.

Dopamine agonists

Bromocriptive has been reported to reduce craving in 'alcoholics' (Borg, 1983). Tiapride was used in a clinical sample where it was shown to improve abstinence in anxious or depressed 'alcoholics' (Shaw *et al.*, 1987).

Drugs used to treat psychiatric disorders associated with alcohol dependence

Anti-depressants

Depressive symptoms commonly occur in patients with drinking problems, particularly during the alcohol-withdrawal phase. Treatment with antidepressants (tricyclics, SSRIs) should be delayed until the 'depressed' patient has been abstinent for at least 10–14 days.

Lithium

Despite early promise, lithium therapy does not appear to be of direct benefit in the treatment of alcohol dependence (Dorus *et al.*, 1989). However, this drug is effective in stabilising mood among patients with manic-depressive (bipolar affective) illness.

Buspirone

A non-benzodiazepine tranquilliser with no dependence liability, buspirone has been shown to reduce alcohol consumption in anxious 'alcoholics' and to improve treatment retention (Kranzler *et al.*, 1994).

Amethystic agents

The search for a drug to reverse alcohol intoxication dates back to the time of Greek mythology. However, no effective and safe alcohol antagonist has been found to date.

The present position

In this chapter we have attempted to outline the main special approaches available today in the treatment of drinking problems. We hope that this discussion will stimulate the reader to explore these treatments further and in actuality. However, effective treatments cannot be imparted without a good therapist and it appears that therapist characteristics are often as important as well as the treatment approach chosen. Here as elsewhere the qualities of empathy, non-possessive warmth and genuineness on the part of the therapist are likely to facilitate improvement (Rogers, 1957). Support, training, and prevention of burnout are important (Brown & Brooke, 1991). The fundamental position taken in this chapter is that choosing the best treatment for the individual patient is a skilled and highly responsible undertaking that needs to be negotiated and later reviewed with the patient, guided by clinical experience, and illuminated by a critical understanding of what an evolving research base can tell.

References

Annis, H. M. (1986). A relapse prevention model for treatment of alcoholics. In *Treating Addictive Behaviours: Processes of Change*, ed. Miller, W. R. & Heather, N., pp. 407–33. New York: Plenum Press.

Azrin, N. H. (1976). Improvements in the community-reinforcement approach to alcoholism. *Behaviour Research and Therapy* **14**, 339–48.

Azrin, N. H., Sisson, R. W., Meyers, R. & Godley, M. (1982). Alcoholism treatment by disulfiram and community reinforcement therapy. *Journal of Behaviour Therapy and Experimental Psychiatry* **13**, 105–12.

Beck, A. T., Wright, F. D., Newman, C. F. & Liese, B. S. (1993). *Cognitive Therapy of Substance Abuse*. New York: Guilford Press.

Bien, T. H., Miller, W. R. & Tonigan, J. S. (1993). Brief interventions for alcohol problems: a review. *Addiction* **88**, 315–36.

Borg, V. (1983). Bromocriptine in the prevention of alcohol abuse. *Acta Psychiatrica Scandinavia* **68**, 100–10.

Bowers, T. G., & Al-Rehda, M. R. (1990). A comparison of outcome with group/marital and standard/individual therapies with alcoholics. *Journal of Studies on Alcohol* **151**, 301–9.

Brown, C. & Brooke, D. (1991). Protecting your assets: caring for the therapist. In *The International Handbook of Addiction Behaviour*, ed. Glass, I. B., pp. 269–73. London: Routledge.

Chick, J., Gough, K., Falkowski, W., Kershaw, P., Hore, B., Mehta, B., Ritson, B., Ropner, R. & Torley, D. (1992). Disulfiram treatment of alcoholism. *British Journal of Psychiatry* **161**, 84–9.

Daley, D. C. (1991). *Kicking Addictive Habits Once and for All: A Relapse Prevention Guide*. Lexington: Lexington Books.

Davidson, R. (1992). Prochaska and DiClemente's model of change: a case study? *British Journal of Addiction* **87**, 821–2.

Davison, S. (1996). Psychotherapy: why do some need more and some need less? In *Psychotherapy, Psychological Treatments and the Addictions*, Edwards, G. & Dare, C., pp. 77–93. Cambridge: Cambridge University Press.

Dorus, W., Ostrow, D. G., Anton, R., Cushman, P., Collins, J. F., Schaefer, M., Charles, H. L., Desai, P., Havashida, M., Malkerneker, U., Willenbring, M., Fiscella, R. & Sather, M. R. (1989). Lithium treatment of depressed and non-depressed alcoholics. *Journal of the American Medical Association* **262**, 1646–52.

Drummond, D. C. & Glautier, S. (1994). A controlled trial of cue exposure treatment in alcohol dependence. *Journal of Consulting and Clinical Psychology* **62**, 802–17.

Elkins, R. L. (1980). Covert sensitization and alcoholism: contributions of successful conditioning to subsequent abstinence maintenance. *Addictive Behaviours* **5**, 67–89.

Falkowski, W. (1996). Group therapy and the addictions. In *Psychotherapy, Psychological Treatments and the Addictions*, ed. Edwards, G., Dare, C., pp. 206–19. Cambridge: Cambridge University Press.

Fuller, R. K., Branchey, L., Brightwell, D. R., Derman, R. M., Emrick, C. D., Iber, F. L., James, K. E., LaCoursiere, R. B., Lee, K. K., Lowenstam, I., Maany, I., Neiderhiser, D., Nocks, J. J. & Shaw, S. (1986). Disulfiram treatment of alcoholism: a Veterans Administration co-operative study. *Journal of the American Medical Association* **256**, 1449–55.

Heather, N. (1993). Disulfiram treatment for alcohol problems: is it effective and, if so, why? In *Treatment Options in Addiction. Medical Management of Alcohol and Opiate Abuse*, ed. Brewer, C., pp. 1–18. London: Gaskell.

Heather, N. (1995). *Treatment Approaches to Alcohol Problems*. World Health Organisation Regional Publications European Issues No. 65. Copenhagen: World Health Organisation.

Holder, H., Longabaugh, Miller, W. R. & Rubonis, A. V. (1991). The cost effectiveness of treatment for alcoholism: a first approximation. *Journal of Studies on Alcohol* **52**, 517–40.

Hughes, J. L. & Cook, C. C. H. (1997). The efficacy of disulfiram: a review of outcome studies. *Addiction*, **92**, 381–95.

Hunt, G. M., Azrin, N. H. (1973). A community-reinforcement approach to alcoholism. *Behaviour Research and Therapy* **11**, 91–104.

Institute of Medicine (1990). *Broadening the Base of Treatment for Alcohol Problems*. Washington DC: National Academy Press.

Kranzler, H. R., Burleson, J. A., Del Boca F. K., Babor, T. F., Korner, P., Brown, J. & Bohn, M. J. (1994). Buspirone treatment of anxious alcoholics. *Archives of General Psychiatry* **51**, 720–31.

Litten, R. Z. & Allen, J. P. (1991). Pharmacotherapies for alcoholism: promising agents and clinical issues. *Alcoholism: Clinical and Experimental Research* **15**, 620–33.

Littleton, J. (1995). Acamprosate in alcohol dependence: how does it work? *Addiction* **90**, 1179–88.

Litman, G. (1986). Alcoholism survival: the prevention of relapse. In *Treating Addictive Behaviours: Processes of Change*, ed. Miller, W. R. & Heather, N., pp. 391–405. New York: Plenum Press.

Marlatt, G. A. & Gordon, J. R. (1985). *Relapse Prevention*. New York: Guilford Press.

Miller, W. R. & Hester, R. K. (1986). The effectiveness of alcoholism treatment: what research reveals. In *Treating Addictive Behaviours: Processes of Change*, ed. Miller, W. R. & Heather, N., pp. 121–74. New York: Plenum Press.

Miller, W. R. & Rollnick, S. (1991). *Motivational Interviewing: Preparing People to Change Addictive Behaviour*. New York: Guilford Press.

Miller, W. R. & Sanchez, V. C. (1993). Motivating young adults for treatment and lifestyle change. In *Alcohol Use and Misuse by Young Adults*, ed. Howard, G. S. & Nathan, P. E., pp. 55–81. Notre Dame: University of Notre Dame Press.

Monti, P. M., Abrams, D. B., Kadden, R. M. & Cooney, N. L. (1989). *Treating*

Alcohol Dependence. New York: Guilford Press.

Oei, T. P. S. & Jackson, P. R. (1982). Social skills and cognitive behavioural approaches to the treatment of problem drinking. *Journal of Studies on Alcohol* **43**, 532– 47.

O'Farrell, T. J. (1993). A behavioural marital therapy couples group program for alcoholics and their spouses. In *Treating Alcohol Problems: Marital and Family Interventions*, ed. O'Farrell, T. J. New York: Guildford Press.

O'Farrell, T. J., Choquette, K. A., Cutter, H. S. G., Brown, E. D. & McCourt, W. F. (1993). Behavioural marital therapy with and without additional couples relapse prevention sessions for alcoholics and their wives. *Journal of Studies on Alcohol* **54**, 652–66.

O'Malley, S., Jaffe, A. J., Chang, G., Schottenfeld, R. S., Meyer, R. E., & Rounsaville, B. (1992). Naltrexone and coping skills therapy for alcohol dependence, a controlled study. *Archives of General Psychiatry* **49**, 881–7.

O' Malley, S., Jaffe, A. J., Chang, G., Rode, S., Schottenfeld, R., Meyer, R. E. & Rounsaville, B. (1996). Six-month follow-up of naltrexone and psychotherapy for alcohol dependence. *Archives of General Psychiatry*, **53**, 217–24.

Paille, F. M., Guelfi, J. D., Perkins, A. C., Royer, R. J., Steru, L. & Parot, P. (1995). Double-blind randomised multicentre trial of acamprosate in maintaining abstinence from alcohol. *Alcohol Alcoholism* **30**, 239–47.

Proschaska, J. O. & DiClemente, C. C. (1986). Towards a comprehensive model of change. In *Treating Addictive Behaviours: Processes of change*, ed. Miller, W. R. & Heather, N., pp. 3–27. New York: Plenum.

Prochaska, J. O., DiClemente, C. C. & Norcross, J. C. (1992). In search of how people change: applications to addictive behaviours. *American Psychologist* **7**, 1102–14.

Rogers, C. R. (1957). The necessary and sufficient conditions for therapeutic personality change. *Journal of Consulting Psychology* **21**, 95–103.

Sass, H., Soyka, M., Mann, K. & Zieglgänsberger, W. (1996). Relapse prevention by acamprosate. Results from a placebo-controlled study on alcohol dependence. *Archives of General Psychiatry* **53**, 673–80.

Shaw, G. K., Majumdar, S. K., Waller, S., MacGarvie, J. & Dunn, G. (1987). Tiapride in the long-term management of alcoholics of anxious or depressive temperament. *British Journal of Psychiatry* **150**, 164–8.

Sutton, S. (1996). Can 'stages of change' provide guidance in the treatment of addictions? A critical examination of Prochaska and DiClemente's model. In *Psychotherapy, Psychological Treatments and the Addictions*, ed. Edwards, G. & Dare, C., pp. 189–205. Cambridge: Cambridge University Press.

Volpicelli, J. R., Alterman, A. I., Hayashida, M. & O'Brien, C. P. (1992). Naltrexone in the treatment of alcohol dependence. *Archives of General Psychiatry* **49**, 876–80.

Wanigaratne, S., Wallace, W., Pullin, J., Keaney, F. & Farmer, R. (1990). *Relapse Prevention for Addictive Behaviours. A Manual for Therapists*. Oxford: Blackwell Scientific Publications.

Whitworth, A. B., Fischer, F., Lesch, O. M., Nimmerrichter, A., Oberbauer, H., Platz, T., Potgieter, A., Walter H. & Fleischhacker, W. W. (1996). Comparison of acamprosate and placebo in long-term treatment of alcohol dependence. *Lancet* **347**, 1438–42.

18

Working towards normal drinking

It is sensible to remember the varied nature of the population coming for help with drinking problems. Not everyone who turns for help because of their drinking is suffering from alcohol dependence, but with greater public understanding, people with earlier and lesser problems are increasingly asking for help, especially within the primary care or general hospital setting. To propose one exclusive goal for everyone, be it normal drinking or abstinence, is therefore not sensible (Heather & Robertson, 1981). We need, as always, to plan treatment in terms of flexible responses to multiple needs. To claim that no one who has experienced trouble with drinking will ever be able to drink in a trouble-free way is not true (Sobell & Sobell, 1973, 1976, 1987). However, it is unhelpful to make 'normal drinking' into a slogan or heedlessly to attack AA's position. The probability of successful long-term controlled drinking among the kind of patients who usually present to specialised centres is not high (Davies, 1962; Edwards,1985, 1994; Helzer *et al.*1985). A sense of balance is needed when considering these questions (Heather, 1984; 1995).

Much that was said in Chapter 15 about abstinence-oriented approaches is equally applicable to the normal drinking goal, for instance, the relevance of the patient-therapist relationship and those general points will not be repeated. The discussion of special techniques in Chapter 17 also bears on present considerations. In this chapter, the phrases 'normal drinking' and 'controlled drinking' are used synonymously.

What is 'normal' drinking?

If a patient or client is to aim for normal drinking, how is 'normality' to be defined in practical and recognisable terms? It is no good leaving the definition vague, for only when a goal is closely specified is goal-setting possible. The matter is made difficult by society's latitude with regard to what constitutes an ordinary way of using alcohol. Getting drunk once a month is to some people the expected way to drink, while for others even one episode of mild intoxication would transgress expectations. For goal-setting, normality must be considered in terms of at least two different criteria.

(1) *Objectively normal drinking: quantity/frequency dimensions*. The upper limit which is to be permitted needs to be agreed with the patient. About 16–20 g of alcohol on any one drinking occasion (say one pint of beer, a double of spirits, two glasses of wine) is a reasonable ceiling for anyone who is working toward control of a drinking problem, but may perhaps initially be rather too high. As for frequency, it is wise to agree that drinking should not be reinstated on a fixed daily schedule: there should be breaks and variation. Normality in these terms certainly implies avoidance of intoxication.

(2) *Subjectively normal drinking*. Someone who is drinking alcohol, normally, should be no more apprehensive about this activity than if they were drinking coffee or tea. They should know their usual intake level without having to monitor their drinking behaviour and without a sense of effort. If at a certain point they say: 'Not another, thank you', this should be without the conscious exertion of iron will. They should be able to think about the company and the conversation rather than their thoughts being preoccupied with drinking, the next drink, or not having the next drink. Such easiness in the relationship between the drinker and what they drink is characteristically lacking when moderate or severe alcohol dependence has been established. The patient who has progressed even to mild dependence will, when they have brought their drinking back to objective normality, often at first still experience subjective unease. Subjective normality usually therefore takes longer than objective normality to attain, and sometimes considerably longer. 'Normal' drinking in the true and complete sense has not been won until the two elements have come together, and when there has only been an objective change the patient's position remains precarious. This probable two-stage nature of recovery should be discussed with, and understood by, the patient (Edwards *et al.*, 1986; Booth, 1990).

Other dimensions could also be added to provide a more complex definition of normality, for instance, limitations in the speed of drinking, or limitations on the circumstances in which alcohol is taken.

Who is a candidate for a normal drinking goal?

There are many patients for whom it is inappropriate to attempt such a goal. For those with a history of fully developed alcohol dependence, abstinence is the only feasible objective (Edwards *et al.*, 1983). Equally, there are instances where no one could doubt that for at least a trial period it is sensible to go along with and support the patient's wish to ameliorate rather than abstain (Sanchez-Craig *et al.*, 1984; Booth *et al.*, 1992), and this would often be true of the patient who has been drinking too heavily only recently and intermittently, and who is not manifesting significant dependence symptoms. The following considerations often contribute to the decision-making (these matters are summarised in Box 18.1).

Box 18.1. Factors relevant to the choice of a normal drinking goal

Factors unfavourable to a controlled drinking goal	Favourable factors in support of a controlled drinking goal
Severe dependence dependence	Mild or absent signs of
Previous failures at controlled drinking	Recent sustained normal drinking
Strong preference of the client or patient for abstinence	Strong preference of the client or patient for normal drinking
Poorly developed capacity for self-control in other areas	Mature and determined person with evidence of strong self-control in other areas of life
Concomitant diagnosis of mental illness or drug misuse	No evidence of mental illness or drug misuse
Severe alcohol-related organ damage	Mild or no physical complications of alcohol misuse
Heavy drinking family or friends; Heavy drinking at work; Social isolation	Supportive family and friends
Employment jeopardised by drinking problems at work	Drinking has not affected employ ment or work performance
Serious violence when drinking	Not violent when drinking

Degree of dependence

The importance of this factor has just been mentioned. In practical terms, if the patient has never experienced withdrawal symptoms of such severity as to demand morning relief drinking, then (other things being equal), normal drinking is an option. If the patient has experienced withdrawal symptoms and drunk intermittently in the morning but only for the last six months or less, normal drinking is possible but questionable. If, for 6 or 12 months or longer, the patient has not only experienced withdrawal symptoms but has repeatedly engaged in morning relief drinking, a return to normal drinking is unlikely to be achieved. The guidelines are, however, to be read as examples of ways in which the evidence may be examined rather than as fixed rules.

Evidence of recent sustained normal drinking

If within the last couple of years the patient has been able to drink in a relaxed and controlled manner continuously for two to three months, this may indicate that they retain a capacity for a normal style of drinking, and that this capacity may now with due care be strengthened and extended. The circumstances in which this drinking occurred should be examined. The evidence must, however, be approached warily. Careful questioning may reveal that this previous period of 'sustained normal drinking' was less sustained and less normal than the patient at first suggested, and it may have been only a slide towards reinstatement of dependence.

The patient personally wishes to attempt a normal drinking goal

A patient who wants to return to normal drinking may be deluding themselves, and it is then the therapist's responsibility to try to help them to accept abstinence rather than conniving in the delusion. On the one hand, some patients will frankly declare that drinking other than for intoxication seems to them a purposeless use of alcohol. On the other hand, a patient may be right in believing they can control their drinking and be strongly committed to attempting this goal.

Personality

The mature and determined person who is good at exercising self-control is more likely to succeed in drinking normally than the person whose capacity for self-control is in general not well developed.

Underlying mental illness

The patient who is suffering from any type of mental illness and as a result uses alcohol to relieve unpleasant feelings is not in a good position to attempt normal drinking. Whatever its nature the underlying disorder has first to be treated, but there is always the danger that a relapse into that illness will precipitate loss of control over drinking, although equally it may overthrow an intention of complete abstinence. Underlying brain damage or learning disability usually suggests that normal drinking will not be possible, and a concurrent drug dependence, which has not been dealt with successfully, also rules out a return to safe use of alcohol. Pathological gambling may threaten maintenance of control over drinking – the euphoria of the win, the depression of the loss, or the tension associated with continuous gambling, all rather easily invite a return to heavy use of alcohol.

Alcohol-related physical illness

The decision in this instance must be made in relation to the actual type and degree of illness, but alcohol-related physical illness usually suggests that the patient would be wise to avoid any further drinking and risk of progressive tissue damage.

Social and family support

The patient or client who is socially isolated and without a family will probably find it more difficult to drink normally again than the person whose behaviour is being monitored and influenced by close support. However, a certain type of family network may positively encourage excessive drinking. Occupation has similarly to be taken into account. Someone who has no job, much time on their hands and no structure to their day may find it hard to control their drinking, while jobs that involve exposure to heavy drinking may make it difficult to pursue a controlled drinking goal.

The clinical skill thus lies in knowing how to weigh and integrate these and other factors when assessing the feasibility of a normal drinking goal, and in learning how to feed information to the patient to help their own decision-making. But whatever the therapist proposes, it is finally the patient who makes the decision.

An interval of sobriety as first step

For some patients normal drinking emerges directly out of more chaotic drinking. Suddenly or gradually the new pattern supersedes the old. To begin with there may be occasions when drinking is at a social level with frequent occasions where limits are broken, but after a few months the 'bad occasions' are averted. Alternatively, the story may be of a shorter or longer initial period of abstinence, followed by a tentative move towards moderate drinking. That move may have been planned at the outset as a step that would be taken after a certain interval of sobriety, or the patient may start to drink again while feeling anxious about breaking the rules. When drinking follows a period of sobriety the therapist has the responsibility of working out with the patient whether this is a sadly familiar story of unguardedness and self-deception foreshadowing major relapse, or whether this is indeed the evolution of re-established control.

Whether the patient who is aiming at controlled drinking does best to do so directly or by the pathway of initial abstinence is not an easy question to answer. Different strategies suit different people. But if the drinking is chaotic and surrounded with problems, in general the patient is likely to do better if they start out afresh from a less chaotic base.

Techniques for establishing and maintaining control

Patients are themselves often very inventive in designing ways to keep their drinking within a limit, and it is always useful therefore to explore and encourage these personal strategies. A variety of methods which may be employed (Marlatt & Gordon, 1985; Heather *et al.*, 1987; Alden, 1988; Connors, 1993; Saunders, 1994) are described below.

Full initial discussion with the patient

The first step in setting a treatment programme for the individual patient who is aiming at controlled drinking must be to clarify what is being expected of the treatment and the precise goal that is to be achieved, the methods of working, and the mutual level of commitment.

Limiting the type of beverage

Shifting from one type of alcoholic drink to another is often dismissed as the typical strategy of the drinker who refuses to face up to the fact that their problem lies not in the specific drink but in their relationship with any sort of alcohol – the whisky drinker who believes that 'beer will be safe' is classically warned that alcohol is simply alcohol, whatever the label on the bottle. The therapist has to distinguish between self-delusion and sound strategy, but the patient who is going to effect a successful return to normal drinking may often spontaneously discover that a change of beverage is helpful. They choose what they may term as a 'social drink' – beer instead of wine perhaps or wine instead of beer, but in any case a beverage free of old associations.

Limiting the quantity and frequency of intake

The importance of strictly defining with each patient what is to count as 'normal' has already been mentioned. If the patient is making their definition in terms of 'a single of . . .', or 'a glass of . . .', or other such familiar but often rather vague measures (a 'single' is usually a very uncertain quantity of alcohol if the patient is pouring their own drink at home), then properly objective measures have to be agreed.

Speed of drinking

A patient may learn to pace their drinking. This may be in terms either of not drinking faster than a slow-drinking companion or of pacing against the clock.

Motivations for drinking

The patient may discover that it is unwise for them to drink in response to mood, for instance when they are angry, depressed, or bored. They do better to drink only when they do not 'need' a drink.

Circumstances and company

Drinking is at first often best limited to situations in which that individual's previous experience has shown that control is more likely to be maintained, while drinking situations that can be identified as leading to loss of control are best avoided. For instance, the patient may decide that they will drink with their spouse on Tuesdays in the pub at the corner, but will 'avoid the Saturday night crowd'. They will never drink at work during the day, and will not drink when they are on business trips away from home. When guests come to dinner, control will mean no drink before dinner or after dinner, but only with the meal (and within explicit limits).

311

Identifying 'competing activities'

The client may usefully identify activities that can immediately be engaged in to prevent the risk of uncontrolled drinking. For instance, if a housewife knows that she is likely to start drinking in an uncontrolled fashion when she is alone in the middle of the afternoon, then she has to find and plan activities that can divert her from drinking at this time of the day. She may decide on a simple strategy like doing some shopping in the afternoon or calling on a friend, and so on. If the dangerous circumstances which particularly invite uncontrolled drinking can thus be neutralised by competing activity, practice in normal drinking can then be restricted to occasions when the chances of success are more real.

Individual behavioural analysis

The headings above provide ideas about the kinds of strategies that might be suggested for any patient. Essentially what is being learnt is self-control. It may in addition be useful to carry out an individual and more detailed behavioural analysis of the patient's drinking. The aim is to identify the circumstances in which a particular patient tends to drink excessively, using recent instances and the experiences that evolve during treatment. General statements such as 'I drink when I am bored' are not to be discounted, but are usually of far less value to the planning of treatment than minute analysis of the immediate antecedents and circumstances of, say, last Friday's drinking binge. The analysis identifies the *cues* that are related to excessive drinking, both in internal (mood) and external (event and situation) terms. It is necessary to form an idea of how such cues interact rather than seeing them only in isolation, and to understand the sort of *pathway* that the individual is apt to move along when they indulge in excessive drinking. Such material is then used in planning the package of strategies that go to make up the individual drinking programme.

How testing should the programme be?

The patient must identify risky situations (Marlatt & Gordon, 1985), although it may then be difficult for them to avoid many of these. They may, for instance, have to go away on business trips knowing that a lonely weekend in a hotel is particularly likely to invite heavy solitary drinking. However, not only may exposure to such a risky situation be unavoidable, but for the real effectiveness of treatment such exposure to temptation may be highly desirable. The patient should not make impossible demands on their own strength and determination, but the essence of therapy is that they should experience some sense of struggle, of temptation, and perhaps of craving to drink excessively, *and that temptation and craving should then be successfully resisted*. It is the repeated exposure to the relevant cues and the repeated resistance to an excessive drinking response that will in the end extinguish the potency of those cues. Without experience of craving there can be no long-term extinction of craving. In terms of a familiar analogy, a child who is afraid of dogs is unlikely to overcome that fear simply by avoiding all dogs; such a normal fear is dealt with in terms of ordinary family wisdom by introducing a dog to the child, and then by praise and close support persuading the child on this occasion not to run away. The objective behaviour towards dogs changes and then more slowly the anxiety experienced at the approach of a dog begins to fade out.

In similar fashion the patient who only avoids risk will probably only achieve an objective recovery; their drinking will be objectively within acceptable social limits, but it will still be associated with subjective unease. Subjective recovery comes about when there has been repeated exposure to cues, and repeated resistance to an excessive drinking response. Treatment will, however, suffer a reverse if on too many occasions the patient does in fact drink excessively – the potency of the risky cue is confirmed rather than extinguished. Cue exposure is also discussed on p. 289.

Involving the spouse

The spouse has an important part to play in supporting the patient's work on dealing with the problem. They are often accepted as a direct and useful restraining influence and as the person within whose company normal drinking may most safely be attempted. If, however, their help is effectively to be enlisted, the views of the spouse should be taken into account. Therapy will be handicapped if the spouse's reservations about their partner's normal drinking goal have not been discussed.

Seeing it through

The patient who is aiming at normal drinking is likely to need quite close support over some months. Treatment which aims at return to normal drinking is far from being a cheap option in terms of service costs, and if such a treatment is to be given its place within the range of what is offered by a treatment service, it cannot be on a casual, unplanned, and understaffed basis that fails to provide the proper follow-through of support and which risks irresponsibility.

Monitoring of progress must firstly involve the patient's own regular objective and subjective report at follow-up treatment sessions, and these sessions should probably be at not less than two-weekly intervals. Verbal reports may usefully be supplemented by asking the patient to keep a drinking diary, and thus to engage in self-monitoring. The spouse should also be seen regularly both for them to share in the discussion and planning of treatment and for their contribution to monitoring.

One of two alternative decisions will then at some point have to be made in the light of progress and monitoring:

Termination of successful treatment

A successful outcome may be assumed when over about 12 months the patient has achieved both objective and subjective normality in their drinking. Judgement of 'success' is as ever provisional, but at some point, treatment and frequency of visits should be wound down. The patient may be left with an open invitation to return if they encounter further difficulties, or it may be wise to offer widely spaced (say six-monthly) follow-up appointments and 'booster' discussions over the next year or two.

Termination of unsuccessful treatment

The patient who is failing to make progress should not immediately and without review be told to abandon the normal drinking goal. Lack of progress is to be taken in the first instance as a matter for careful analysis of the causes of the difficulty, and on that basis some planned shift in the strategy may be possible. But if the patient still fails in any way to progress, there comes a moment when there is no profit in encouraging them in a frustrating and perhaps damaging pursuit of normal drinking. They may now be persuaded by experience that it is better to opt instead for an abstinence goal, either as the short- or longer-term solution.

A final word of caution

The decision to advise a patient to aim for total abstinence may sometimes result in that person alternating sobriety with explosive and damaging relapses, rather than their learning how to control their drinking or attenuate relapse. Choice of the abstinence goal does not by itself guarantee anyone's safety. Treatment of every new case is an experiment that requires the patient's informed consent and professional and ethical decisions on the therapist's behalf, and that is so whatever the drinking goal.

That having been said, there are special problems which can attach to working towards normal drinking. What is to be done if in the therapist's experienced judgement normal drinking is for a particular patient likely to lead only to further postponement of the necessary decision to stop drinking? Depending on the circumstances two different types of response can be envisaged:

(1) *Supporting a normal drinking goal on an experimental basis and in the short-term.* If there are no pressing dangers it may be acceptable to work along with the patient and let them determine whether normal drinking is attainable. In the process and in one way or another something useful will have been learnt.

(2) *Stating firmly that abstinence is for carefully explained reasons probably the only feasible goal.* One is dealing here with probabilities rather than certainties but the therapist may feel that for this patient and on strong balance of probabilities normal drinking is likely to be unattainable and dangerous in its pursuit. That then should be said. In the long-term it may be better for a patient at least temporarily to break contact but take with them an unambiguous, honest, and accurate message, rather than the therapist being drawn into a course of action which they see as against the patient's best interests. It may be the moment for challenge rather than connivance.

Ten years ago discussion of how treatment can assist return to normal drinking might have been seen as heterodox. Today, with the growing awareness of the need to provide help for people whose drinking problems are of many different degrees and kinds, a discriminating ability to work with some patients or clients towards a normal drinking goal is a necessary therapeutic skill.

References

Alden, L. (1988). Behavioral self-management: controlled drinking strategies in a context of secondary prevention. *Journal of Consulting and Clinical Psychology* **56**, 280–6.

Booth, P. G. (1990). Maintained controlled drinking following severe alcohol dependence – a case study. *British Journal of Addiction* **85**, 315–22.

Booth, P. G., Dale, B., Slade, P. D. & Dewey, M. E. (1992). A follow-up study of problem drinkers offered a goal choice option. *Journal of Studies on Alcohol* **53**, 594–600.

Connors, G. J. (1993). Drinking moderation training as a contemporary therapeutic approach. In *Innovations in Alcoholism Treatment: State of the Art Reviews and their Implications for Clinical Practice*, ed. Connors G. J., pp. 117–34. New York: Haworth Press.

Davies, D. L. (1962). Normal drinking by recovered alcohol addicts. *Quarterly Journal of Studies on Alcohol* **23**, 194–204.

Edwards, G. (1985). A later follow-up of a classic case series: D.L. Davies's 1962 report and its significance for the present. *Journal of Studies on Alcohol* **46**, 181–90.

Edwards, G. (1994). D. L. Davies, and 'Normal drinking in recovered alcohol addicts': the genesis of a paper. *Drug and Alcohol Dependence* **35**, 249–59.

Edwards, G., Duckett, A., Oppenheimer, E., Sheehan, M. & Taylor, C. (1983). What happens to alcoholics? *Lancet*, **ii** 269–71.

Edwards, G., Brown, D., Duckitt, A., Oppenheimer, E., Sheehan, M. & Taylor, C. (1986). Normal drinking in a recovering alcohol addict. *British Journal of Addiction* **81**, 127–37.

Heather, N. (1984). Controlled drinking treatment: where do we stand today? In *Addictive Behaviours: Prevention and Early Intervention*, ed. Loberg T., Miller W. R., Nathan P. E. & Marlatt G. A.,pp. 31–50. Amsterdam: Swets and Zeitlinger.

Heather, N. (1995). The great controlled drinking consensus: is it premature? *Addiction* **90**, 1160–2.

Heather, N. & Robertson, I. (1981). *Controlled Drinking*. London, Methuen.

Heather, N., Robertson, I., Macpherson, B., Allsop, S., & Fulton, A., (1987). Effectiveness of a controlled drinking self-help manual: one year follow-up results. *British Journal of Clinical Psychology* **26**, 279–87.

Helzer, J. E., Robins, L. N., Taylor, J. R., Carey, K., Miller, R. H., Coombs-Orme, T. *et al.* (1985). The extent of long-term moderate drinking among alcoholics discharged from medical and psychiatric facilities. *New England Journal of Medicine* **312**, 1678–82.

Marlatt, G. & Gordon J. (1985). *Relapse Prevention*. New York: Guilford Press.

Sanchez-Craig, M., Annis, H. M., Bornet, R. & MacDonald, K. R. (1984). Random assignment to abstinence and controlled drinking. Evaluation of a cognitive-behavioural program for problem drinkers. *Journal of Consulting and Clinical Psychology* **52**, 390–403.

Saunders, B. (1994). The cognitive-behavioural approach to the management of addictive behaviour. In *Seminars on Alcohol and Drug Misuse*, ed. Chick, J. & Cantwell, R., pp. 154–73. London: Gaskell.

Sobell, M. B. & Sobell, L. C. (1973). Individualized behaviour therapy for alcoholics. *Behaviour Research and Therapy* **4**, 49–72.

Sobell, M. B. & Sobell, L. C. (1976). Second-year treatment outcome of alcoholics treated by individualized behaviour therapy: results. *Behaviour Research and Therapy* **14**, 195–215.

Sobell, M. G. & Sobell, L. C. (eds.) (1987). *Moderation as a Goal or Outcome of Treatment for Alcohol Problems: a Dialogue*. New York: Haworth Press.

19

When things go wrong, and putting them right

Every attempt has been made in previous chapters of this book to present a perspective on drinking problems that is close to reality, and not to give an idealised view of the therapeutic process as an operation smoothly and inevitably moving forward to success as each patient responds to our wise and well-planned interventions. This chapter seeks to correct any such accidental caricature and considers some workaday clinical problems as they may arise in anyone's office or consulting room, and in the homes of our patients or clients.

Going wrong

The person who wishes to treat alcohol problems must develop an appreciation of the ways in which treatment can go wrong. He or she must train their eyes quickly to recognise these situations, and they must be aware of the familiar patterns of events against which to interpret the latest instance of something going wrong. They must learn to examine the extent to which the therapist is going wrong, and the extent to which it is the patient, and most particularly to analyse what is amiss in the interaction. They must learn not to be discouraged or defeated by such events, but to turn them so far as possible to good therapeutic advantage. One cannot treat alcohol dependence without things very often going wrong and the essence of treatment is usually a series of trials and errors rather than a straight-line advance. Such a statement is not to be read as a license for complacency – true, things will go wrong and we must not be too flustered by that fact, but equally true is the insistence that the situation must be recognised and an effort made to put it right.

This chapter does not attempt a consideration of all possible eventualities. Anyone who has experience of this field will see ways in which the list might be extended, and a personal listing of cases where therapy went wrong (a list kept, as it were, on mental file) is a valuable working tool.

Losing the balances

Much of therapy is a matter of finding balances (and of readily shifting balances), and things often go wrong because balance has been lost. Let's give this statement meaning by considering balance in terms of a number of different paired factors.

Emphasising the drinking/emphasising all else

It is possible to go wrong because the treatment has become so exclusively focused on the individual's drinking that the man or woman doing that drinking in a complex personal and social setting is overlooked – the drinking is everything. The complementary imbalance is a sensitive awareness of that individual's total life situation, but with the reality of alcohol as a destructively pervasive aspect of that situation discounted – the drinking is hardly anything. This problem has already been noted in an earlier chapter (p. 255). To set the balance right is often difficult, and at a certain stage of learning and experience it is particularly the sensitive, open-minded therapist who is apt to fall into the trap of underestimating the seriousness of the drinking problem – the admirable desire to see the whole person and to respect the complexities of that individual's life must not be put in opposition to awareness of the true threat of the drinking.

> A man aged 44 years had experienced a deprived and troubled childhood. Despite this he managed to contract a seemingly happy marriage and for 16 years all had appeared to go well. Then his wife had an affair, and his world fell to pieces. All his fearful beliefs as to the inevitability of separation and betrayal were proved to be well-founded. His feelings towards his wife were unforgiving. He determined that an unhappy episode should be the occasion for catastrophe and he divorced, threw in his job, sold his house, gave up his friends and moved to a new city. A couple of years later he overdosed with barbiturates and consequently came under the care of a psychotherapist who spent a year exploring with this patient his problems relating to a rejecting mother. He frequently turned up for interviews drunk, and this was duly interpreted. He was then admitted to hospital for a further and more serious suicidal attempt. The psychi-

atrist who saw him forthwith instituted a course of ECT for what he diagnosed as a severe and untreated depressive illness. He noted that the
patient had 'recently engaged in some secondary relief drinking'. The
evening following the first ECT the patient developed an acute confusional state – it was one of the night nurses who made the diagnosis of
delirium tremens.

Both the psychotherapist and the psychiatrist had focused on important
aspects of this man's condition, but each had over-focused, and seen
things comfortably in terms of their own predilections. Neither had
bothered to take a drinking history. It seems likely that the patient was
not so much covering up the seriousness of his drinking as that those
who came in contact with him were almost wilfully turning a deaf ear
to what he was telling them. A careful reconstruction of the history later
suggested a drinking problem going back to the early days of marriage,
a marriage much affected by drinking, and a wife who finally moved
out because she could no longer tolerate the drinking and the violence.
The next move must not be the substitution of an exclusive alcohol focus
and a new imbalance for old, but ensuring that treatment of this man's
alcohol dependence is accorded its balanced place within the total strategy of his treatment.

There are many different ways of falling into error through seeing the
patient as 'an alcoholic' and believing therefore that all the patient's
problems are to be understood and treated within that definition alone.
A short extract from another case history should correct any notion that
the error is always in one direction.

A 33-year-old labourer had been admitted to an alcohol treatment unit,
where a diagnosis of alcoholic hallucinosis was made. It was noted that
he had previously been admitted to another hospital with what was now
deemed to be the mistaken diagnosis of schizophrenia; the case-notes
were not borrowed. He was put into the ward therapeutic group but
seemed to spend more time listening to imaginary voices than participating. After six weeks or so he was thought to be 'somewhat improved' and
was discharged to a hostel for drinking problems which was run on intensive therapeutic community lines. He was put into an encounter group on
the evening of his arrival, and shortly thereafter again developed florid
schizophrenic symptoms, and was readmitted to the first hospital rather
than to the alcohol unit. Their case-notes recorded a clear initial attack of
schizophrenia at the age of 17, in a man who did fairly well provided he
was not too stressed and could find a supportive environment. But this
was certainly a patient who over recent years had begun to over-medicate
himself with alcohol.

The staff of the alcohol treatment unit had so specialised a perspective
that when a case of schizophrenia presented to them they reacted in

terms of a predetermined psychological set, and the consequent diagnosis led to a package of group therapy and confrontation being given to a man whose needs were quite otherwise.

So much for two rather extreme cases to illustrate the poles of imbalance that can occur. The errors are usually on a smaller scale and more subtle. Perhaps the mass of general agencies tend to underrate the importance of the drinking while the specialised alcohol agencies run the risk of being too alcohol focused.

Too ambitious/too unambitious goals

Sometimes things go wrong because the therapist (and the patient) have got the balance wrong as to reasonable expectation of what changes may be achieved, or the pace of such change. This dilemma can occur at any stage of treatment. The mistake may be that too great a therapeutic pace is being set which can readily force the patient into breaking contact, but equally the problem may be in the direction of inertia.

> A 60-year-old man stopped drinking but continued to treat his wife in a curmudgeonly fashion, was at cross purposes with his grown-up children, and had no leisure activities other than watching television and grumbling about the quality of the entertainment provided. At the end of a further year he was still sober and still regarding the world with unrelenting enmity.

What is the community psychiatric nurse (CPN) to do next time they call round on this family and the man purposely turns up the volume on the television, while otherwise angrily staring ahead and not acknowledging the caller's presence? The wife offers a cup of tea in the kitchen and says, 'He's always been that way and I suppose he won't change – a real old misery I call him'. What is the right balance of treatment ambition?

The reality may indeed be that a man of 60 who has for most of his existence defined the world as antagonistic and who has built up his self-image largely in terms of afflicted righteousness, is unlikely radically to change his ways. His wife's assessment of the situation may be just about right, and she does not seem too put out by his ill-grace. Her father was much like that anyhow, and this husband's behaviour is in accord with what she expects of men. She is happy enough that he is no longer running her short of money.

And yet it seems sad to leave it at that. There is the lingering feeling that the goal is being set too low, that more happiness for two people should be possible than is seen here. The answer is perhaps for that CPN to try setting a moderately more ambitious goal on a trial basis. The goal had better be expressed concretely, and the starting point must be the identification of something which patient and wife themselves at least half-hint at being wanted. In this particular instance the wife let drop 'and he never takes me on holiday of course'. The 'of course' was an important part of the statement; it was clear that the wife's communication with her husband often carried the implication that she expected his response to be negative. A modestly realistic goal in these circumstances was to see if this couple could go away for a week's holiday together and come home with the feeling that they had enjoyed themselves. Working at first through the wife and suggesting that she might for once expect the answer 'yes' from her husband, the holiday was booked. The couple went for a week to the seaside, and although the holiday provided much cause for grumbling, in sum the week provided a real sense of shared reward. Beyond the immediate happening a small shake-up had occurred in negative patterns of interaction, and the basis established for the possibility of further, small changes. The question which is being dealt with here relates to the issue of the 'quality of sobriety' (p. 258).

Too indulgent/too hard

There is a balance to be struck regarding the degree to which the relationship offered by the therapist to the patient or client is to be supportive and non-judgemental, as contrasted with one that emphasises elements of tough-minded expectation and hard confrontation. To put the matter in terms of absolutes and contradictions is an over-simplification, but it may be useful to examine this particular idea in terms of two contrasting examples. Firstly, imbalance in the direction of indulgence.

> A social worker of rather little professional experience became highly committed to helping this family. The 30-year-old man was not alcohol dependent, but seemed to use drink to enhance his passivity and incompetence. He seldom worked. He borrowed, pawned, and stole. The wife who was faced with this chronically difficult situation tried to prop up the family as best she might. The social worker soon became no more than a provider of gifts, and she protected the man from the consequence of his having cheated on welfare payments. She found him good second-hand clothes so that he could go for a job interview, and when he sold the clothes and did not go to the interview she treated him as an amusingly naughty child.

The social worker was operating on the hypothesis that this patient was deprived and was testing out her 'goodness'; she believed that she 'must not reject him'. Where she may have gone wrong is in her assumption that the opposite to indulgence is rejection.

As an example of the tough-minded imbalance, the following case is illustrative – it relates to consequences of a stance that is quite commonly taken by helping agencies in their attempt to screen-out the 'unmotivated' patient.

A man with a drinking problem was to be discharged from prison and it had been agreed that he should then be admitted to hospital. He was homeless. However, the decision was made 'to test this man's sincerity'. The consultant in charge of the treatment unit decided that the man would not be admitted straight away, but should find himself lodgings, go to AA, and then present at a ward group for assessment by the other patients. Coming out of prison after four years the man was anxious, a little bit elated, very lost, and he immediately made his way to old friends. He was drinking again within hours, and within days had once more committed his familiar offence of breaking and entering. The consultant was confirmed in his sense of wisdom, and took these events as evidence that the patient was 'insufficiently motivated'.

There are occasions when it is therapeutically useful to be nurturing and there are others when it is kinder and constructive to challenge openly. This is another dimension where the question of balance has to be kept under review in all therapeutic dealings.

Too directive/too afraid of a position

The alternative to forcing one's opinion on a client is not necessarily the pretence of having no opinions at all. A therapist may have difficulty in treating drinking problems because they give their clients the impression of lacking confidence at a time when that person badly needs to borrow some certainties – an orthodox therapeutic detachment is for instance inappropriate in a situation where someone needs very practically to be helped by the therapist's knowledge of how to deal with a drinking crisis, while a dictatorial attitude will be equally counter-productive. Here is an example which bears on this particular and difficult aspect of balance.

A 40-year-old woman who over a two-year period had begun to move towards severe alcohol dependence in the setting of a depressive illness was visited on the ward by her husband. The husband made himself unpopular with the staff by his unsympathetic and scolding attitude towards his wife. One of the junior nurses exclaimed to the patient, 'I don't see how living with that man you could ever stay sober – you should go and live with that son of yours who seems so fond of you'

In the treatment of drinking problems more than in the treatment of many other conditions, the therapist is faced with the problem of directiveness because it often appears glaringly obvious that the patient is engaging in wrong-headed and self-destructive behaviour, is revealing a chaotic inability to make good decisions and order their life well, and manifestly does not know what is best for their own good. This area of practice seems therefore to pose a specially acute challenge to the orthodox notion of the therapist's need to maintain neutrality. The nurse felt that she knew what was good for the patient, and said what she thought. Discussion of this incident in the staff group would usefully bring into the open wider issues related to the limits of directiveness, but the conclusion in this particular instance could only be that the balance had gone wrong. The nurse knew too little about the marriage to give directive advice and she certainly knew too little about that patient's son.

Defeated by defences

That the patient's defences have to be identified, their utility for the patient understood, and their existence adequately dealt with, are ideas common to the treatment of many conditions other than a drinking problem, and the defences which the drinker may deploy are by no means specific to this particular condition. The therapist who is going to work with drinking problems will, however, do well to cultivate a lively awareness of how defences can manifest themselves on this scene. An inadequate response to the patient's defences is one of the more common reasons for things going wrong.

Denial in pure or mixed form

By *denial* is meant a defence against the threat of reality which is based on a refusal to admit the existence of that reality; it is oneself rather than others who have to be deceived. In pure form the mechanism is pictured as operating at a subconscious level, with denial thus differentiated from a conscious untruth which is aimed at the deception of other people. Often the patient's initial difficulty in facing up to the threat posed by their drinking is a manifestation both of denial in the classic sense and of prevarication. In practice, it is often difficult to determine the extent to which the two different elements are contributing to a given presentation, and conscious and unconscious processes commonly seem to merge.

In the popular image the 'alcoholic' is frequently pictured as someone who insists on drinking themselves to death while maintaining that no drop of alcohol ever passes their lips. Such crude and primitive defensiveness is relatively uncommon, but when it reaches extreme proportions it can be baffling and a block to all progress, despite every therapeutic stratagem Here is a case abstract which shows the kind of problems that can be set by entrenched denial.

> A 50-year-old accountant was brought to a psychiatric clinic by his business partner, who said that unless something was done his colleague would have to be pensioned off. The patient's breath smelled heavily of drink, his liver was mildly enlarged and he had bruises from several recent falls. He charmingly acknowledged his gratitude to the partner for taking this trouble, but said that the poor man was overworked, worried, and getting things out of proportion. The patient admitted to having an occasional beer at lunch-time, but that was the limit of his drinking. He was then seen with his wife, who said that he was permanently intoxicated, that he was frequently incontinent, that he had recently fallen down stairs when drunk, and that empty bottles were falling out of every cupboard. He said that his wife was a dear woman but a terrible worrier, that of course he was often tired at the end of the day (who wasn't), and as for falling down those steps there had been a loose stair rod.

Given that one does not at this point surrender hope entirely, the best approach might first be to try to get some insight into the reasons that could lead a patient to engage in this stonewalling. Usually there are several reasons rather than one. For instance, some people make life-long use of certain favoured defensive mechanisms (in sickness and in health), and this man may under stress be reaching for his personally most available coping mechanism out of a limited repertoire. Another explanation may be that this stance is a passive–aggressive response to what he conceives as an attack on his integrity. He sees his partner and his wife (his father and mother) as out to dominate him, and he reacts with angry and childish stubbornness.

With these guesses in mind the therapist might then sit down alone with the patient, with the other actors out of the room. With no implication of attack, the therapist will start a discussion on the basis of an openly stated assumption that both he and the patient know that reality is being denied. The therapist will furthermore immediately lay ground-rules for the interaction by stating that the interview will not be allowed to degenerate into a useless cross-examination which could offer no fruitful result but only further entrenchment. The aim is thus not frontal assault on the defensive position, but to get behind the defence. It can be put to the patient that a lot of people find difficulty in talking openly about the degree of worry and trouble which their drinking is causing – they may be afraid of attack and afraid of being demeaned – and in such circumstances to try to insist that the worrying facts do not exist can be a natural response. The therapist might try to convey that he or she sees this situation from the patient's point of view, and then offer possible alternative solutions. It can be put to the patient that if, for example, a man drives his car off the road and someone comes up and asks questions, the driver may well respond defensively if he thinks that it is a policeman who is questioning him, but it will make no sense to treat the person who is offering first-aid as if they were a policeman, and hence bleed to death.

The defensiveness may still remain absolute. The patient may take the line that the therapist is a nice person whom it is a privilege to meet, but that the clinic's valuable time is being wasted on the basis of a most unfortunate mistake – everyone is getting hold of absolutely the wrong end of the stick. What to do next?

It may be possible as a temporary measure to go on leaving the defence in place, as it were, but to take no notice of it – to allow the patient to hold to the assumption that he has no drinking problem, while the therapist works on the assumption that there is a serious problem which has to be treated. Such a peculiar agreement to differ is unlikely to continue happily for long; either the patient will slide into accepting the therapist's definition of reality or contact will be unprofitable. Another and rather simple approach, which may sometimes be promising, is to concentrate for the time being on the patient's physical health. The patient may find it acceptable that they are in need of advice on their physical health (an alcohol-free diet for their liver's sake), without any of the loss of face which they fear would result from fully admitting his dependence on alcohol.

If none of these approaches pays dividends, the only course may be to leave the patient with an unambiguous message as to the need for them to open their eyes, and a factual warning of the dangers which will stem from the denial and prevarication continuing, and then not to make any offer to see the patient again for a period of some months, unless they so asks. The spouse meanwhile may well need help or support in their own right.

The occasional baffling intractableness of deeply entrenched denial should not itself be denied. The temptation is almost literally to raise one's voice in the hope that the patient will actually hear, or to confront them with every sort of proof positive and hope that the high walls of their defences will then dramatically collapse. The temptation is, in short, to resort to the battering ram. Sadly, the consequences of that attack will probably only be the patient strengthening the wall of defence.

The 'defence' of sickness'

Sometimes a client will claim that they continue to drink because they are indeed 'an alcoholic'. They are suffering from an illness, which is the explanation of their behaviour, and the responsibility for curing this illness rests with the therapist – the client may be intending to continue drinking with the position nicely established that the therapist is to blame. Things go wrong if this position is accepted, but they go equally wrong if the therapist automatically assumes that this person is playing games or working some kind of intentional trickery. They may be taking up this particular version of the sick role because they truly believe that they are sick, damaged, and no longer able to control their own behaviour. They are then not so much displaying a defence as manifesting symptoms of learned helpfulness. The two different possible meanings of outwardly similar presentations have therefore to be distinguished. In the wrong circumstances, cutting the drinker down with an aggressively neat analysis of the game they are playing is likely to result in the therapist being rid of a difficult client, but nothing else. It may be more useful to try to move this person towards a realisation that they can indeed start to take responsibility for not drinking, that they have more resources than they supposed, and that it would be misleading if anyone else were to pretend to be able to take over the responsibilities for them. The job is to work for increased self-efficacy and strengthening of motivation.

Absolution

Patients may be able to defend themselves from the pain that would otherwise force them to change their behaviour if they can find a doctor or counsellor who can be persuaded to offer regular absolution. At the same time they may present a picture of pseudo-insight. Intellectually they know what suffering they are causing to themselves and others, but they are able to divorce this insight from any deep feelings, provided they are given regular doses of forgiveness. They are, in fact, seeking the therapist's connivance as actor in a repetitive and unproductive play. Here is a case extract that illustrates one such presentation.

> The patient settled into a chair and said that he knew he was an 'alcoholic', had been going to AA for years, and knew that all he now had to do was to get through one day without drink. His wife was threatening to leave him, and after this last 'slip' and all that she had been through, he entirely saw her point of view and did not blame her in the least. He was most dreadfully sorry and knew that he had behaved to her like a swine.

Furthermore, he had let the doctor down again, and was thoroughly ashamed of himself. He had said exactly the same thing on at least a dozen previous occasions with a similar show of contrition coupled with detachment from real feeling.

Things go wrong if the therapist falls into the position of aiding and abetting this cycle of behaviour. Such a story is not uncommon and the patient may sometimes be a long-term AA attender who has managed to get little out of AA. One may suspect that they have used the AA meetings in much the same way as they would employ the interview with the psychiatrist, and they are nowhere near grasping the real AA message. For the therapist to continue contact on this non-therapeutic or anti-therapeutic basis is useless. It is more helpful to throw the responsibility back on the patient and refuse to be the confessor. An element of challenge and confrontation may produce new possibilities, but there is always the risk that the patient will instead go off and find another therapist who will at least temporarily provide the absolutions.

The romantic defence

Drinking peculiarly lends itself to a romantic defence, an identification with famous drinking poets and playwrights. The following is an abstract from a referral letter.

> This lady is a successful artist and you will certainly know of her husband who is the novelist. She has led a truly amazing life, and if she gets round to telling you about her years in Paris you will find it fascinating. Everyone in her set drinks, and I think one has to accept that drinking is for her essential to the creative life. Recently she has been hitting the bottle and she was seen by someone last year who rather annoyed her by calling her an alcoholic. She cannot accept help which is conditional upon her giving up drinking.

In this instance the patient's defence has overwhelmed the judgement of an experienced physician, who had been seduced into accepting drinking as symbolising 'the creative life'. That the drinking was profoundly affecting this woman's ability to work and threatened to destroy her was being screened out.

If this position is accepted things will very certainly go wrong, with the patient continuing to drink and the therapist effectively neutralised as an amused and admiring spectator of a fascinating way of life, but with the therapeutic position lost. At the start of the contact the therapist has therefore to hold to the position that drinking must be de-symbolised and seen in its reality. The patient may have an immediate sense of relief if they find that they can discard the act that self-destruction is romantic fun.

Endless argument

The problems set by intellectual defence are familiar in any area of psychotherapy. In work with drinking problems the intellectualisation is likely to go off in certain special directions – the patient will divert the discussion away from any real therapeutic content towards making the interview a symposium either on the definition of alcohol dependence or on the determinants of drinking behaviour, or both. The therapeutic response should be to steer the patient away from consideration of generalisations and back to the immediacy of their own position. Otherwise the therapist will find themselves engaged in a lengthy analysis of 'the disease concept' while the patient continues to drink.

The patient who knows someone who drinks much more

A block to treatment, which can be no more than a minor distraction but which may sometimes be employed as a major stratagem to escape the reality of the threat that drink imposes, is the claim made by the patient that they know someone who drank much more than they ever did themselves, or who drank a great deal and never came to harm.

> All right, I drink my share. But I'll tell you this, my old father died at 86 and he drank much more heavily than I have ever done. Absolutely routine, he'd never go outside the house without putting a bottle of whisky in his pocket, just like picking up his tin of tobacco.

To enter a debate with such a patient as to whether their drinking is more or less than the father's is bound to be defeating. The data on the patient's drinking is probably at that stage uncertain and the data on the father's drinking much falsified, so the patient is in a position to prop up their defence by revising all elements of the comparison at will. If one agrees to enter this debate, one gets involved in a kind of pub conversation, with wildly unlikely but incontrovertible assertions being heaped one on the other. 'Look at Winston Churchill. He had the best part of a bottle of brandy every morning before he got out of bed. Greatest Englishman who ever lived . . .'. The best way to avoid entanglement in this unproductive argument is to say that it is not the patient's father nor Winston Churchill who has come for the consultation and that they will be left outside the room.

Box 19.1. When things go wrong: the positive therapeutic response to case problems

- Problems should be shared. Talk through the situation with a colleague

- Problems can be two-way. Try to understand your own behaviour, attitudes, and expectations as well as those of the patient

- Identify blocks – in particular the therapeutic approach losing its balance or the unhelpful defence mechanisms which the patient may be using to negate progress

- Motivation is essential to change – does further work need to be done on readiness to change?

- Check back on the original assessment and formulation, review the case, and get a purposive plan in place again with the patient participating, recover the therapeutic situation

- Remember, no one is omnipotent and therapist have rightful needs

When everything goes wrong

Box 19.1 sets out some ideas on ways of getting the therapeutic block unstuck. There are times in treating drinking problems when everything seems to go wrong at once, and this is not just in terms of happenings relating to one particular patient but with several patients getting into serious difficulties over the same few weeks. One's most hopeful patient relapses, another seems bent on destroying themselves with their continued drinking, and a patient for whom the therapist had especially warm feeling dies and there is an element of self-blame. These periods occur, and it is necessary for the therapist who runs into such a patch of trouble to remember (or be reminded by colleagues) that this kind of practice will inevitably at times be a fraught and perplexing business. Sometimes the therapist may have been selecting for themselves all the more difficult cases, and there is the possibility that they have become over-stretched, overtired, or careless. But it is more probable that events have randomly clustered and that the therapist needs their self-confidence supported more than being invited to blame themselves. Sometimes things go wrong because of forgetfulness and oversight – the need for a physical examination is overlooked, the spouse is not seen, what the patient is trying to say is not heard. Perhaps more dangerously, things go amiss when the therapist becomes over-confident, fails to entertain doubts and assumes that they know all, and that if the patient fails to respond what is needed is more medicine of the same kind. On occasions, the way in which the treatment system is working may also need to be scrutinised and it may, for instance, be evident that difficulties stem from staff liaison being in poor repair or there are personal tensions between staff members.

Treating the person with a drinking problem is about moving that individual by every available strategy towards alliance with his or her own recovery. The richest arena for learning is the actuality of contact, the experience of things sometimes going wrong, and the discovery that with patience, flexibility, and mutual effort things often very happily come right.

Every individual and team should explore the question of how, within their practice circumstances, they are going to address such problems positively and effectively, so as to help the patient through and themselves to learn in the process. Both the younger and the more experienced therapist equally have needs in this regard, and male and female staff members may at times have different kinds of support need. Sharing of problems rather than a drift to isolation is vital and the availability for staff support of an experienced therapist from outside the team can be valuable. There should be an open and unashamed willingness to see oneself as needy rather than yielding to the destructive belief that one can endlessly give without being given.

20

Treatment settings, professional roles, and the organisation of treatment services

Treatment is provided for people with drinking problems in varied settings, by diverse professionals and by non-professionals. Many of the organisations and individuals that provide this treatment have different goals as well as different conceptions of the underlying problem, and they aim to help the problem drinker in different ways. This diversity offers advantages and pitfalls that need to be understood both by helping agencies and treatment purchasers.

In this chapter we shall consider the way in which different settings and different professional roles contribute to the treatment of the problem drinker, as well as the ways in which treatment services can be integrated and organised.

Treatment settings

Help may be offered to the patient or client in an almost infinite variety of settings by a wide range of people. Such help is given by the spouse who encourages a partner to seek help, the employer who counsels an employee regarding drunkenness in the workplace, the publican who refuses to serve a customer who has already had too much to drink, and the policeman who arrests someone who is 'drunk and disorderly'. The home, the workplace, premises on which alcohol is served, and even a public space may all, therefore, be settings in which help is provided.

Not only the spouse, but also the treatment professional, may find that treatment begins in the home of the person with a drinking problem. The primary care physician or social worker, for example, may identify evidence of a drinking problem when visiting the home to see another member of the family.

In the context of this broad view of treatment beginning in the community, it is helpful to consider in detail some of the more formal settings in which professionals are likely to work on a day to day basis (see Box 20.1). Each of these settings has its own particular opportunities, as well as certain drawbacks, for the provision of help to the problem drinker.

Box 20.1. Treatment settings

- Primary care

- Community alcohol team

- Specialist alcohol treatment unit

- Residential rehabilitation

- Self-help groups

- General hospitals

- Psychiatric hospitals

- Criminal justice system

- Industry

Primary care

Provision of primary medical care varies considerably around the world. In some countries it may include provision of care by staff with minimal training. The World Health Organisation has made great progress in trying to remedy this (Edwards & Arif, 1980), but even so the traditional healer, or the priest or shaman, and a belief in folk medicine may play a more significant role than that of orthodox Western medicine. Such cultures pose a particular challenge to the management of drinking problems. However, primary care will be taken here to refer principally to the non-specialist provision of medical care in the community by a physician and a variable team of professionals drawn from a background of nursing, social work, counselling, and other disciplines.

The doctor working in primary care has a unique perspective that accommodates both the family and the long-term context, as well as a good overall medical history of his or her patients. This offers the opportunity for early detection of a range of alcohol related harms, which might not be obvious to others or which might not warrant specialist referral. It also offers opportunities for interventions including brief counselling, support, and education in a setting that is non-stigmatising. The effectiveness of early interventions offered in primary care has been demonstrated by research (Kristenson *et al.*, 1983; Wallace *et al.*, 1988).

Where specialist referral is required, the physician working in primary care is in a good position to know what resources are available, and which ones might be most appropriate for a given patient. It is increasingly clear that the role of many specialist agencies, such as community alcohol teams, should be to support the management of problem drinkers within the primary care setting. Thus they may offer advice and support to the primary health care team, or arrange clinics to be held within the buildings of the health centre or surgery. Furthermore, there is evidence that the majority of patients can be treated as effectively in primary care as by a specialist service, in respect of improvements in both drinking behaviour and alcohol related problems (Drummond *et al.*, 1990). However, it is important that the primary health care team are provided with adequate support by the specialist agency.

The community alcohol team

In recent years, in many countries, there has been a trend towards providing substance misuse services in the community rather than in a residential or 'in-patient' setting. This partly stems from the economic benefits of such an approach to treatment, but it also reflects a realisation that in many cases in-patient treatment is no more effective than out-patient treatment. There is much research evidence to support this approach. A large proportion, if not the great majority, of alcohol dependent patients can be detoxified safely and successfully in the community (Hayashida *et al.*, 1989; Collins *et al.*, 1990; Stockwell *et al.*, 1991). There is evidence that out-patient treatment for drinking problems is as effective as in-patient treatment (Edwards & Guthrie, 1967) and even that brief advice is as effective as intensive (Edwards *et al.*, 1977) or extended (Chick *et al.*, 1988) treatment for many patients. Furthermore, treatment in the community avoids much of the stigma associated with the old mental hospitals.

To some, it may seem that the community alcohol team is simply a relocated out-patient clinic, and in certain cases this may be true. However, at its best, the community team is far more flexible in its

333

ability to liaise with the primary health care team, as well as the community mental health team and other agencies. It is also able to provide services in a series of geographically convenient locations and, where necessary, conduct domiciliary assessments.

The range of treatments offered by the community alcohol team is likely to vary depending upon contractual obligations, local need, and the experience and interests of staff. However, in principle, most patients with drinking problems can be offered most treatments in this setting. Brief and longer term counselling, relapse prevention and behavioural treatments, individual and group psychotherapy, pharmacotherapy and detoxification can all be provided by this route. A day programme may be available.

The specialist alcohol treatment centre

This kind of facility may take many forms. In some cases it will be difficult to distinguish the therapeutic environment from that found in non-medical therapeutic communities or other forms of residential rehabilitation (see below). However, the 'specialist alcohol treatment centre' will be taken here to refer to the facility that has a multi-disciplinary staff, including medical and other professionals, with or without an in-patient unit, a day centre, an out-patient clinic, and possibly a community team (see above). It may be able to offer urgent assessment or treatment in any of these settings.

The functions of such a unit are the diagnosis or management of the difficult case, including where necessary specialist physical, psychological, or psychiatric investigation and management. The centre is also likely to offer support and advice to other services, and may offer a teaching or educational programme. Liaison with primary care (see above), the general hospital (Glass-Crome et al., 1994), and mental health services may be an important function of the specialist alcohol treatment centre. It may also offer assessment or management of patients awaiting trial for, or convicted of, criminal offences (see below).

In many communities a facility of this sort may not be available at all. Where it is available, it may or may not offer in-patient care. In-patient facilities are particularly expensive to run, and as mentioned earlier there is reason to believe that out-patient services may be equally effective for many patients. However, the in-patient unit clearly offers certain advantages where it is available. Some patients cannot be safely detoxified in the community (see Chapter 14), and others may require admission for the assessment or treatment of comorbid psychiatric disorders. It is also recognised that many patients fail to respond to out-patient interventions and, in a minority of cases, it appears reasonable to attempt a period of in-patient treatment where all else has failed. An in-patient unit offers access to more intensive psychotherapy, occupational therapy, and medical care than is available in the community.

The specialist alcohol centre is not associated with the stigma that discourages patients from attending psychiatric services. It is also important to maintain and develop expertise in a field that is still often not popular with, or well understood by, generic staff in medical or psychiatric facilities (MacDonald & Patel, 1975; Potamianos *et al.*, 1985).

Residential rehabilitation

This usually occurs in a non-medical setting, and the form that it takes reflects the underlying philosophy of the particular organisation. Such settings are extremely varied, both in respect of the particular programme that is offered and also the underlying beliefs concerning alcohol related problems. However, most offer some sort of therapeutic community approach (Kennard, 1983), with counselling or psychotherapy seen as an important part of the rehabilitative process. Staff are often, although not invariably, drawn from recovering alcoholics or addicts who have graduated from the programme. The therapeutic goal is almost always towards total abstinence, and this is usually taken to include abstinence from all addictive substances, not just alcohol.

In the United States, and to a lesser extent in many parts of Europe, most of these centres are based upon the Twelve Step programme of AA. In these facilities, problem drinking (or 'alcoholism') is treated alongside other forms of substance misuse (or 'chemical dependency') using a common approach to treatment often known as the 'Minnesota Model' (Cook, 1988a, b). This form of treatment is discussed further in Chapter 16.

On a worldwide basis, the next most frequently encountered type of residential rehabilitation would probably be that based upon a religious philosophy. In most cases, such centres operate from a Christian foundation, and the Salvation Army is particularly active in this area of work. However, such centres are much less homogenous in terms of programme content than are the Minnesota Model facilities. Group work is less central and contribution to the running of the community through practical chores is more frequently emphasised. In some cases, religious devotions may also be given priority, although most such communities do not demand adherence to the Christian faith as a prerequisite for residents.

Self-help groups

The role of AA and related organisations is discussed in Chapter 16. Although the self-help model strictly excludes consideration of this as a 'treatment' setting, it is still a very important source of help to many people with drinking problems. It also provides a reminder that people with drinking problems receive help in many settings other than those which involve interaction with treatment professionals. Patients staying on alcohol treatment units, or in residential rehabilitation, may be encouraged to travel to attend such meetings off site. Many people in the community will attend such groups in addition to any other professional help that they are receiving. For others, AA will provide their only source of help, and large numbers have achieved abstinence through this route alone, with no professional help at all.

General hospitals

Alcohol related problems are encountered in every department of the district general hospital, and there is evidence that they contribute a significant proportion of the morbidity seen in many such wards (Jariwalla et al., 1979; Jarman & Kellett, 1979; Barrison et al., 1982) and clinics (Persson & Magnusson, 1987). Physicians and surgeons are thus in an excellent position to advise their patients about sensible drinking limits, and about the effects that alcohol consumption is having upon their physical health. Nurses also have an important role to play in counselling problem drinkers in this setting, the potential efficacy of which has been demonstrated by research (Chick et al., 1985). Similarly, staff in the Accident and Emergency (A & E) department will see many of the traumatic and other consequences of alcohol use. It may be difficult to offer counselling amidst the hectic activity of a busy A and E department, and therefore liaison with specialist services is particularly important (Holt et al., 1980).

The opportunities for helping problem drinkers in the general hospital setting will be lost unless steps are taken to identify them. It is thus vital that an alcohol history becomes a routine part of medical and nursing assessments in this setting (Barrison et al., 1980). It is to be hoped that stories such as the following will become increasingly rare:

> In the course of an epidemiological study of a general medical ward, a consultant physician declared that 'he never saw alcoholism'. There was on that day a patient on his ward, admitted for treatment of a bleeding ulcer, who was rapidly going into delirium tremens. The notes showed no evidence whatsoever of enquiry into the patient's drinking history, and a look at further case-notes showed that on that treatment service it was quite exceptional to ask about a patient's drinking.

At least one recent study, looking at patients who had taken an over-dose, revealed that an alcohol history is still often neglected by medical staff (Shepherd *et al.*, 1995).

Psychiatric hospitals

In many areas, there may not be specialist in-patient alcohol facilities and often there is an expectation that patients with drinking problems will be admitted to the general psychiatric ward instead. This setting offers certain advantages where patients suffer from comorbid psychi-atric disorders in addition to their drinking problem. It should also provide opportunities for pharmacotherapy, counselling, psycho-therapy, and occupational therapy. However, many general psychiatric wards are now reserved for acutely psychotic or suicidal patients, and such an environment is particularly unsuitable for the management of patients with drinking problems.

Criminal justice system

The association between crime and alcohol has been discussed in Chapter 4. The large number of alcohol related offences committed each year indicates an opportunity to identify, and intervene in, drinking problems amongst offenders.

Treatment as an alternative to sentencing

It has long been recognised that neither society nor the offender benefit from the continued fines or custodial sentences that result from a long series of drunkenness offences. Various systems have been operated, in different countries, in an effort to avoid this scenario. The police may take the street drunk to a detoxification centre rather than to a police cell, and possibly thus avoid a court appearance altogether. Alternatively, the courts may impose treatment in place of or in addi-tion to a punitive sentence.

Treatment imposed by courts

Having recognised the existence of a drinking problem, and having found a person guilty of a crime, a court may decide to impose treat-ment as a condition of probation, or as an alternative to a punitive sen-tence, or else in addition to any other sentence that is imposed. Alternatively, the court may take into consideration treatments which are being undertaken on a voluntary basis. All of these arrangements offer the opportunity for a person to enter treatment when they might not otherwise have done so. However, this can also create difficulties. Some patients may enter treatment purely as a means of attracting a more sympathetic response from the courts. Other patients may be reluctantly referred for treatments with which they do not want to engage. Surprisingly, however, it seems that these instances do not necessarily prejudice treatment outcome (Laundergan et al., 1979). Occasionally, a patient may be compulsorily admitted to hospital in order to protect the public from violence or other serious crime. However, it is rarely if ever appropriate that admissions of this sort should be made to an alcohol treatment centre.

Drink-driving offenders

Drink-driving is itself an important alcohol related problem, and drink-drivers will include many who have also experienced other alcohol related problems. Yet, it is a feature of the 'prevention paradox' (see Chapter 1) that many drink-drivers will not be very heavy drinkers or experience other alcohol related problems. Two drink-driving convictions, however, are much more likely to be indicative of a serious underlying drinking problem (McMillen et al., 1992).

Educational and therapeutic interventions should be made available for those who have been convicted of drink-driving offences. Increasingly, in some parts of the world, they are being offered by courts as an alternative to punitive sentences. However, the research evidence for the benefits of such programmes is modest, and it would seem best that they are offered in addition to, rather than instead of, punitive measures such as fines, licensing restrictions, and prison sentences (Peacock, 1992; Edwards et al., 1994).

Treatment in prison

Many people in prison, and on a worldwide basis probably most people in prison, receive no help for their drinking problem. However, a few prisons have provided special facilities for problem drinkers and AA groups may hold meetings in prisons. In some places individual counselling is available and the prison doctor or chaplain are in a position both to identify the need for such interventions and to ensure that they are provided.

Prison provides a most unusual environment in so far as it generally (although not always) ensures enforced abstinence for the duration of a sentence. Whilst this may appear to offer advantages to the problem drinker in the short-term, in the longer term perspective it denies the opportunity to learn coping skills that are relevant to an environment in which alcohol is freely available. Furthermore, release from prison is in itself a stressful life event which may easily precipitate relapse. This would therefore appear to be a treatment setting in which relapse prevention work could offer benefits.

338

Industry

The workplace provides particularly good opportunities for preventive measures to combat problem drinking, combined with opportunities for early detection and intervention for problems that do arise. Whilst the interface between employment and healthcare poses ethical and policy dilemmas, the need to maintain employment also provides a strong incentive for the problem drinker actively to engage in treatment.

Workplace alcohol programmes are often combined with programmes to address drug misuse and other health or welfare needs. In North America, and increasingly in Europe, such programmes are referred to as Employee Assistance Programmes (or EAPs). As with other treatment programmes, EAPs may be strongly influenced by a particular approach to treatment, such as the 12 steps of AA.

There are a number of issues that all such programmes need to address if they are to be effective; these are discussed below.

Policy

It is vital that written workplace alcohol policies should be established through a written policy agreed by employers and unions in order to clarify what is and is not allowed in respect of drinking and work. In some cases this will need to be very strict, particularly where public or employee safety is concerned.

A written workplace alcohol policy will be needed to document the procedures for identifying and managing the employee with an alcohol problem, and it may specify the implementation of an alcohol screening programme (see Chapter 12).

Provision of help

Large organisations may have their own services through which help may be offered to the employee with an identified drinking problem. In smaller organisations arrangements may be made for it to be provided by local primary care services, or specialist alcohol agencies. Whatever the size of the organisation, a separation of medical treatment provision from occupational health will in any case usually be necessary for ethical reasons (British Medical Association, 1980).

Confidentiality and ethical issues

The occupational physician, counsellor or nurse is in an unusual position in comparison with others of their profession. Whereas confidentiality of information divulged by a client or patient would normally be absolute, in the occupational setting there is also a duty to the welfare of the entire workforce, and possibly also to the general public, as well as to the employer. These dual allegiances can sometimes lead to ethical dilemmas. Staff are unlikely to confide in a nurse or counsellor who will 'tell all' to the employer. Neither does an employer have a right to expect that all information obtained through such channels should be made available to them. However, in so far as information is obtained that affects safety in the workplace, confidentiality may be over-ridden. It must be made clear at the outset that this is the case, and written agreement should be obtained from employees for the passing of medical information to the employer.

The occupational physician should also not usually offer treatment to an employee, but this should be arranged by, or in consultation with, the patient's own GP (British Medical Association, 1980).

An example

A patient was referred by an occupational physician to a specialist alcohol unit for assessment and advice. He had for several years shown evidence of minor liver damage attributable to drinking, which was above the recommended limits (see chapter 8). The company policy indicated that his continued employment would not be allowed unless he had received a period of in-patient treatment for his alcohol problem. This hard line had been taken because of the risk to public safety that was involved. However, it was clear to the specialist that this employee's alcohol problem was relatively minor, that it had never impaired his performance at work, and that in-patient treatment would never normally be considered appropriate for such a patient. The occupational physician was able to provide continued monitoring of the problem on an out-patient basis, the correct treatment was offered to the patient for his drinking problem, public safety was ensured, and the patient retained his job.

Professional roles

As already discussed, the broader context of treatment involves diverse individuals operating in diverse settings. Many of those who may significantly influence the treatment of a problem drinker are not themselves treatment professionals. Thus, the important roles of the spouse, the friend, the AA sponsor, and others should not be underestimated. However, in this section, we shall focus primarily upon the roles of different professionals involved in the treatment of problem drinkers (see Box 20.2).

The provision of a comprehensive service for people with alcohol-related problems requires a range of skills and experience which is beyond the boundaries of any one profession and arguably beyond the capacity of any individual. It is therefore essential that treatment is seen in the context of a multidisciplinary team provision, albeit some relatively isolated professionals may find themselves working outside any formal team structure.

Box 20.2. Professional roles

- Medical practitioners

- Nursing

- Social work

- Occupational therapy

- Psychology

- Counselling

- Psychotherapy

- Teamwork

Medical practitioners

There will be few doctors who do not encounter alcohol related problems in their day to day clinical practice. Medical advice is taken seriously by most patients, and doctors are therefore in a strong position to influence their patients' alcohol consumption. Simple advice on the adverse effects of alcohol consumption upon liver function, intellectual capacity, mental state, heart disease, and hypertension can all be very effective in persuading a patient to cut down or discontinue alcohol consumption.

In addition to providing education and care for patients with alcohol related physical or psychiatric disorders, doctors have other important roles to play in the treatment of alcohol dependence and alcohol misuse. A range of pharmacotherapies have been shown to influence alcohol consumption or reduce relapse rates (see Chapter 17). Alcohol withdrawal is a potentially serious medical condition that requires appropriate medical treatment and supervision (see Chapter 14). Psychiatrists specialising in various forms of psychotherapy can contribute usefully to the psychological management of patients with drinking problems.

341

Nursing

Almost all nurses will have opportunities to offer education, advice, and counselling to their patients regarding alcohol consumption and alcohol related problems. Some patients may feel more able to speak freely to a nurse than to a doctor, and more time may be available for them to do this.

On an in-patient alcohol unit, nurses will fulfil the traditional nursing roles of dispensing medication, observing and recording clinical signs (such as severity of withdrawal, pulse and blood pressure, etc.), and planning and providing 24-hour care. However, as with most other areas of psychiatric nursing, these traditional functions are a relatively small part of the task that the nurse faces. A nurse working with this group of patients, particularly, requires skills in counselling and psychotherapy.

Much of the counselling and psychotherapeutic work associated with specialist alcohol work, in the community or in a residential setting, is ideally suited to the suitably trained nurse. Thus community alcohol teams, hospital liaison services, specialist alcohol units, and even non-medical alcohol agencies may all find that nurses comprise a large proportion of their staff.

Social work

Social workers, including probation officers, are well equipped to engage the problem drinker in appropriate counselling and psychotherapeutic work, especially in the family context, as well as to offer help with the practical issues of housing, benefits, employment, and legal matters. Their training offers a different perspective on these activities to that provided by most nursing and other medical staff. However, it is important that their expertise is not diverted solely towards the adverse social consequences of alcohol misuse, whilst denying opportunity to address the drinking itself.

Alongside their other responsibilities, social workers in some countries are entrusted with statutory duties in respect of matters such as child-care and mental health legislation. Whilst these duties may have only an indirect relevance to working with problem drinkers, they can assume great importance in individual cases. For example, the suitability of a parent with drinking problems to care for children may be in serious doubt (see Chapter 4), or comorbid psychotic illness may necessitate assessment of the need for formal admission to a psychiatric unit under the terms of national mental health legislation.

Occupational therapy

Although occupational therapy offers a vital contribution to general psychiatric and medical services, it is surprising and disappointing that this discipline is often neglected in specialist alcohol treatment services. Occupational therapists help individuals to learn or relearn behaviours necessary in daily life, including social skills (Royal College of Psychiatrists & College of Occupational Therapists, 1992).

A dependent drinker who becomes abstinent will find that they have to fill time which was previously spent drinking. The occupational therapist should play a part in the assessments and treatments offered by any comprehensive alcohol treatment service. However, it is important that other members of staff do not see the role of the occupational therapist as 'simply filling time'. The concern of the occupational therapist is with the occupational and therapeutic purpose of activity, and not simply activity for its own sake.

Occupational therapists, along with most of the other disciplines described here, also have a contribution to make to a broad spectrum of counselling and psychotherapeutic work, especially in the group context.

Psychology

If alcohol misuse is viewed as a learnt behaviour, then the clinical psychologist would appear to be the most appropriate therapist. Many of the psychotherapeutic methods employed in this field have a behavioural psychological basis and ultimately the focus of all such work is on a behavioural outcome – the context, quantity, and pattern of alcohol consumption. A comprehensive behavioural analysis of the context of alcohol consumption can provide a valuable basis for further counselling and treatment. Many psychologists are also interested in cognitive or dynamic therapeutic methods and these can also have a part to play.

Most psychologists would be quick to recognise that they cannot personally conduct all psychological treatments within any department, and the alcohol unit is no exception. The clinical psychologist must therefore expect to play a role in the training of other members of the multidisciplinary team in psychological treatment methods.

The assessment of alcohol induced brain damage is also an area in which the skills of the clinical psychologist are required. In addition, the industrial psychologist may make a contribution to identifying alcohol related problems in the workplace, and the educational psychologist may encounter the adverse effects of parental drinking upon children and teenagers.

Counselling and psychotherapy

A contribution to counselling and psychotherapy is a role for all of the other professional groups listed above. Counselling in this sphere of activity also attracts counsellors of a type not seen in many other areas of work. These are the addicts and 'alcoholics' who have themselves achieved sobriety and who have felt a calling to help others who suffer as they did. In many cases these people have found help through AA and NA and their principles of working thus draw much from the twelve steps and the Minnesota Model. Their experience is varied, and their training even more so. However, standards of training and practice are improving, and many of these individuals now combine a sound theoretical knowledge with the insights of their personal experience. In most centres, a mandatory minimum period of abstinence (usually two years or more) is expected before such a counsellor will be employed on the staff team.

The advantages and disadvantages associated with employment of 'ex-alcoholic' counsellors in a treatment team have been discussed in detail elsewhere (Blume, 1977), and the idea of employing such staff is not new (Anderson, 1944). Whilst they offer a sound role model to patients, personal experience of the problems associated with drinking, and a thorough understanding of the AA programme, there may also be problems associated with their employment. Competition and conflict with other staff can arise. Such counsellors may also over-identify with clients. However, on balance, there is more to be gained than lost from the incorporation of this kind of experience within the multidisciplinary team.

Teamwork

In planning an alcohol treatment service, thought should be given to the composition of the multidisciplinary team. If 20 nurses are employed alongside a single occupational therapist it is likely that the latter individual will either become deskilled, or else isolated and ostracised. If a service is provided to an area in which unemployment and homelessness are prevalent, the skills and experience of a social worker are likely to be required. If the service is in a non-medical setting, thought must be given to who will provide medical advice and care. In any setting, individuals should be chosen who display an ability to work with and learn from, rather than fight against, the different perspective of other professions.

The appointment of the right individuals will not in itself ensure a happy outcome. Good communication must be built into the working week in the form of business meetings, clinical reviews (or 'ward rounds'), staff groups, and individual staff supervision. The final ingredient is clinical leadership and management, without which even the best team can become inefficient and lose sight of its objectives.

Integration and organisation of services

Often the different treatment settings described above are planned and operated separately. Funding may come from the health service, social services, and charitable or private sources. However, at some level, an overview of these different services is required in order to ensure that they provide for the total needs of the community and that they work efficiently together. This overall perspective of treatment provision should be seen in the broader context of a public health policy in which prevention plays the major role (Edwards *et al.*, 1994). Depending upon the national and local setting, this overview may be achieved by political authorities, by purchasing authorities, or by health service planners.

Assessment of need

In an ideal world, the planning of alcohol services would always start with an assessment of need. Sadly this is often neglected or given a lower priority than it deserves. In many countries the true prevalence of alcohol related problems is still unknown, and even in a relatively small community, research into the true extent of the problem may be costly and time consuming. However, in most cases, at least some information may be obtained relatively easily.

Figures may be available for the numbers of people attending existing alcohol services (if any exist), and it may be possible to estimate the numbers of people with alcohol related problems who attend other medical or social services. Similarly, information on alcohol related offences and convictions, such as drink-driving, may indicate the scale of the problem.

Purchasing decisions

Whether or not a detailed assessment of need is available, it is inevitable that treatment resources will be limited, and that decisions must be made as to purchasing priorities. The good news for purchasers of services is that brief interventions are cheap and effective (Bien *et al.*, 1993; Freemantle *et al.*, 1993), and the good news for health departments is that there are also cost-effective means of prevention of alcohol related

345

problems (Edwards *et al.*, 1994). A cornerstone of planning should therefore be to introduce such measures.

There are, however, significant numbers of individuals who do not readily respond to simple interventions. These people, and their families, suffer considerably as a result of their drinking and cannot be ignored. What treatments should be purchased for this group of problem drinkers?

Research has generally supported the conclusion that there is no general advantage of in-patient treatment over out-patient treatment, of longer programmes over shorter ones, or of more intensive treatments over less intensive ones (Miller & Hester, 1986). It would therefore seem sensible, on an economic basis, to purchase shorter, less intensive, out-patient treatments for as many problem drinkers as possible. However, some recent studies have provided evidence of superior efficacy for in-patient programmes (see for example Walsh *et al.*, 1991; Bunn *et al.*, 1994), and a recent review has suggested that there may be a need to re-evaluate the evidence on the influence of treatment setting on outcome (Finney *et al.*, 1996). Other reviewers have also pointed out that, whilst many may benefit from cheap and brief interventions, we must still recognise the need for intensive in-patient services for a minority (Godfrey, 1992; Heather, 1996). It is therefore important that in-patient services are retained for those problem drinkers with serious medical and psychiatric conditions, those with few social resources, those whose environments are not conducive to recovery in the community, and possibly also those with severe dependence or other severe alcohol related problems.

Diversity of services: choice, competition, and co-operation

The different arrangements for providing healthcare in different countries will result in different approaches to drinking problems. Culture and social trends will also render some approaches more or less popular than others. However, in many countries there is a combination of provision by the state, by private organisations, and by voluntary organisations or charities. The extent to which each of these sectors provides help will vary considerably from place to place.

This diversity of provision should be seen as a strength rather than as a problem, and efforts should be made to try to match patients or clients with the most appropriate source of help. Unfortunately, whilst research suggests some benefits in patient–treatment matching (Lindström, 1992) there can be no universal guidance as to which are the most important patient characteristics upon which such selections should be made. Professionals working in the field need to be willing to recognise

the limitations of their own services and to be ready t
sources of help where this seems appropriate.

Audit and research

In view of the limited knowledge of how to choose the best treat.....
for any given patient and the limited funding available for services, it is
important that all alcohol services are subject to audit and research. At
the same time, the self-sufficiency of AA, which accepts no outside
financial support, may be seen as an impressive form of cost-efficiency.

Any comprehensive assessment of outcomes should seek to address
at least some items from each of the three dimensions of alcohol
consumption, alcohol related problems, and level of dependence. A
quantitative estimate of the actual levels of consumption, problems, and
dependence, is to be preferred. These assessments should be conducted
before, and at intervals after, any intervention or treatment that is
offered. Assessments of change can be useful.

An independent assessment of outcome, based upon the account of a
spouse, or repeated measures of a suitable laboratory test (see Chapter
12) adds valuable corroboration to the account of the patient or client.

More detail on outcome studies is provided in a recent review (The
Plinius Maior Society, 1994). However, it should not be imagined that
good outcome data are easily obtained. A comprehensive and valid
assessment is both expensive and time consuming.

References

Anderson, D. (1944). The place of the lay therapist in the treatment of alcoholics. *Quarterly Journal of Studies on Alcohol* 5, 257–66.
Barrison, I. G., Viola, L. & Murray-Lyon, I. M. (1980). Do housemen take an adequate drinking history? *British Medical Journal* 281, 1040.
Barrison, I. G., Viola, L., Mumford, J., Murray, R. M., Gordon, M. & Murray-
Lyon, I. M. (1982). Detecting excessive drinking among admissions to a
general hospital. *Health Trends* 14, 80–3.
Bien, T. H., Miller, W. R. & Tonigan, J. S. (1993). Brief interventions for alcohol
problems: a review. *Addiction* 88, 315–36.
Blume, S. B. (1977). Role of the recovered alcoholic in the treatment of alco-
holism. In *Treatment and rehabilitation of the Chronic Alcoholic*, ed. Kissin, B. &
Begleiter, H., *The Biology of Alcoholism*, vol. 5, pp. 545–65. New York:Plenum.
British Medical Association (1980). *The Handbook of Medical Ethics*. London:
British Medical Association.
Bunn, J. Y., Booth, B. M., Loveland Cook, C. A., Blow, F. C. & Fortney, J. C. (1994).

The relationship between mortality and intensity of in-patient alcoholism treatment. *American Journal of Public Health* **84**, 211–14.

Chick, J., Lloyd, G. & Crombie, E. (1985). Counselling problem drinkers in medical wards: a controlled study. *British Medical Journal* **290**, 965–7.

Chick, J., Ritson, B., Connaughton, J., Stewart, A. & Chick, J. (1988). Advice versus extended treatment for alcoholism: a controlled study. *British Journal of Addiction* **83**, 159–70.

Collins, M. N., Burns, T., Van den Berk, P. A. H. & Tubman, G. F. (1990). A structured programme for out-patient alcohol detoxification. *British Journal of Psychiatry* **156**, 871–4.

Cook, C. C. H. (1988a). The Minnesota model in the management of drug and alcohol dependency: miracle method or myth? Part I. The philosophy and the programme. *British Journal of Addiction* **83**, 625–34.

Cook, C. C. H. (1988b). The Minnesota model in the management of drug and alcohol dependency: miracle method or myth? Part II. Evidence and conclusions. *British Journal of Addiction* **83**, 735–48.

Drummond, D. C., Thom, B., Brown, C., Edwards, G. & Mullan, M. J. (1990). Specialist versus general practitioner treatment of problem drinkers. *Lancet* **336**, 915–18.

Edwards, G. & Arif, A. (Eds.) (1980). *Drug Problems in Socio-Cultural Context.* Geneva: World Health Organisation.

Edwards, G. & Guthrie, S. (1967). A controlled trial of in-patient and out-patient treatment of alcohol dependency. *Lancet* **1**, 555–9.

Edwards, G., Orford, J., Egert, S., Guthrie, S., Hawker, A., Hensman, C., Mitcheson, M., Oppenheimer, E. & Taylor, C. (1977). Alcoholism: a controlled trial of 'treatment' and 'advice'. *Journal of Studies on Alcohol* **38**, 1004–31.

Edwards, G., Anderson, P., Babor, T. F., Casswell, S., Ferrence, R., Giesbrecht, N., Godfrey, C., Holder, H. D., Lemmens, P., Mäkelä, K., Midanik, L. T., Norström, T., Österberg, E., Romelsjö, A., Room, R., Simpura, J. & Skog, O.-J. (1994). *Alcohol Policy and the Public Good.* Oxford: Oxford University Press.

Finney, J. W., Hahn, A. C. & Moos, R. H. (1996). The effectiveness of in-patient and out-patient treatment for alcohol abuse: the need to focus on mediators and moderators of treatment settings. *Addiction* **19**, 1773–96.

Freemantle, N., Gill, P., Godfrey, C., Long, A., Richards, C., Sheldon, T., Song, F. & Webb, J. (1993). *Brief Interventions and Alcohol Use.* Effective Health Care No. 7, University of Leeds.

Glass-Crome, I. B., Jones, P. & Peters, T. J. (1994). A joint problem drinking clinic: the King's College and Maudsley hospitals initiative. *Alcohol and Alcoholism* **29**, 549–54.

Godfrey, C. (1992). *The Cost Effectiveness of Alcohol Services: Lessons for Contracting?* YARTIC Occasional Paper, 2. York: Centre for Health Economics, University of York.

Hayashida, M., Alterman, A. I., McLellan, A. T., O'Brien, C. P., Purtill, J. J., Volpicelli, J. R., Raphaelson, A. H. & Hall, C. P. (1989). Comparative effectiveness and costs of in-patient and out-patient detoxification of patients with mild-to-moderate alcohol withdrawal syndrome. *New England Journal of Medicine* **320**, 358–65.

Heather, N. (1996). *Treatment Approaches for Alcohol Problems.* Copenhagen: World Health Organisation.

Holt, S., Stewart, I. C., Dixon, J. M. J., Elton, R. A., Taylor, T. V. & Little, K. (1980). Alcohol and the emergency service patient. *British Medical Journal* **281**, 638–40.

Jariwalla, A. G., Adams, P. H. & Hore, B. D. (1979). Alcohol and acute general medical admissions to hospital. *Health Trends* **11**, 95–7.

Jarman, C. M. B. & Kellett, J. M. (1979). Alcoholism in the general hospital. *British Medical Journal* **2**, 469–72.

Kennard, D. (1983). *An Introduction to Therapeutic Communities.* London: Routledge and Kegan Paul.

Kristenson, H., Öhlin, H., Hultén-Nosslin, M.-B., Trell, E. & Hood, B. (1983). Identification and intervention of heavy drinking in middle-aged men: results and follow-up of 24–60 months of long-term study with randomised controls. *Alcoholism, Clinical and Experimental Research* **7**, 203–9.

Laundergan, J. C., Spicer, J. W. & Kammeier, M. L. (1979). *Are Court Referrals Effective? Judicial Commitment for Chemical Dependency in Washington County, Minnesota.* Minnesota: Center City, Hazelden.

Lindström, L. (1992). *Managing Alcoholism: Matching Clients to Treatments.* Oxford: Oxford University Press.

MacDonald, E. B. & Patel, A. R. (1975). Attitudes towards alcoholism. *British Medical Journal* **B**, 430–1.

McMillen, D. L., Adams, M. S., Wells-Parker, E., Pang, M. G. & Anderson, B. J. (1992). Personality traits and behaviors of alcohol-impaired drivers: a comparison of first and multiple offenders. *Addictive Behaviors* **17**, 407–14.

Miller, W. R. & Hester, R. K. (1986). In-patient alcoholism treatment: who benefits? *American Psychologist* **41**, 794–805.

Peacock, C. (1992). International policies on alcohol-impaired driving: a review. *International Journal of the Addictions* **27**, 187–208.

Persson, J. & Magnusson, P.-H. (1987). Prevalence of excessive or problem drinkers among patients attending somatic out-patient clinics: a study of alcohol related medical care. *British Medical Journal* **295**, 467–72.

The Plinius Maior Society (1994). Guidelines on evaluation of treatment of alcohol dependence. *Alcoholism* (Supplement), **30**.

Potamianos, G., Winter, D., Duffy, S. W., Gorman, D. M. & Peters, T. J. (1985). The perception of problem drinkers by general hospital staff, general practitioners, and alcoholic patients. *Alcohol* **2**, 563–6.

Royal College of Psychiatrists; College of Occupational Therapists (1992). *Occupational Therapy and Mental Disorders.* London: Royal College of Psychiatrists & College of Occupational Therapists.

Shepherd, R. M., Dent, T. H. S., Alexander, G. J. M. & London, M. (1995). Prevalence of alcohol histories in medical and nursing notes of patients admitted with self-poisoning. *British Medical Journal* **311**, 847.

Stockwell, T., Bolt, L., Milner, I., Russell, G., Bolderston, H. & Pugh, P. (1991). Home detoxification from alcohol: its safety and efficacy in comparison with in-patient care. *Alcohol and Alcoholism* **26**, 645–50.

Wallace, P., Cutler, S. & Haines, A. (1988). Randomised controlled trial of general practitioner intervention in patients with excessive alcohol consumption. *British Medical Journal* **297**, 663–8.

Walsh, D. C., Hingson, R. W., Merrigan, D. M., Levenson, S. M., Cupples, A., Heeren, T., Coffman, G. A., Becker, C. A., Barker, T. A., Hamilton, S. K., McGuire, T. G. & Kelly, C. A. (1991). A randomized trial of treatment options for alcohol-abusing workers. *New England Journal of Medicine* **325**, 775–82.

Author index

Subject index

C f 17